THE COMPLETE GUIDE TO

yinyoga

PHILOSOPHY + PRACTICE

THE COMPLETE GUIDE TO
yinyoga
PHILOSOPHY + PRACTICE

BERNIE CLARK

FOREWORD BY SARAH POWERS

A WILD STRAWBERRY PRODUCTION

First edition: 2011

Second edition: 2019

Printed in the United States

Clark, Bernie, 1953-

The complete guide to yin yoga: the philosophy and practice of yin yoga / by Bernie Clark.

Includes bibliographical references and index.

ISBN 978-0-9687665-8-3 (pbk.)

ISBN 978-0-9687665-9-0 (ebook)

Second printing 2020

Credits for Art and Photography

Chapters 3, 4 and 7: Photographs of Cherise Richards are by Christy Collins. Copyrighted 2011 by Bernie Clark. Photographs of Bernie Clark, Carla Johnson, Chervelle Richards, Diana Batts, Lisa Papez and Nathalie Keiller are by Tom Belding (www.tombelding.com). Copyrighted 2019 by Bernie Clark.

Chapter 6: p. 218: "Collagen Fibers," reprinted, by permission, Matthew P. Dalene and the Rensselaer Polytechnic Institute; p. 221: "Connective Tissues," reprinted from *Gray's Anatomy, 38th Edition, The Anatomical Basis of Medicine and Surgery*, p. 76, by Pearson Professional Limited 1995 and with their kind permission; p. 226: "Types of Synovial Joints," reprinted, by permission, Produnis of the Wikimedia Share Commons.

Cover and interior design by Alex Hennig (www.alexhennig.ca)

For Nathalie, who has come to
share my belief that yin is truly in!

CONTENTS

PREFACE
TO THE SECOND EDITION

Yin is certainly in! In the 8 years since I wrote the first edition of *The Complete Guide to Yin Yoga*, the practice of Yin Yoga has expanded tremendously. It seems today that most studios in North America now offer at least one Yin Yoga class each week, and many have several on their schedules. It takes a long time to become an overnight success, and the pioneering work by Paul Grilley and Sarah Powers, spanning 3 decades now, has borne a mighty fruit. Yin is everywhere, which is very gratifying because balance is needed everywhere.

The first edition of *The Complete Guide to Yin Yoga* was a follow-on from my first book, *YinSights*. As time goes on, we learn new things and develop new perspectives. Years after writing *YinSights*, I felt the need to expand upon what I had written, to include more about the practice of Yin Yoga and de-emphasize the general philosophy and history of yoga. In the second edition, this evolution continues apace. You will find much more about the practice of Yin Yoga, including new sections on: how and why to use props in your practice; a more functional approach, emphasizing the concept of targeted areas; why Hot Yin is not an oxymoron and may be very beneficial for many people; the importance of stress in reducing fragility; understanding the nature of creep and the importance of counterposes, with a revised list of effective counterposes, including a full description of the lovely Golden Seed flow Paul and Suzee Grilley created; many new photographs of the postures and their variations for different body types; a current overview of the physiology of tissues and the energy body, reflecting new understandings in the science of fascia and cellular signaling; and many other updates too numerous to catalogue here.

Diminished in this edition are the stories of the developers and early teachers of Yin Yoga: Sarah Powers, Paul Grilley and his teacher Hiroshi Motoyama. Their stories are still available, but to make space for the new material, Paul Grilley suggested that I move these personal stories to the Web. So for interested readers wanting to learn more about Paul, Sarah and Dr. Motoyama, please visit www.YinYoga.com or their own websites. Also missing from this edition is one particular asana that never really resonated with me: the Camel. In my view, it is too yang to really be used as a yin posture, so I removed it (with Paul's blessing—although it is still available on the website for those Camel fans who do love it). In its place, I added the Bridge, which I have come to love as a very yin-like backbend. Hopefully, you will love it too.

Another significant change is the de-emphasis of the traditional benefits listed for each posture. Benefits are still important, of course, but many yoga teachers over the centuries have made claims for the practice that are not borne out or are pure hyperbole. At best, the claims refer to anecdotes, which can be acceptable as evidence but are not considered strong science.

A woman once approached me after a Yin Yoga class. She had been coming every Sunday night for a year and was eager to share something important. "A year ago," she said, "I had very bad, chronic back pain. Nothing I tried helped me. And now, after doing your Yin Yoga classes for a year, my back is completely healed, like new!" I smiled at her beaming face and marveled with her at this wonderful news. However, as she happily went away, I had to wonder, "What cured her?" I would love to believe it was the practice of Yin Yoga or my teaching, but in reality—I just don't know. Maybe what cured her was learning to be mindful of sensations. Maybe it was calming her breath. Maybe it was getting away from her partner one night a week. Or being in a community. I cannot say that Yin Yoga cures back pain based on this one anecdote, but there is no doubt that her back pain had been cured. That was real. There is something about the practice that heals, even if we can't prove scientifically exactly what it is.

In the evolution of my teaching, I now prefer to cite benefits only where there is good reason to support the claim, rather than repeating time-honored beliefs that do not withstand scrutiny. The good news is that science does stand behind many benefits. Recent investigations into fascia have shown numerous pathways to optimal health. Likewise, studies have been conducted into the risks of certain postures, and where these have been documented, I have included them in this new edition.

"Anicca," stated the Buddha. "Things change." Impermanence is the only constant. The practice of yoga continues to evolve, as does our understanding and teaching of it. Who know what the next edition of this book may include, but I am sure that however the future unfolds, yin will still be in.

PREFACE
TO THE FIRST EDITION

Many readers of my previous book, *YinSights: A Journey into the Philosophy & Practice of Yin Yoga*, wrote to tell me how much they enjoyed reading it and how valuable they found the practice of Yin Yoga. Along with many emails, there were also requests posted in the YinYoga.com Forum, asking for even more information: how to get into the poses described in the book and how to safely come out of them, how to do Yin Yoga for the upper body, whether Yin Yoga would be helpful for unique, special situations, and lots of other questions. Many readers asked about the Daoist history that also informed and influenced the development of Yin Yoga. The demand grew for a second edition of *YinSights* that would cover these and other details of the practice of Yin Yoga.

Unfortunately, a technical challenge arose: adding to the information already presented in *YinSights* would make the book unwieldy. *YinSights* was already over 400 pages long, and extending it to answer all the questions being raised would make the book too bulky. A second edition did not seem like a good idea. Fortunately, the opportunity arose to solve this problem by creating not a second edition of *YinSights*, but a new book focused more tightly on the practice of Yin Yoga and its benefits and less on the philosophy and evolution of yoga in general. The result is what you are reading right now.

The Complete Guide to Yin Yoga borrows heavily in many places from *YinSights*, but it extends what was presented in the earlier book considerably. Yinsters familiar with *YinSights* will find a few sections repeated entirely, but they will also find an expanded description of the Yin Yoga postures, more flows following broader themes, and postures designed to work the upper body. Special situations are also covered, such as how to modify your Yin Yoga practice if you are pregnant, or what to do to help you become pregnant. There is a more complete examination of the effects of Yin Yoga on our fascia and our muscles.

Of course, the benefits of Yin Yoga go far beyond the physical, and this book will also describe the considerable mental, emotional and energetic benefits we can receive through the practice of Yin Yoga. I hope previous readers will enjoy *The Complete Guide to Yin Yoga* as much as they did *YinSights* and that new readers will be inspired to take a walk on the yin side. After all, yin is in!

FOREWORD

The practice of yoga has always been evolving, but essentially yoga is the cultivation of attention. What we attend to and the attitude with which we attend greatly influence how we experience ourselves and our life. In yoga, we concentrate on both form (our bodies and tissues) and formlessness (our breath, energy channels and mind states). These interconnected aspects of reality are in constant interplay, they are the yin and yang of life, and in yoga, we develop and balance these polar complementarities within our body/mind experience. For most of us, beginning with that which is most tangible, the body (yang), is a common doorway into the practice. As we become less distracted and healthier physically, most students eventually become interested in that which is more hidden. This can be called the yin aspect of reality, which relates with that which is subtle. It is only by paying attention in a relaxed and attuned way that this yin aspect of yoga is revealed.

When students first begin a yoga practice, perhaps to reduce stress or to get in shape, or maybe just to accompany a friend, they will often be guided to place the largest percentage of their attention on the shape of the poses they are trying to do. This keeps the practice safe, and as we learn postural integration, our body-based experience becomes more joyous and healthy and the postures more fun to inhabit. Eventually, with skillful guidance, sincere practitioners become interested not only in the outer forms of yoga, but also in the inner revolution that yoga can offer—or as Bernie might say, they start to go *yin-side*. It is here that the deeper aspects of yoga are revealed.

Paying attention to the fluctuations of the breath, noticing the sensations ebbing and flowing in the physical body, tracking the changing feelings in the emotional body, and recognizing the space of the mind as well as the thoughts in the mental body are all part of yoga. This yoking or joining of the body, heart and mind provides health benefits beyond simply being more flexible or stronger. The word *health* is derived from an Old English word meaning "whole." Yoga re-establishes our natural wholeness—the balanced integrity of our yin and yang nature.

Adding a yin or quieter aspect to our yoga practice can introduce us to the possibility of physical/emotional/mental equilibrium by marrying the softer, contemplative modes of being in life to the stronger activities we are so often compelled by. This helps reduce the compulsive extremes of behavior that cause us to lose balance, lose focus and diminish our joy of living. Yang energy is needed to bring vitality to our yin interior, but it is the gentler yin qualities within us that balance our yang intensities. If you have felt that life is too often not how you would like it to be, then learning the ancient art of deep listening, tuning in to the internal, non-conceptual, softer aspects of your yin nature may be the healing direction.

Yin Yoga, when taught skillfully, can provide this opportunity to go within and realign our orientation. It will also affect our physical body in ways that may surprise us. It is simple, but often challenging. It will provide us with ample periods of stillness within, when we can start to pay attention to what is really happening, right here, right now. It can provoke insights that may move us to make significant changes in our life or allow us to accept that what is happening right now is exactly what ought to be happening right now. We may discover ourselves opening up to and connecting with our experience as it is, rather than holding on to resistance and feelings of victimization.

For anyone seeking to learn and benefit from the practice of yoga, this book will be an invaluable guide. Bernie has been a student and friend of mine for many years. I know him to be a thoughtful and dedicated teacher who has helped many through his workshops, website and writings. Through this book, he is sharing his own practice for all our benefits, seeking to help anyone who desires genuine health and wholeness. Within these pages, you will find explorations on the physical benefits of Yin Yoga and explanations on the ways Yin Yoga helps us energetically as well as emotionally and mentally. The practice of Yin Yoga is described in detail, and the various *asanas* are reviewed in a simple way, allowing them to be fully experienced. For those interested, the evolution of yoga in general and Yin Yoga specifically is also presented.

It is with heartfelt encouragement that I invite you to experience opening within through the study and practice of Yin Yoga.

Sarah Powers

New York

September 2011

ACKNOWLEDGMENTS

Showing the way fearlessly and compassionately,
the stream of all our Ancestral Teachers,
to whom we bow in gratitude.

From "*Touching the Earth*," a *gatha* of the
monastics of Plum Village, France

Writing a book begins as a solitary endeavor, but never one that starts without encouragement. Along the way, through all the stops and starts, friends appear who give us the strength to continue. There are many people I wish to thank for helping make this book a reality. Firstly, I would like to thank Paul Grilley for suggesting the project in the first place and for introducing me to the concepts presented in this book. My eternal thanks to my first Yin Yoga teacher, Sarah Powers, who helped me understand how to slow down and mindfully practice yoga. Of course, I would not even be in a position to write about Yin Yoga if it were not for all my other teachers, to whom I bow in gratitude.

Producing a book requires the dedicated support of a team working anonymously in the background. I have many people to thank for their participation and assistance. To the models who posed for the many photographs: Carla Johnson, Cherise Richards, Chervelle Richards, Diana Batts, Lisa Papez and Nathalie Keiller—thank you! To the photographers: Christy Collins and Tom Belding—thank you! To the owners of the studios where we took the photographs: Gloria Latham of Semperviva Yoga Studios, Vancouver, B.C. and Emily Le Bihan of Yoga Spirit and Wellness, Burnaby, B.C.—thank you! To Pilar Wyman who created the index—thank you! To Dania Sheldon for editing the text numerous times—thank you! To Tania Cheffins for the rounds of proofreading—thank you! Again, to Nathalie Keiller for reviewing the early drafts—thank you! And to Alex Hennig for all her work on designing and laying out the text, the book cover and the relaunch of the www.YinYoga.com website—many thanks!

Finally, my blessings and thanks to all the students who have allowed me the honor of teaching them: the best way to learn a subject is to try to teach it. Indeed, my students have been my greatest teachers.

ACKNOWLEDGMENTS

PLEASE NOTE! Before embarking on this practice, please make sure you are able to do so: check with your doctor or health-care professional before starting any yoga practice. The guidance given in this book is not meant to replace medical advice and should be used only as a supplement if you are under the care of a health-care professional. While care has been taken in compiling the guidance in this book, we cannot take any responsibility for any adverse effects from your practice of yoga. When you are not sure of any aspect of the practice, or feel unwell, seek medical advice. Please read the contraindications for each pose before you try the pose, so that you will know whether this particular posture is a good one for you to try. Be aware of the many options available to make each pose more accessible. Practice with both intention and attention.

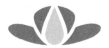

INTRODUCTION

Modern yoga has sprung from a figurative forest of many different styles of yoga with many varied intentions. One particular tree germinating in this fertile forest about 1,000 years ago is called Hatha Yoga, which means the forceful yoga. Hatha Yoga, distinct from the other trees in the yoga forest, was primarily designed to strengthen the body and prepare it for other forms of yoga; these forms could be the meditative practices that lead to liberation and enlightenment, but Hatha Yoga could also be a path toward developing darker arts and black magic. Many Hatha yogis were famed for their prowess as warriors and were hired as mercenaries.

Today, we mostly know of Hatha Yoga in the West as the practice that makes us healthier and calmer. Not too many practitioners of yoga today are aiming for spiritual awakening, although if that happens, that might be nice. The intentions for attending a yoga class today may range from seeking health to seeking companionship. The fact that you can actually take a yoga class today is very new: there were no classes in ages past—you learned by sitting at the feet of your guru. If you were lucky, he would impart to you everything he had learned from his guru, but this transmission would take many years of dedicated study and practice.

The Hatha tree sprouted many stout branches. Far more than the physical postures, or asanas, the original practice emphasized the breath and energetic circles formed by the hands and body, called mudras. In the last 100 years, asanas have moved into the spotlight in the evolving Western versions of Hatha Yoga. There are dozens of branches now; some of the oldest are called Iyengar Yoga and Sivananda Yoga, while some of the newest and smallest shoots have names such as aqua yoga, dance yoga, goat yoga and wine-and-chocolate yoga. Most of these modern forms of Hatha Yoga emphasize health and wellness physically, mentally and emotionally.

With the modernization of Hatha Yoga, some things have been lost. The original forms of Hatha Yoga equally emphasized strong muscular activities, which can be characterized as yang practices, and the softer activities that open our deeper tissues, such as the joints, which can be characterized as the yin practices. The yin side of yoga was de-emphasized and hidden inside a few softer styles, such as restorative yoga, and in the meditation practices, which very few people are drawn to. This was an unfortunate omission because it robbed the student of the chance to develop enhanced health for the whole body, heart and mind.

This book is an investigation into that missing half: Yin Yoga. The investigation will take you into the philosophical underpinnings of yin versus yang and will explain the benefits of adding a yin perspective to your yoga practice. These benefits are considerable and are found in all aspects of our life, from our physical well-being to our mental and emotional well-being.

The practice of Yin Yoga is explained in detail, but a book is never a substitute for a teacher. If you are drawn to investigate this part of the yoga forest further, you are encouraged to seek out a Yin Yoga teacher whom you can relate to. Like all yoga practice, theory alone is insufficient: you must actually do the practice. It is entertaining and educational to read about how and why you might do Yin Yoga, but the real value comes in getting down on the floor. So...as you begin to read this book, get off your couch or out of your chair, place a cushion on the floor, and begin to read while sitting or lying on the ground. Move around all you want, but stay on the floor for as long as you can. You are already beginning the practice.

1

YIN YOGA DEFINED

Our goal in life is not to become perfect:
our goal is to become whole.

Modern yoga is deeply rooted in Eastern mysticism, was fertilized by 19th-century gymnastics and wrestling, and has been shaped by Western sensibilities.[1] Today, yoga as practiced in the West is totally unique and has never existed anywhere else: we practice Western yoga for the benefits that Westerners desire. These benefits are considerable and will be explored in this book. If you have been doing yoga for a while, you might discover that you have been experiencing only part of the practice and achieving just some of the available benefits.

Yin Yoga is the other half. Most forms of yoga today are dynamic, active practices designed to work only half of our body, the muscular half, the "yang" tissues. Yin Yoga allows us to work the other half, the deeper "yin" tissues of our ligaments, joints, deep fascial networks and even our bones. All of our tissues are important and need to be exercised so that we can achieve optimal health and vitality.

Exercise our joints?! Isn't that dangerous? Yes and no. It depends on how we do it; we can exercise our joints safely if we do so intelligently. If we exercise them incorrectly, we can definitely hurt ourselves, but we can say that about any form of exercise.

Saying that Yin Yoga is the other half, that it works the deeper tissues of the body, is just the beginning of defining what Yin Yoga is all about. We need to look at the definitions of the underlying principles of yin and yoga to examine the intention behind engaging in a yoga practice, and to explore the benefits and methodologies used in a Yin Yoga practice.

There are numerous reasons for beginning a yoga practice; obtaining optimum physical health is just one. Many people are drawn to yoga to help reduce the effects of stress in their lives. Others wish to deepen their meditation practices or to simply become more present in their daily lives. As you will discover, yoga in general and Yin Yoga in particular provides physical, mental, emotional and energetic benefits and, for some, spiritual ones. Which benefits you enjoy will depend greatly upon your intention when you practice.

How you practice is just as important as what you practice. There is a yin aspect to life and a yang aspect. There is a yin way to practice yoga and a yang way that go beyond the actual movements and postures employed in a yoga session. Yin is yielding, allowing and nourishing. Even within an active, sweaty yang practice, we can adopt a yin sensitivity that will help us gain much more from our yoga practice. Even within an active yang lifestyle, we can adopt a yin awareness and acceptance that will help us gain contentment in our lives.

Yin Yoga can have the same goals and objectives as any other school of yoga. What we do will be different, but *how* we do it will be the biggest difference. Why we do yoga really comes down to our own unique, particular intentions. Knowing the benefits of the Yin Yoga style will help you clarify the intentions for your practice.

Some students initially find this style of yoga quite boring, passive or soft, but they quickly discover that it can be quite challenging due to the long duration of the poses. Yin Yoga is simple, but simple does not mean easy. We can remain in the postures anywhere from 1 to 20 minutes!

» *PLEASE NOTE! Yin Yoga as described here is* **not** *restorative yoga. If the tissues you are targeting for exercise are damaged in some way, please give yourself a chance to heal before resuming your regular practice.*

YIN AND YANG

Patterns define our lives. Look around you right now and you will notice the patterns surrounding you. Look up; you will see things that are high. Look down; you will see things that are low. Listen; you will hear things close by, and you will hear things far away. Bring your attention inward; you may feel the tip of your nose or the top of your head. Now you may be feeling the tips of your toes. Up, down … near, far … these are just some of the adjectives we can choose to describe the patterns of life, of existence. All patterns are formed by contrasts. The pattern on a chessboard is formed by the contrast of dark and light. The pattern of your life, when reflected upon, has displayed a contrast of good times and bad. For the Daoist, harmony

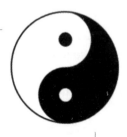

1.1

The taijitu or yin and yang symbol

and health are created when conditions arise where the contrasting aspects are in balance.

Balancing is not a static act. Imagine the typical depiction of weighing scales: two plates held by a common string suspended at a point halfway between them. When two equally weighted objects are placed upon the scales, there is a slight swaying motion, like a pendulum. If one side is too heavy, the scales tip and balance is lost. When both sides are equal, there is still a slight oscillation around the middle position. This rebalancing is the return to wholeness and health.

The ancient Chinese called this middle that we return to the Dao.[2] The Dao is the tranquility found in the center of all events, and the path leading to the center. The center is always there, even if we are not always there to enjoy it. When we leave the center, we take on aspects of yin or yang.

Yin and yang are relative terms describing the two facets of existence. Like two sides of one coin, yin cannot exist without yang, nor yang without yin. They complement each other. Since existence is never static, what is yin and what is yang are always in flux, always changing.

Yin	Yang
Dark	Light
Cold	Hot
Passive	Active
Inside	Outside
Solid	Hollow
Slow	Rapid
Dim	Bright
Downward	Upward
Substance	Function
Water	Fire
Matter	Energy
Mysterious	Obvious
Female	Male
Moon	Sun
Earth	Heaven
Night	Day
Even	Odd
Dragon	Tiger
Plastic	Elastic

3

The ancient Chinese observed that everything has yin or yang attributes. The terms existed in Confucianism and in the earliest Daoist writings. The yin character refers to the shady side of a hill or stream. Yang refers to the sunny side. Shade cannot exist without light, and light can only be light when contrasted with darkness. And so we see how, even in the earliest uses of these terms, patterns are observable.

There is no absolute yin or absolute yang. A context is always required: in the context of light, darkness and brightness define yin and yang. In a number of other contexts, yin describes that which is relatively denser, heavier, lower, more hidden, more yielding, more feminine, more mysterious and more passive. Yang describes the opposite conditions: what is less dense, lighter, higher, more obvious or superficial, more masculine and more dynamic. The table on this page shows a more complete list of comparisons. There is no limit to the relative contexts in which yin and yang can be applied.

Yin Contains Yang

Look again at the symbol for yin and yang at the beginning of this section. Do you see the white dot within the dark paisley swirl? Even within the darkness of yin, there is a lightness of yang and vice versa. In the context of temperature, we say that hotter is yang and cooler is yin; but hot water is yin compared to boiling water, which is yang. In the other direction, cold water is yang compared to ice, which is yin.

In our yoga practice, there are very active asana workouts, which we may call yang, but even within these yang practices we can find yin aspects; watching our breath mindfully while we flow through a vigorous vinyasa[3] is just one example.

Yin Becomes Yang Becomes Yin

Just as we detect yin elements within the yang aspects, we can also notice how yin becomes yang, and yang can transform into yin. These transformations may be slow and subtle, or they may be devastatingly quick. The seasons roll slowly by, changing imperceptibly. The yang of spring and summer transforms day by day into the yin of fall and winter. It is not possible to pick the exact moment at which one season becomes another, astronomical observations notwithstanding. But the transformation may also come quickly: the eye of a hurricane quickly brings calm, and just as quickly the eye moves on and the other half of the storm strikes.

In our own lives, we often experience both the slow and the quick transformations of yin into yang and yang into yin. We wake up in the morning; yin becomes yang. Sometimes our awakening is slow, leisurely; this is a slow transformation. Sometimes we wake with a start and jump out of bed, perhaps because we overslept. When we work long hours for many weeks or months in a row (a very yang lifestyle), our body may seek balance by suddenly making us too sick to work (a very yin lifestyle), or it may gift us with a severe migraine to slow us down. Yang is quickly transformed into yin.

Yin Controls Yang

In this last example, we can see that if we stay too long in an unbalanced situation, the universe acts to restore balance. It throws us to the other side: our health may suffer and our lives may change. If we do not heed the need for balancing yin and yang, this transition can be devastating. A heart attack could be the balancing force applied to us. These imbalances are often referred to as an excess or a deficiency. We can have an excess or a deficiency of either yin or yang. The cure is to apply the opposite quality to address the imbalance.

In the Eastern world of the yogis[4] of India and the alchemical Daoists of China, the need for balance is well known and understood.[5] In the West, while we do not use the terms yin and yang, the need to pay attention and balance our opposing natures has been realized by many astute observers of our psychological landscape. Carl Jung recognized his dark side, which he termed "the shadow," and discovered that if left unattended, these dark, repressed energies will wreak havoc in one's life. The oppositions within create a dynamic tension that can lead to destruction or amazing creativity. For Jung, the way to work with these opposing energies is to integrate them, or individuate.[6] He, and his followers after him, developed many tools to achieve this integration. Shadow work can include active imagining or creating rituals that honor both energies within us.

Spiritual	Practical
Losing	Winning
Outgo	Income
Fasting	Eating
Passivity	Action
Giving	Earning
Poverty	Possession
Repose	Activity
Celibacy	Sex
Observation	Decisiveness
Obedience	Freedom
Duty	Choice
Ecstasy	Sobriety
Vision	Focus
Less is more	More is better

Notice the differences and the similarities between the first table describing yin and yang characteristics with the table on this page, taken from Robert Johnson's book *Owning Your Own Shadow*.[7] Here, Johnson shows the many opposing values we are subjected to in Western cultures.[8] One set includes the religious or spiritual beliefs required of us, and the other set is what we need to survive and thrive in our secular life and the business world. Note the yin-like qualities and the opposing yang-like energies. How we reconcile the opposing energies of Sunday morning versus the rest of the week will lead to either a breakdown or a breakthrough, a revelation. The latter is only possible if we do the work required, if we do our yoga, whether with Western or Eastern techniques.

In the West, true understanding of yin and yang is uncommon. We don't think in these terms; our lifestyles rarely reflect the need for balance. We seek it only when the universe forces us to pay attention, when we suffer the breakdown that avoiding our dark side creates. Only then do we seek help to regain balance. Only when we become exhausted or sick do we take time off. Only when we injure our bodies do we slow down and look for gentler ways to exercise. We can be yang-like for only so long before crashing. We can be yin-like for only so long before stagnating. We need balance in all things.

YIN TISSUES AND YANG TISSUES

As mentioned, yin and yang are relative terms and need a context to be appropriately applied. They can be used as adjectives, although they are often used as nouns. Within our bodies, if we use the context of position or density, the yang tissues can be seen as our muscles, blood and skin, compared to the yin tissues of ligaments, bones and joints. The contexts of flexibility or heat can also be used: muscles are elastic, but bones are plastic;[9] muscles love to get warm, while ligaments generally remain cool.

Yang styles of yoga generally target the muscles and employ rhythmic, repetitive movements to stress the muscle cells. Being elastic and moist, the muscles appreciate this form of exercise and respond well to it. Yin tissues, however, being dryer and much less elastic, can be damaged if stressed in this way. Instead, our more plastic tissues appreciate and require gentler pressures, applied for longer periods of time, in order to be stimulated to grow stronger. This is why orthodontic braces must be worn for a long time with a reasonable (but not always comfortable) amount of pressure to reshape the jaw bones.

Our joints can be seen simply as spaces between the bones where movement is possible. Stabilizing a joint are ligaments, muscles, tendons and fascia, which bind the bones together. Generally, one of the muscles' jobs is to protect the joint; if there is too much stress on the joint, the muscles will tear first, then the ligaments, and then finally the joint itself may be damaged. In this regard, yang yoga is designed to *not* stress the joint. This is why so much care is taken to align the body and engage the muscles correctly before coming into asanas in the yang practice. However, Yin Yoga is specifically designed to exercise the ligaments and to regain space and strength in the joints.

An example can help explain the different roles of the muscles and ligaments. Place your right index finger in your left hand. Extend the finger and tighten the muscles and, with your left hand, try to bend the finger upward. Notice that there is virtually no movement. The muscles' job is to bind the bones together and limit the range of motion allowed in the joint. Next, relax the finger completely. Shake it out for a moment. Now, keeping the muscles passive, try to push the finger upward. Notice the difference? The relaxed finger can move 90° or more. When the muscles are relaxed, the stress is moved to the ligaments and the joint capsules. We can summarize this understanding of the safest way to target our joints:

- When a joint is bearing a load, stiffen the joint muscularly.
- To enhance a joint's range of motion, reduce the load and relax the muscles.

Stability and Mobility

Remember the white dot within the paisley swirl of the yin and yang symbol? Within yang there is yin and vice versa. This also applies to our tissues. Consider muscle, which we just described as a yang tissue. Even here we will find yin within yang: 30% of what we call our muscle is actually fascia. As we will discover, the fascia within our muscles governs the muscles' range of movement, while our muscle cells govern their strength. Yang yoga is great at developing the yang attribute of strength within our muscles but, surprisingly perhaps, it is the yin part of our practice, the holding of the pose, that develops length.

Within our yin tissues, we also find yang elements. In our fascia and ligaments, which are predominantly yin-like, there are contracting fibers, just like within our muscles. We also find elastic fibers called elastin within our yin tissues. So there is yang within yin here too: our connective tissues can contract and shorten.

Physiologically, through our yoga practice, we build stability and mobility. If we look at the arc of aging, which everyone follows, albeit at faster or slower rates, we begin life completely yang-like: our mobility is greater than it will ever subsequently be, but we have no stability. Newborn babies have to be handled carefully because they have no internal stability. Then we start to stiffen, to become more yin-like. We gain stability as we age. When we are youngsters, we don't need to work on gaining more mobility because we are already so yang-like; we need to work on building our muscles and gaining strength. This is a yang time of life, so we need yang forms of exercise.[10] Somewhere around our mid-20s to mid-30s, we reach the optimal balance between yin and yang, between mobility and stability. But the arc of aging must be followed: we continue to become more yin-like as we age, until eventually we end up completely rigid, as rigor mortis sets into our dead bodies. As we get older, more yin-like, we need a yin form of exercise to keep us mobile.

The Theory of Exercise

All forms of exercise share two features:

- First, we must stress the tissues.
- Then, we must let the tissues rest.

Yang tissues do better when stressed in a yang manner, and yin tissues do better when stressed in a yin way. Stress has many negative connotations in our culture because we forget the "rest" part of the theory. But to have little or no stress in our life is just as damaging as having too much stress. We need to stress the body, and we need to rest it. There is a yin/yang balance here that leads to health. Too much of anything is not healthy.

Yang exercise targets the yang tissues: the muscles. They love to be rhythmically and repetitively moved. Any static holds are brief.[11] The muscles are elastic and can take this type of exercise. However, applying yang exercise to yin tissues can damage them. Yin tissues, being more plastic, require gentler but long-held stresses. Imagine bending a credit card back and forth 108 times every morning, over and over again. It wouldn't take many mornings of this for it to snap in half. The credit card is plastic, just as our ligaments are. To rhythmically bend ligaments over and over again, as some students do when dropping back from standing into the Wheel or moving from Up Dog to Down Dog, can, over time, damage the ligaments, just like the credit card. The warning here is: **Do not apply yang exercise techniques to yin tissues!**

Applying a yin exercise to yang tissues can also be damaging. Holding a muscle in a contracted state for a long period of time is called "tetany" and may damage it.[12]

Is it better to tighten muscles (yang) or relax them (yin)? That depends on your intention. We tighten our muscles to protect our joints. We relax our muscles so we can exercise our joints. What is your intention in the pose you are doing?

Many health-care professionals shudder at the thought of exercising joints, as they have the mistaken view that all exercise is yang exercise. Nonetheless, it is possible to exercise ligaments, bones and joints in a yin way. In fact, such exercise is necessary.

However, because they are yin tissues, we must exercise them in a yin way. And please remember the important second part of this theory—we must rest![13] There is a lot of research proving the importance of stress and rest for more than just developing physical strength, but it is beyond the scope of this journey to go into this further.

Stretch versus Stress

We need to define a couple of terms that many yoga teachers use rather loosely: stress and stretch. These are not synonyms. Technically, stress is the tension that we place upon our tissues, while stretch is the elongation that might result from the stress. We often say we are stretching our muscles, but to be more precise, we are applying a stress to our muscles that may or may not result in a stretch. For example, in isometric exercises, we stress the muscles, but there is no change in their length.

We can also stress tendons, ligaments and other fascial systems, especially in Yin Yoga, but because many fascial materials are more plastic and less elastic than muscles, that stress is less likely to result in a stretch. (Even the tightest ligaments stretch a little, but some ligaments can and should stretch a lot![14]) We are *not* trying to *stretch* our ligaments or joint capsules with Yin Yoga. We *are* trying to *stress* them. Over time, the tissues may become longer, thicker and stronger, but in any single Yin Yoga session, we are not necessarily trying to lengthen these particular tissues. Said another way, in yoga, the key is the stress, not the stretch. If a stretch happens and there is no pain during the pose, or when coming out of the pose, or even over the next 24 to 48 hours, so be it. Let these areas stretch. The key remains the amount of stress we are generating.

When we use the term *stretch* in this book, it will either refer to a lengthening of the tissues (for example, we will stretch a muscle to make it longer) or indicate that the intention of the applied stress is to lengthen the tissues. For our Yin Yoga practice, we mostly will not use the term *stretch* but will stick to the term *stress*.

ORIGINAL YIN

Hatha Yoga, the most common form of yoga practiced today in the West, is a physical practice. The intention of Hatha Yoga, which blossomed around the 10th century, was to prepare the body for the more advanced yoga practices of meditation and insight. Hatha Yoga arose out of the earlier Tantra Yoga style, which in turn drew from the Classical Yoga of around 2,000 years ago.

There has never been one yoga from which all other yogas have evolved. There is no yoga tree that one can create to show the interrelationships between all the various forms and expressions of yoga over the millennia. Rather, we would need to draw a forest of yoga trees to really understand yoga's full and varied history. We do know that Hatha Yoga as a specific practice is not itself thousands of years old but does have roots going back that far. It is also known that ancient yogas from many lineages incorporated some basic physical practices, such as sitting in meditation.

If you have ever tried to sit for even one hour at a time, you know this is not easy. To sit for hours upon hours every day requires special training of the body and the mind; the back muscles need to be strong, the posture needs to be correct, the hips need to be open, and the mind needs to be focused. While there are no extant texts from 2,000 years ago or earlier that describe how these ancient meditators prepared their bodies for these exertions, we can safely assume that they did prepare. One of the best ways to prepare for a specific yoga pose is to do that specific pose! So one way to best prepare ourselves for sitting is to sit. Sitting quietly for a long period of time is a yin practice. We can speculate that most, if not all, of the earliest asana practices were yin-like in nature. However, things did not stay that way.

A small number of texts describe how Hatha Yoga was taught in the 10th to 18th centuries: the *Hatha Yoga Pradipika*, the *Gheranda Samhita*, the *Shiva Samhita* and a few others. However, none of these ancient texts were meant to be read alone; all required the guidance of a guru to ensure understanding. The books were used more like notes—shorthand reminders of the actual teaching. Much of the real knowledge was deliberately kept hidden; only when the teacher felt the student was ready was the knowledge revealed. We cannot tell simply from reading these old texts how the physical practice of yoga was performed. What we can say, as mentioned earlier, is that the purpose of the physical practice was to prepare the student for the deeper practices of meditation.

In the earliest spiritual books of India, the *Vedas*, yoga is not described as a path to liberation, and asana practice is not described at all. Rather, *yoga*, among its many other meanings, means discipline, and the closest word to *asana* is *asundi*, which describes a block upon which one sat in order to meditate. By the time the *Yoga Sutra* was compiled, yoga was defined as a psycho-spiritual practice aimed at ultimate liberation.[15] Asana, however, was still a very minor aspect of the practice. The *Yoga Sutra* mentions asana twice[16] in all its 196 aphorisms, and only to say that it should be *sthira* and *sukham*: steady and comfortable. These are very much yin qualities compared to the style of asana we see performed today in yoga classes. When we are still and the mind is undistracted by bodily sensation, meditation can arise.

The point of yoga practices is to enter into a meditative state from which realization or liberation may arise. Historically, different schools of yoga have had different techniques for achieving this. Some even claimed that one cannot become liberated while in the body. The goal in these early dualistic schools was to get out of the body as fast as possible, but this had to be done in the right way. Other schools rejected that approach and suggested that since we can only meditate and practice yoga while in the body, we must treat the body well and keep it healthy. The focus of the Hatha Yoga schools was to build a strong, healthy body that would allow the yogi to meditate for many hours each day. In Hatha Yoga, the practice of asana began to take on a new, broader importance. However, the ultimate goal was still to be able to sit comfortably and steadily for hours.

The *Hatha Yoga Pradipika* was written around the 14th to 15th centuries by Swami Swatmarama.[17] It is almost twice as long as the *Yoga Sutra* and has generated a lot of commentary since its writing. It is one of the oldest extant documents we have describing Hatha Yoga. Compared to today's practices, however, it too contains very little asana practice. Only 15 asanas are listed, and of these, 8 are seated postures.[18] These are quite yin-like in their nature, but many of the other postures are definitely yang-like. The Peacock (*Mayurasana*) is prescribed, and if you have seen this posture performed, there is nothing relaxing or yin-like about it. We are told that one of the 15 postures is supreme; once one has mastered *Siddhasana*, all the other postures are useless.[19] Siddhasana is a simple, yin-like seated posture.

The *Hatha Yoga Pradipika* claims that Lord Shiva taught the Hatha Yoga sage Matsyendra 84 asanas.[20] Other myths claim there are 84,000 or even 840,000 asanas. Regardless, only 15 are listed in the *Pradipika*, and the instruction is to practice them to gain steady posture, health and lightness of the body.[21] None of the Hatha texts mention how long to hold a pose. This is where a guru's guidance is necessary. However, we can assume that the seated postures were meant to be held a long time, while the more vigorous poses, such as the Peacock, were held for briefer periods. It is in the seated postures that the *vayus* (the winds or the breath) become trained through *pranayama*. The Lotus (*Padmasana*) is the prescribed pose for conducting pranayama.[22]

As time went on, later texts expanded the number of asanas explained. The *Gheranda Samhita*, written perhaps in the late 1600s,[23] describes 32 asanas, of which one-third could be said to be yin-like and the others more yang-like. A trend had begun: more yang asanas than yin asanas. Later, the *Shiva Samhita* listed 84 asanas. By the time of the British Raj, when England began to colonize Indian culture and change the school system, asanas were beginning to become blended with forms from the gymnasiums. Wrestling, gymnastics and other exercises were cross-fertilizing the asana practice. Something entirely new started happening in the early 20th century: the asana portion of Hatha Yoga practice was being extracted from the private one-on-one teachings received by a student from his guru into secular offerings in a small classroom setting. The intention of asanas evolved from preparing the body to sit for long periods in meditation to cultivating a healthy physical body. Another innovation occurred at this time: Sun Salutations, which had been completely separate practices from yoga, were incorporated into asana practice.[24] The era of yang yoga was upon us.

It is not that the more yin-like poses disappeared, but they were diminished: B.K.S. Iyengar, in his 1966 book *Light on Yoga*, suggests that the pose Supta Virasana should be held for 10 to 15 minutes.[25] That is Yin Yoga; he just never used that terminology. The American Theos Bernard, a very popular Hatha Yoga teacher in the mid-20th century, also recommended long holds of various postures. The problem arose that, despite yin-like poses remaining in the lexicon of asanas, they were marginalized in favor of the more yang-like postures. One is not better than the other; they are simply different. To sit for long periods of time in deep, undisturbed meditation requires a body that is open and strong. This opening, especially in the hips and lower back, is developed through a dedicated yin practice. However, there is certainly nothing wrong with working the heart and making our muscles longer and stronger too.

While the late 19th and early 20th centuries saw more and more yang postures emphasized, yin poses are not new and neither are they found only in a yoga practice. Throughout the ages, athletes, dancers and gymnasts have been utilizing long-held static stress in their training to help build mobility and range of motion. Yin Yoga as a separate practice is due to the genius of Paul Grilley, who in the 1990s realized the yin postures could be extracted from a generalized yoga class into a separate class on its own. He was the first person to create an entirely Yin yoga class, complete with opening meditation, counterposes, contraindications and ending Shavasana. Until Paul came along, yin postures were embedded into asana practice simply as additional postures to perform. Paul was the first to work out how to teach Yin Yoga on its own, and he also worked out why this was so valuable.

As with all things in life, harmony comes through balance. By combining yin and yang styles, progress in practice is more assured. But why do we call this "Yin" Yoga? Yin is not an Indian term; it is a Chinese word. Where did this crossover come from? Let's look at the parallel development of physical practice from a Chinese, or Daoist, perspective.

DAOISM

Ten thousand years ago, throughout all cultures, shamans blazed the spiritual paths. In India, the shamanic traditions evolved into the yogic practices and philosophies we have been investigating. But this evolution was not confined to the valleys of the Indus, Sarasvati (now gone) and Ganges rivers. In Europe (especially in Greece), the Middle East and China, the same discoveries were being made. Over centuries, despite the distance and difficulty of travel, knowledge filtered out and was shared between cultures. It is not surprising that we find similar concepts discussed in the spiritual practices and philosophies of each region. However, the models and metaphors were modified to fit the local cultural landscape.

The concept of spirit (breath) in the European world had its counterpart in prana (breath) in India. In China, life energy was known as *chi*. Chi is just one of several concepts central to Chinese medical practices. These concepts evolved out of native spiritual practices grouped together under the name Daoism.[26]

There are many forms of Daoism and many ways to practice the teachings. The Dao is sometimes personalized as a god, but most often it is impersonalized as a benevolent but disinterested power: the way of the universe. Live in harmony with the way, and you will benefit. Struggle against the way things are, and you will suffer.

Most Westerners know of the Dao through an ancient book by Lao-tzu called the *Dao De Ching: The Way of Virtue*.[27] In the *Dao De Ching*, we are taught that the Dao is the source of everything. It is nameless because whenever you try to capture the essence of the universe in a concept, you miss the totality of what you are trying to name. The Dao is infinite and inexhaustible. Only the Dao is unchanging and unchangeable.

Since everything is part of the Dao, it follows that the earth, sky, rivers, mountains, stars and humans are also part of the Dao. Humanity is not outside of all this but part of it.[28] In the *Dao De Ching*, the message is: "Get involved! Help, but help in a non-intrusive way. When finished, retire." Yang is acting. Yin is retiring. The Dao is the balance between the two.

In the Daoism of Lao-tzu, the sage is one who cultivates life. The sage learns physical techniques to do this: regulating the breath, honing the body, garnering health, and managing the internal energies, including sexual energy. Along with physical techniques, sages follow ethical principles and regulate their minds through meditation. Diet is also an important part of building and maintaining health. Through all these practices, the sage seeks to change body and mind to recover youth and vitality and live in peace.

The Five Major Systems

There are 5 main systems in Daoism. These are sometimes contradictory and confusing, especially to people of different cultures. Many of the practices of one system are used in the other systems. Thus, the lines between these systems are not fixed and final.

1. **Magical Daoism**: This is the oldest form of Daoism still practiced today. In this practice, the powers of the natural elements and spirits are invoked and channeled through the practitioner to gain health, wealth and progeny.

2. **Divinational Daoism**: This is based on understanding the way of the universe and seeing the great patterns of life. Knowing how the universe works allows us to live in harmony with those universal forces—as in heaven, so on earth. Divinational Daoism utilizes the study of the stars and patterns found on earth to help us live harmoniously. The *I-Ching* (the book of changes) is a divinational book.

3. **Ceremonial Daoism**: Daoism was originally a spiritual practice. Unlike yoga, which remained a personal spiritual practice, this branch of Daoism evolved into a religion and includes daily and significant life rituals, such as marriages and deaths.

4. **Action and Karma Daoism**: Through proper action, we accumulate merit. Following the introduction of Buddhism into China, ethics took on a greater role in spiritual practice. But it did not start there; Confucius also taught the value of proper behavior and morality. Good deeds result in rewards in both this life and the next.

5. **Internal Alchemy Daoism**: Immortality is the goal of this practice. The seeker works to change his or her mind and body to achieve health and longevity. In this practice, chi became recognized as the key to health and long life. Chi is gathered, nurtured and circulated through very strict practices. Incorrect practice is dangerous, and this path of Daoism requires an expert teacher. It is mostly from this system that Chinese medicine evolved.

While an investigation of all these forms of Daoism is beyond the scope of this book, the really interesting branch for our purposes is internal alchemical Daoism.[29]

Internal Alchemy Daoism

The Indian yogis were seeking spiritual immortality: liberation from samsara, the endless cycles of death and rebirth. The Daoist yogis (if we can mix our terms and call them that), who practiced alchemical Daoism, were seeking physical immortality: they wanted to live forever in this body. The form of alchemy we are talking about is not the transformation of base materials to gold but of a normal body to a perfect body. Changing lead to gold is a metaphor for the real goal. There was a period when external alchemy was tried, which involved a lot of poisonous substances such as mercury, but after hundreds of years of poisoning seekers to death, this form of alchemy was dropped in favor of an internal method—change from within.

To become physically immortal, one needed to become really healthy, and that required a lot of dedication and hard work. It could be done! Or at least, it was believed that a few amazing individuals had achieved immortality, but these Daoist immortals were not easy to find, and we can assume they were mythological beings. Certainly, many believe that the real immortality alchemical Daoists seek is spiritual immortality after this mortal coil has been shuffled off. In either case, spiritual immortality or physical immortality, the practice of the internal alchemical Daoists is every bit as challenging as the Indian yogis' practices.

The first priority of an internal alchemist is to conserve his or her energies. When we are born, we are given a certain amount of 3 main kinds of energy: generative energy (called jing), which feeds our sexual desires; vital energy (the commonly known chi energy); and spirit energy (called shen). While these energies are filling us up as we grow in our mother's womb, the mind and the body are already starting to separate. When we are born, due to our ignorance we begin to dissipate our main energies. We lose our generative energy any time we even think about sex. Our chi leaks out through our emotions, and our shen is lost when our thoughts flow. These leakages weaken us, cause illness, and lead ultimately to our death.[30] Through alchemical practice, through internal transformation, our original stores of energy can be rebuilt and we can regain health and longevity.

Alchemical Daoism focuses on the stimulation and balancing of energy in both its yin and yang aspects. The yin energy is the dragon; the yang energy is the tiger. To unify yin and yang we must remove all blockages throughout the body so that these energies can unite in 3 cauldrons, called the tan-t'iens.[31] The process of stimulating these energies involves our breath. Fast breathing will direct yang fire to the middle and upper cauldrons, while slower and softer breathing will stimulate yin energy to incubate our internal energies.

Transformation also involves physical and mental exercises to change our skeletal structures and our mental formations. Before working on the mental changes, we must master the physical changes. Tools here include a host of exercises designed to hone the body: tendon-changing practices, massage, martial arts and the more widely known t'ai chi ch'uan and ch'i-kung practices. Once this basic training is successful, the alchemist moves on to transforming his internal energy. Refining and transforming generative energy, which is stored in the Kidneys, into vital energy involves physical work in the abdomen area, as well as mental practices to minimize sexual desires. Care now must be taken not to dissipate our vital energy through negative emotions, such as anger, fear, frustration or sadness. Now the alchemist is ready for the final stage: transforming vital energy into spirit energy. This requires meditation. The mind must become empty of thoughts, and all signs of duality must be extinguished. Now, there is no division between subject and object, thinker and thought.

When the alchemist is sufficiently advanced, he or she is ready to begin to circulate energy through a practice known as the microcosmic orbit, which is described in Chapter 7. The alchemist will not be successful if all the blockages to the flow of energy have not been cleared or if the mind or senses are stimulated. In the 1930s,

Richard Wilhelm[32] described the benefit of the circling of light in his translation of *The Secret of the Golden Flower, a Chinese Book of Life*. This ancient text had been transmitted orally for centuries before being written down in the 8th century. Wilhelm, a friend of Carl Jung, wrote:

> If the life forces flow downward, that is, without let or hindrance into the outer world, the anima is victorious over the animus; no "spirit body" or "Golden Flower" is developed, and, at death, the ego is lost. If the life forces are led through the "backward-flowing" process, that is, conserved, and made to "rise" instead of allowed to dissipate, the animus has been victorious, and the ego persists after death. It is then possessed of shen, the revealing spirit. A man who holds to the way of conservation all through life may reach the stage of the "Golden Flower," which then frees the ego from the conflict of the opposites, and it again becomes part of Tao, the undivided, Great One.

Success at last! Immortality is achieved through the inner alchemical practice of changing the body, managing energy and meditating. Along the way, many herbs and other dietary rules are followed. Lifestyle changes are also required. This is not an easy path.

Cultivating the Body

Tendon changing? What the heck is that? How do we change our tendons and why is that so important? Good questions. The Daoists use terms that sound familiar to our Western ears, but they don't quite mean what we think. For example, the word organs to a Western mind refers to physically differentiated tissues that perform specific functions, located in one specific area of the body. To the Daoist, however, Organs[33] refers not only to the physical organs as we know and love them in the West but also to an Organ function dispersed throughout the body. Similarly, Blood to our Daoist friends doesn't just flow through our veins, it flows through our meridians and nourishes our Tendons. Tendons are more than simply the connective tissues that join a muscle to a bone. In Daoism, Tendons include ligaments and muscles, fascia and nerves, as well as other soft body tissues.[34]

Tendon-changing practices are ones that target a wide range of tissues and involve stressing, strengthening and massaging these tissues. Of interest to our exploration is that Tendon changing deliberately targets not just the muscles, but also the joints and ligaments; the intention is to regain our natural, dynamic state, our original or optimal ranges of motions. The Daoist practices for cultivating the body include both yin and yang forms of exercises, just as the original Hatha Yoga practices did.

Bone exercises include a technique called "Marrow washing." Fortunately, we don't actually extract our bone marrow and clean it before sucking it back in. This is

Marrow, not marrow. Marrow washing incorporates slow, smooth pressure applied to our joints and bones. This is a yin-like way to stress the bones and joints; there is a more yang-like way, which involves hitting and grinding the bones, but that technique is quite esoteric.

Breath work is also very important to fully cultivate the body. It includes deep abdominal breathing, natural and unforced, breathing through the mouth, through the nose, through both mouth and nose, through the perineum, and several other more esoteric practices. Tortoise breathing is notable: because tortoises live so long, they must be doing something right. They breathe very lightly when they are huddled inside their shells. In fact, they barely breathe at all.[35]

No doubt you are already familiar with some of the classical exercises performed in Daoism called t'ai chi ch'uan and ch'i-kung. These practices look like slow-motion calisthenics, but really they are designed to move energy internally. They combine stretching, breathing and meditation. They can be performed while sitting, standing and even walking. If our Tendons are healthy and soft, if our energy channels are open, then these practices will facilitate the flow of inner energy.

Endnotes

1 For the fascinating story of how Western physical fitness culture influenced modern yoga asana practice, read Mark Singleton's *Yoga Body: The Origins of Modern Posture Practice* (Oxford: Oxford University Press, 2010) and Elliott Goldberg's *The Path of Modern Yoga: The History of an Embodied Spiritual Practice* (Rochester, VT: Inner Traditions, 2016).

2 This concept of the Dao is not unique to China; it has been observed in many cultures throughout history. In India it is Dharma, the law that holds the universe together. In ancient Egypt, it was called Ma'at, a scale whose cosmic balance would weigh a man's soul at the end of his days; without Ma'at, there would be only chaos. Logos served a similar role for the Greeks: it was the underlying order of the universe.

3 A vinyasa is a sequence of postures or asanas that flow smoothly from one to the next. It literally means "to place in a special way."

4 The term yogi refers to a person who practices yoga and so is gender neutral. When we wish to refer specifically to a male practitioner, we use yogin, and to a female practitioner, yogini.

5 The yogis have similar words for yin and yang, tha and ha, which together form the word hatha, after which the well-known school of yoga is named.

6 Individuation is the process of making the individual whole psychologically. In this respect, it is similar to several yogic concepts, but individuation is applied in the psychological realm, whereas yoga is applied to the spiritual realm. We need both: as Georg Feuerstein once said, "Enlightenment is no substitution for integrating one's personality."

7 Robert Johnson was a Jungian analyst, a lecturer and an author of several books on Jungian concepts and relationships, such as *He: Understanding Masculine Psychology, She: Understanding Feminine Psychology* and *We: Understanding the Psychology of Romantic Love.* He studied in Switzerland at the Jung Institute and in India at the Sri Aurobindo Ashram.

8 From Robert Johnson, *Owning Your Own Shadow* (New York: HarperCollins, 1993), 78.

9 Elastic materials return to their original shapes once the stress upon them ends. Plastic materials retain the new shape.

10 In other words, for physiological reasons, children do not need to do Yin Yoga. Some kids may benefit from some of the energetic or meditative aspects of the practice, but it is not really recommended for children. Childhood is a time to play, not to sit still and meditate.

11 Brief can mean 5 or 8 breaths or up to 1 to 2 minutes.

12 Tetany is an involuntary cramping of a muscle. Cramps are not fun! We really don't want to deliberately cramp up our muscles by keeping them contracted for long periods of time.

13 This theory applies beyond the tissues of our body. We need to have stress, and then rest, in all areas of our life in order to be healthy, including our relationships, mental abilities and even our immune systems.

14 Many tendons, ligaments and other fascial structures are elastic and are meant to stretch; this elasticity returns energy back to the body when movement occurs in the opposite direction. For example, our Achilles tendons are elastic and help us to run and jump. There are ligaments along the back of our spine, such as the ligamentum flavum, that can stretch 50% or more of their resting lengths, which is a good thing for our spines. For more information, see Bernie Clark, *Your Spine, Your Yoga: Developing Stability and Mobility for Your Spine* (Vancouver, BC: Wild Strawberry Productions, 2018), 132.

15 The *Yoga Sutra* was compiled somewhere between 200 and 300 and is mythically attributed to a sage named Patanjali. See David Gordon White, *The Yoga Sutra of Patanjali: A Biography* (Princeton University Press, 2014).

16 *Yoga Sutra*, lines II-29 and II-46.

17 Georg Feuerstein, *The Shambhala Encyclopedia of Yoga* (Boston: Shambhala, 2000), 121.

18 The *Pradipika* actually describes other positions, which are used for pranayama or mudra work, but these are not listed specifically as asanas.

19 Swami Swatmarama, *Hatha Yoga Pradipika* (Seattle, WA: Pacific Publishing Studio, 2011), I-43.

20 Ibid, I-35.

21 Ibid, I-19.

22 Ibid, II-7 and 8.

23 Feuerstein, *Shambhala Encyclopedia*, 105.

24 See Goldberg, *The Path of Modern Yoga*.

25 In the Yin Yoga style, Supta Virasana is called Saddle Pose; see B.K.S. Iyengar, *Light on Yoga* (New York: Schocken Books, 1979), p. 125.

26 Daoism is often spelled "Taoism," but since it is pronounced more with a "d" than a "t" sound, I am adopting the former spelling.

27 Dao is the way or path. De means "virtue" but is often translated as "power." Ching is a book or story.

28 This philosophy is echoed in many teachings east of Iran, but in Western religions, it is blasphemy. In these Western religions, humanity is part of creation, not of the Creator: we sit apart from the Creator. This is a dualistic view of creation. In the East, for the most part, the philosophies espouse the non-dualistic view that humanity is part of the Creator and the Creator is within each of us.

29 We are using Eva Wong's definitions for the 5 systems of Daoism. If you would like to study this fascinating field, her book *Taoism: An Essential Guide* (Boston: Shambhala, 2011) is a good place to start.

30 Eva Wong, *Shambhala Guide to Taoism* (Boston: Shambhala, 1996), 173.

31 The lower tan-t'ien is found in the belly, around the navel. It is the home of the generative energy. Thanks to the fire (yang energy) found in the abdominal area, the generative energy is transmuted into vital energy. The middle tan-t'ien is located in the chest region. Here the vital energy is transmuted into spirit energy. The upper tan-t'ien, located where the Indian yogis place the sixth chakra, is between the eyebrows. Here the spirit energy is gathered, stored and eventually merged with the original vapors of the Dao itself.

32 Wilhelm was called the Marco Polo of the inner world of China.

33 Note the capitalization of the first letter here. To distinguish between the Western use of a word and its close, but not exact, Daoist equivalent, we will capitalize the Daoist terms.

34 Wong, *Shambhala Guide to Taoism*, 212.

35 Curiously, there is an understanding in Indian yoga that one is born with just enough breaths to allow us to live to be 108 years old. However, if we breathe too quickly, we will use up our allotment of breaths too soon, and we won't reach that nice ripe age. Many people have recognized slowing the breath down as a key to longevity—just as with the turtle. We will return to this topic in Chapter 7 when we look at breath work during Yin Yoga.

2

THE PRACTICE
OF YIN YOGA

How we practice is much more important than what we practice. Too often, yoga students force themselves into contorted positions with no regard for whether what they are doing is helping them or hurting them. Their egos are in control, and the ego wants to look good in front of others. Yoga has never been a competitive sport:[1] it is an inward practice designed to build awareness, non-attachment, equanimity and contentment. We do not use the body to get into a pose; we use the pose to get into the body. Practiced correctly, yoga can provide numerous physiological benefits while offering the deep inner calm and insights treasured by the yogis of old. We simply have to practice mindfully, with attention and intention.

In this chapter, we will look at the question of *how* to practice Yin Yoga. In Chapter 3 we will then be ready to look at the asanas most commonly used in Yin Yoga. Not nearly as many asanas are required in the yin style of yoga as are found in the more active practices. There are perhaps 36 postures, at most (excluding variations). We will discover the most common poses and examine them in detail, including variations, options and some contraindications.

Before embarking on this practice, please make sure you are able to do so safely. Check with your doctor or health-care professional before starting any yoga practice. The guidance given in this book is not meant to replace medical advice. While care has been taken in compiling the guidance in this book, we cannot take responsibility for any adverse effects from your practice. When you are unsure of any aspect of the practice, or feel unwell, seek medical advice. Please read the contraindications for each pose before you try it, and please note the many options available to make each pose more accessible. Practice with both intention and attention.

In Chapter 4 we will investigate several flows, which are simply a linking together of asanas in a logical sequence with a central theme or purpose in mind. The asanas presented will not exhaust the possible poses one can do in Yin Yoga, and the flows will be even less exhaustive.[2] While Yin Yoga generally targets the lower body, it is possible to apply the philosophy to any area. We will look briefly at some upper body Yin Yoga practices as well as well as, in Chapter 5, special conditions that Yin Yoga may assist with, such as pregnancy, knee issues and low back disorders.

HOW TO PRACTICE YIN YOGA

> Having seated [himself] in … a room and free from all anxieties, [the student] should practice yoga, as instructed by his guru.[3]

Straightforward advice. "What type of room?" you may wonder. Well, the room is easy to come by; simply find

> a small room of four cubits square, free from stones, fire, water and disturbances of all kinds, and in a country where justice is properly administrated, where good people live and food can be obtained easily and plentifully… The room should have a small door, be free from holes, hollows, neither too high nor too low, well plastered with cow dung and free from dirt, filth and insects.[4]

Clearly, advice given in ages past may not be ideal for us now. Having a good teacher who can interpret the teachings and intentions of the gurus of yore and bring the teachings to us in a modern manner is invaluable. In India, where the days were very warm and sometimes scorchingly hot, asana practices were often done very early in the morning. Is that the best time to do Yin Yoga? Let's examine this question.

When to Practice Yin Yoga

There absolutely are no absolutes. The question of when to practice Yin Yoga has no single answer. It depends on what we would like to achieve through our practice. It comes down to our intention.

We could do our yin practice:

- When our muscles are cool (so they don't steal the stress away from the deeper tissues—this will be explained in Chapter 6)
- Early in the morning (when the muscles are more likely to be cool)
- Later in the evening before bed (to calm the mind before sleep)
- Before an active yang practice (again, before the muscles become too warmed up)

- In the spring or summer (to balance a natural yang time of year)
- When life has become very hectic (to balance the yang energies in our lives)
- After a long trip (traveling is very yang, even if we are sitting down a lot)
- During a menstrual cycle (to conserve energies)

We could set an intention to maximize the physiological benefits of our Yin Yoga practice—to work into our joints and connective tissues. Or we could intend to maximize the emotional or psychological benefits—to deepen our mindfulness practice. Or we could decide to work on our energy body—to increase the flows of energy or remove blockages. Depending upon which intention we set, the best time to practice may vary.

Physiologically, Yin Yoga targets the deeper connective tissues. If the muscles are warm and active, they will tend to absorb most of the stress of the pose, so we want the muscles to be relaxed. When we do Yin Yoga early in the morning, the muscles have not yet woken up; this is why we sometimes feel stiff when we first wake up.[5] In the same way, doing our yin practice before an active yang practice allows the stress to settle deeper into our tissues.

By the end of the day, our muscles have been warmed up and are at their longest. The physical benefits of a yin practice will be fewer at this time; however, the psychological benefits may be greater. The daytime is yang: a yin practice before going to sleep may balance this energy. Similarly, the spring and summer are yang times of year. When life is busy or when we spend many hours traveling, these are yang times. Balance is achieved when we cultivate yin energies.

However, a yin practice is not recommended when we have already been very placid. After sitting at a desk for 8 hours in the dead of a dull, dark, damp winter's day, a more active practice may create balance much better than a yin practice. Listening to your inner guide may give you the best answer to the question: Is this a time for yin or yang?[6]

Hot Yin

Hot Yin? Does this make any sense? Isn't "Hot Yin" an oxymoron? The temperatures in these studios are not the full-on 105°F (~ 40°C) common in hot yoga classes but rather a "cooler" 78–95°F (25–35°C). Still, at those temperatures, Hot Yin means the muscles will be quite warm, which goes against the idea of doing Yin Yoga when the muscles are cool. So why do so many studios and students love their Hot Yin classes? It again comes down to intention!

While it is certainly true that more stress will reach the ligaments and deeper connective tissues when the body is cooler (see the section in Chapter 6 on cold muscles versus warm muscles), this does not mean there is no benefit at all to stressing our tissues when the body is warm. Even with warm muscles, the ligaments receive some stress. And for many people, only when their body is warmed up can they move deep enough into a posture to achieve a stress in their targeted tissues. In other words, some students need to be warm to get any sensation or stress.

We can generalize and say that the cooler the tissues, the more that the stress from a pose will be experienced by the deeper tissues, but this does not mean that no benefit is gained by stressing a warm body in a yin way. Being warmed up may mean that most students won't get the maximum physiological benefits, but they will still benefit. And for some students, being warmer may be the only time they get those benefits.

Please realize that the benefits from Yin Yoga are not purely physical: students also benefit from the stillness the practice offers. The opportunity to come to an edge, become still and be with sensations is still available even in a hot room. Indeed, there may be more sensations to be aware of in a hot room. The opportunity to practice mindfulness is enhanced by remaining still for 3, 5 or 10 minutes at a time. The temperature of the room need not diminish the quality of the mindfulness practice. Indeed, this is one reason many people are adding Hot Yin to their yoga practice—it is their chance to calm the mind and practice presence.

Another benefit is the energetic stimulation available in Yin Yoga. Whenever an edge is felt, whenever a posture challenges us physically, tissues are being stressed. These stresses create mechanical, electrical and chemical signals that travel through the body and can change the quality of the tissues that transmit these signals. In the East, this is called prana or chi, which flows through nadis and meridians. The Daoists call the mechanical stimulation acupressure. Even in a hot room, the body can experience acupressure, which stimulates energies to flow.

While it is true that more physiological benefits may be available to the student who practices in a cooler environment, it is not true to say that practicing Yin Yoga in a warm room is not healthy or beneficial. The fact that Hot Yin has become popular attests to the fact that people are getting benefits from the practice. Can it be too much? Is there a danger that, in a hot room, the tissues may be stressed too much? Of course! Anything can be overdone. However, this is a risk for a hot yang yoga practice more than for a hot yin practice, because the hot yoga movements are deeper and more dynamic than those used in Yin Yoga. Whether in a hot or cool room, students must always check in and see what their body is telling them, and respect those signals. Inherently, however, there is no reason to avoid Hot Yin—if you like being in a warm room, enjoy it! It is certainly better than not doing any yin at all.

Before You Practice

Even though Yin Yoga is considered a gentler practice than its yang sibling, it is still important to consider the most common precautions. Please note this is not an exhaustive list. If you have questions, please talk to a teacher or your health-care professional.

- If you are pregnant or have serious health concerns such as joint injury, recent surgery, epilepsy, diabetes or any cardiovascular diseases (especially high blood pressure), be sure to discuss with your health-care provider your intention to practice yoga.
- Don't wear perfume or cologne when you practice. Conscious breathing is part of the practice, and you do not want to be deeply inhaling these fumes.
- Do not eat anything for at least 1 to 2 hours beforehand, and avoid big meals for at least 3 hours before you practice. (For yang practice, allow longer waiting times before practicing.)
- Before you begin, it is nice to have a shower. Empty your bowels and bladder. These are all part of the normal morning ritual, which means you won't be doing your Yin Yoga practice right after rolling out of bed. Give yourself at least 30 minutes after rising before starting any yoga practice.
- If you are already physically exhausted, keep the practice very brief and gentle.
- Avoid practice if you have had a lot of sun that day. Prolonged sunbathing depletes the body—let it recover before stressing it further.
- Remove wristwatches and anything metallic that makes a complete circle around the body.[7] If practical, remove glasses too.
- Wear loose, comfortable clothing so that the body is not restricted.
- You will not generate heat internally, so feel free to wear extra layers of clothes and socks. Keep the room a little warmer than normal.
- Have cushions, blocks and blankets handy for padding and to sit up on for most forward bends and meditation.
- Remove obvious distractions: turn off your phone, put the cat or dog in another room, tell family members that you need some quiet time.
- Avoid drafts and cold flowing air.

Above all, practice in a relaxed manner. If you have something to do right after your practice, decide to finish earlier than necessary so you don't feel rushed at the end. Don't expect to have a "great practice"; that kind of expectation can be counterproductive. Expect to do the best you can, and just be present to what arises.

FUNCTIONAL YOGA

Often in a yoga class, a focus on the posture creeps into the teacher's cues. This is understandable because the postures are the tools we use, but the intention behind any posture should be to generate an effect in the body, not to simply perform the posture or look good doing so. This is the main difference between a *functional* approach to yoga and an *aesthetic* approach. When a teacher, or the student herself, starts to judge a pose by what it looks like, rather than what it feels like, then the intention of optimizing health is lost. How you look in a pose is irrelevant: how you feel in the pose is what matters.

An important concept to become familiar with if you wish to adopt a functional approach to yoga is "targeted area." A targeted area can be any part of the body where we want to focus our attention and generate a physical stress. It can be a particular muscle, joint, fascial group, region, or even an internal organ. The concept can be broadened to include nonphysical intentions as well, such as moving energy, paying close attention to sensations, or deepening meditation. By thinking of your yoga practice this way you will naturally evolve a functional approach to yoga over a purely aesthetic or performance-related view. If your goal is to maximize your ability to perform certain postures or gymnastic maneuvers, then by all means continue to follow an aesthetic practice, but if your intention in doing yoga is to regain or maintain optimal health, a functional approach is essential. This applies whether the practice is yin or yang.

Following a functional approach to your yoga practice raises 3 important questions:

1. What targeted areas are you trying to affect?
2. What are you *actually* feeling in the targeted areas?
3. If you are not feeling the pose where you want to feel it, how can you change the pose so that you create the desired feeling?

Moving away from an aesthetically pleasing alignment is allowed! Feel free to wiggle. Move around in any posture to see whether some slight or more dramatic adjustment creates the sensations you are after. (Once you have the desired sensation, then commit to stillness.) Remember, it doesn't matter what you look like—as long as there is no pain present, who cares what you look like? Go to where there is an edge. Sometimes, the adjustment you need may be very minor. Maybe just using a block or a bolster will give you the support needed to find the edge. Other times, all you need to do is back off a little bit. Surprisingly, for some people backing out of a pose a little generates more sensation than going to the ultimate limit of their range of motion. You don't always have to have your legs as far apart as possible in Straddle Pose, for example. Keeping the legs closer together may work some parts of your adductors that you have been overlooking all these years.

If adjusting the posture doesn't work, there may be many other poses that help you get the stress you want in the targeted area. For example, if you just don't feel the outside of your hips in Shoelace, but your targeted areas are the glutes and iliotibial band, maybe Square Pose is what you need. If not the Square, try the Twisted Roots option of Reclining Twist. Experiment until you get the sensations you seek.

THE THREE TATTVAS OF YIN YOGA PRACTICE

A *tattva* is the reality of a thing, or its category or principal nature. Sarah Powers offers us 3 very simple and effective principles for the yin practice:

1. Come into the pose to an appropriate depth.
2. Resolve to remain still.
3. Hold the pose for time.

Remembering these 3 principles as you practice will simplify everything. The first principle, which applies to any yoga asana, is often called "playing our edge."

Playing Our Edge

The first principle of Yin Yoga is this: every time you come into a pose, go only to the point where you feel a significant resistance in the body. Don't try to go as deeply as possible right away. Give your body a chance to open up, and wait to be invited to go deeper. After 30 seconds or a minute, usually the body releases and greater depth is possible—but not always! Listen to your body and respect its requests.

Consider your will and your body as two dancers, moving in total unison. Too many beginning and even experienced yoga students make their yoga into a wrestling match—the mind contending with the body, forcing it into postures that the body is resisting. Yoga is a dance, not a wrestling match.

The essence of yin is yielding. Yang is about changing the world; yin accepts the world as it is. Neither is better than the other. There are indeed times when it is appropriate and even necessary to change the world; other times, it is best to just allow things to unfold. Part of the yin practice is learning this yielding.

This philosophy is reflected well in a prayer that has uncertain roots. It has been circulating the world for perhaps 100 years[8] and speaks to this very challenge of balancing yin and yang:

> *God, grant me the serenity to accept the things I cannot change*
> *Grant me the courage to change the things I can change*
> *And grant me the wisdom to know the difference.*

Harmony or balance in life comes from this wisdom, which must be earned and learned through our own experience. Our first tattva is the opportunity to gain this wisdom. Listen to your body and go to your edge. When and if the body opens and invites you in deeper, then accept the invitation and go to the next edge. Once at this new edge, again pause and wait for the next opening.

In this manner we play our edges, each time awaiting a new invitation. We ride the edges with a gentle, flowing breath, like a surfer riding the waves of the ocean. The surfer doesn't fight against the ocean; she goes with it.

When you come into the pose, drop your expectations of how you should look or be. There is a destructive myth buried deep inside the Western yoga practice: that we should achieve a model shape in each pose—that is, we should look like some model on the cover of a yoga magazine. To dislodge this myth, we should adopt this mantra:

We don't use our body to get into a pose,
we use the pose to get into our body.

Once you have reached an edge, pause. Go inside and notice how it feels. The pose is working if you can feel the body being stretched, squeezed or twisted. Another mantra to adopt in our practice is:

If you are feeling it, you are doing it.

You don't need to go any further if you are already feeling a significant stretch, compression or twist. Going further is a sign of ego; staying where you are is embracing yin.

This is not an excuse to stay back and not go deep into the posture. When we play our edges, we come to the point of significant resistance. This will entail some discomfort. Yin Yoga is not meant to be comfortable; it will take you well outside your comfort zone. Much of the benefit of the practice will come from staying in this zone of discomfort, despite the mind's urgent pleas to leave. This too is part of the practice.

As long as we are not experiencing pain, we remain. Pain is always a one-way ticket out of the pose—a signal that we are tearing the body or close to doing so.[9] Burning sensations, sharp stabbing pains or tingling electrical-like pains are definite no-nos and warrant coming out of the pose immediately. Dull, achy sensations are to be expected, however. No teacher can know what you are feeling, so be your own guru at these times and develop your wisdom.

The Goldilocks Philosophy

Remember the tale of Goldilocks and the Three Bears? Goldilocks found the momma bear's bed too soft and the papa bear's bed too hard, but the baby bear's bed was just right. The Goldilocks Philosophy is not a posture but rather advice about how deep we should go in our poses to ensure we achieve optimal health. Note: we are not talking about maximum performance! That is the trade-off we have to understand. Whenever we practice yoga, we need to be clear about our intentions. Are we striving for optimal health, or are we working toward some performance goal? Athletes, dancers and gymnasts may well be trying to maximize their range of motion, but this does not mean they are getting healthier. Quite the contrary: many athletes and dancers have significant joint issues in later life because they dangerously stressed their bodies to obtain maximum performance when they were younger.

The optimal position for health is given by the Goldilocks Philosophy: not too much and not too little. This can be shown graphically: figure 2.1 shows a classic n-shaped curve that illustrates the danger of being outside the optimal bounds. If we apply too little stress to our tissues, they atrophy. All living things require some stress to be healthy! If we apply too much stress, however, tissues degener-

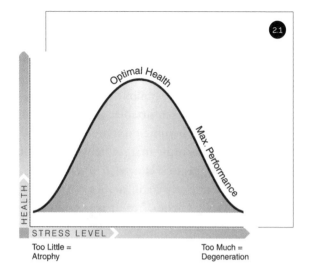

ate. Many scientific studies have verified this n-shaped curve.[10] To obtain maximum health, we need to find that place where the tension in our poses is "just right"—not too deep, which creates degeneration, and not too little, which promotes atrophy.

Antifragility

There are many respects in which human beings can be said to be antifragile. Antifragility refers to a condition whereby an entity gains from randomness, stress and disorder. We can use the example of our bones. Compared to a beam of wood, which breaks down over time (the wood is fragile), our bones get stronger with repeated stress. Bones are antifragile: up to a point, they gain strength with increasing stress. Something fragile suffers from chaos and change. Machines, such as computers or cars, are fragile—they wear out over time and with accumulated stresses. On the other hand, within certain limits, living organisms get stronger with stress.

You are not a machine; stress (up to a point) makes you stronger, not weaker. You are antifragile. This is illustrated in figure 2.2. As stress increases to a limit indicated by point B on the graph, you continue to gain health. If you go past the limit, you become fragile and lose health. However, staying at point A where there is no stress also reduces your level of health. Staying at point A may be comfortable, but it is not healthy. Comfort is the opposite of stress. Modern living tends to seek stress-free conditions, where we are comfortable, but this comes at a terrible cost: fragility. Said another way, comfort is fragilizing!

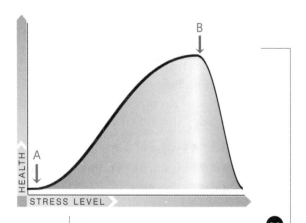

It may seem quite counterintuitive to suggest that someone who is injured should deliberately stress the injured area. The apparently obvious course of action is to rest it, leave it alone and take all stress off the damaged or weakened tissue. While this is comfortable, we pay a price for that comfort: the protected tissues atrophy and become even more unhealthy. We need some stress, but in the presence of injury, the margin between too much stress and not enough stress is very narrow; great care is needed when dealing with injured tissues to ensure we don't go too far, but we still need to subject the tissue to some stress. The Goldilocks Philosophy applies. Yes, it is possible to go too far and damage a joint, but this does not mean that the other extreme is healthier. To never stress a joint is to invite atrophy, pathology and fragility. We have to find the middle path of not too much and not too little. A popular saying summarizes the reality of antifragility: "Use it or lose it!"

Other Edges

Our edges are not only physical—we have emotional and mental edges too. You may be unconsciously holding back from going deeper to avoid a flood of painful memories, thoughts or feelings. You may not be ready for these yet. Honor your edges wherever they appear—and above all, notice them!

Playing our edges is not always a "go further" process. Often, we go forward, pause, maybe back up a little, wait, and then go again or just stop there. Our edges are always changing, and today may be quite different than yesterday. Our bodies change. Some days, we retain more water in our tissues than other days.[11] Water retention affects our flexibility. Our edges will not be in the same place every day. Accept these changes and just take what is offered. Acceptance is the essence of yin.

Resolving To Be Still

The second tattva of the Yin Yoga practice is stillness. Once we have found the edge, we settle into the pose. We wait without moving. This is our resolution, our commitment. No matter what urges arise in the mind, no matter what sensations arise in the body, we remain still.

There are two exceptions to this advice. First, we move if we experience pain or if we are struggling to stay in the pose. Second, we move if the body has opened and is inviting us to go deeper. Unless one of these two arises, we remain still.

We seek 3 kinds of stillness:

1. Of the body, like a majestic mountain
2. Of the breath, like a calm mountain lake
3. Of the mind, like the deep blue of the sky

Stillness of the Body

The body becomes as still as a great mountain, unaffected by the winds and dramas swirling around it. Clouds come and clouds go, rains pelt and snows melt, but the mountain remains.

Stillness in the body means the muscles are inactive. Every time we move, we engage our muscles. The muscles naturally want to take any stretch in the body. One of the muscles' jobs is to protect the joints. Only if we keep the muscles very quiet can we allow the effect of a deep stretch to sink into the joints.

In other words, relax! Why? When we move, our muscles require energy, which is obtained by breathing. When we move, we affect the breath. Stillness of the body leads to a quieting of the breath. Why do we want that?

Stillness of the Breath

Stillness here does not mean cessation. The breath becomes quiet, unlabored and gentle. Like the surface of a mountain lake, unruffled by wayward breezes, the breath is calm. Calm breathing is regular and even, slow, natural and unforced.

Some students prefer a soft *ujjayi* breath during their yin practice.[12] This is perfectly okay, as long as it is soft. The harsher ujjayi found in the yang practices may create waves on the surface of the lake. A soft, rhythmic, ocean sound of the breath will assist with calming the mind.[13]

Your breathing need not be shallow or short, but it should be regular and unforced. You may try to extend each breath to 4 seconds or longer on each inhalation and exhalation. Natural pauses between the inhalations and exhalations may arise. In the pauses between the breaths is the deepest stillness. Allowing the breath to be slow, even, but not necessarily deep is part of allowing this stillness to arise.

Once the breath has become quiet, a deeper stillness arises.

Stillness of the Mind

Long ago, yogis noticed that controlling the mind with the mind is really hard. That is the Zen practice of the samurai warrior and requires tremendous willpower. However, there is a back door to the mind, through the breath. The mind and the breath are like two fish in a school; when one moves, the other moves. If our mind is agitated, our breath is short and choppy. Likewise, if the breath is short and choppy, the mind becomes agitated. However, if we slow the breath down and breathe more evenly, the mind also slows down.

The sky is always with us. Clouds may block our view, but we know with certainty that behind the clouds, the deep blue sky remains. The sky is a metaphor for our true nature. We rarely see who or what we are because so many thoughts and distractions prevent us from seeing clearly what is really there. This vision of our true nature is possible only when the clouds of thoughts have drifted away; stillness of the mind is required for this clarity. Stillness cannot be forced but must arise spontaneously of its own accord. We can, however, create the conditions for this to occur.

To still the mind, the breath must be calm. To calm the breath, the body must be still. When these conditions have been met, deep awareness is possible. This state can be achieved only by commitment and dedication. Commit to stillness and allow whatever arises to be just what it is.

Holding for Time

When we have arrived at our edge and have become still, all that is left to do is to stay. The yin tissues we are targeting are not overly elastic. They do not respond well to constant movement: they are more plastic and thus require long-held, reasonable amounts of traction to be stimulated properly.

Yin tissues don't respond well to maximum stresses held for a short time. Paul Grilley noticed that basketball players, who jump up and down, placing tremendous stresses upon the ligaments of their feet, do not develop fallen arches. Their arches don't fall because the extreme strain is very brief. They are more likely to break bones or tear the ligaments in their feet than to develop fallen arches. However, a 100-pound waitress standing on her feet for 8 hours a day is a prime candidate for fallen arches. She is experiencing a gentle pressure for a long period of time. That is the condition for changing our yin tissues.

Yang postures may be held for as little as 5 breaths or as long as a couple of minutes, depending upon the style of yoga being practiced. Yang tissues require yang exercise. Yin postures are generally held for at least 1 minute and sometimes as long as 20. Yin tissues require yin exercise. Long, gentle pressure coaxes them into greater strength.

It can be dangerous to mix up these forms of exercise. Yang tissues can be damaged by being stressed in a yin manner. No responsible physical trainer would suggest you try to build stronger biceps by holding a heavy barbell in a half-curled position for 5 minutes. Muscles need repetitive movement to grow stronger. Similarly, being stressed in a yang manner can damage yin tissues. Repetitively dropping back from standing into the Wheel Pose can overwork the ligaments in the lower back, eventually wearing them out. We must make sure we exercise yang tissues in a yang way and yin tissues in a yin way.

How Deep?

Each body is different, but in general, every stress on a tissue brings down the tolerance level of that tissue. This is what exercise is all about: we stress tissues to make them weaker, at least initially. Once we release the stress, the tissues recover and become stronger. If we apply too much stress, or hold for too long, or do not allow enough rest, then we are in danger.

The graphs here show how these 3 variables work together. In figure 2.3, the curved line shows the level of stress the tissue can tolerate before becoming damaged. The jagged lines below show the amount of stress being applied repeatedly (or from one prolonged, steady stress). The horizontal axis represents time.

Notice how the amount of stress (the top curve) that our tissues can tolerate decreases with increased stress and time. Eventually, if we continue to stress the tissues to the point where the two lines cross, injury will occur.[14] However, notice figure 2.4. Here we see the recuperative effect of rest, which is also called the refractory period.

If we stress and then rest the tissue, its tolerance level increases above the previous limit. The key then is to not overstress the tissue by having too much stress, applying the stress too frequently or holding it for too long, but rather to allow the tissue enough time to recover and grow stronger.

Follow the Goldilocks Philosophy in all poses, whether yin or yang. Don't go too deep or too much (unless your objective is performance and not health). Don't stay where it is too little, either. From the physiological perspective, in the Yin Yoga practice, time—not intensity—is the magic ingredient. To go deeper in Yin Yoga means to hold longer, not necessarily to move further into a pose.[15]

Also remember that you can do too much of anything. Don't hold your Yin Yoga poses so long that you start to exceed your tissues' tolerance levels. Find the middle path!

How Long?

As important as it is to find the right depth, we also have to consider how long to stay in the pose to get optimal health benefits. Again, each and every body is different, so what might work for a friend could be dangerous for you. Allow yourself time to open up: weeks and even years may be required. In Chapter 3 on asanas, you will

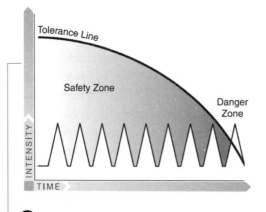

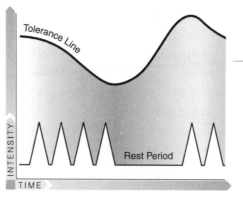

find some recommended lengths of time to hold each pose; beginners should start at the shorter end of the range, except for those who are already quite flexible and open. The range is just a suggestion. Some students can stay much longer, whereas others (such as pregnant students) may need to come out earlier. It all depends upon your unique circumstances and experience while doing the work.

If you are practicing on your own, use a timer or a stopwatch; 3 to 5 minutes may work well for you. If you are just beginning, you may want to start with 1- or 2-minute holds and work your way toward longer periods. You may find that some postures allow you to remain in the pose longer than others; this is alright—reset the timer and stay longer. Our bodies are not uniformly open. It may be better to stay in a challenging pose, such as Saddle, for less time than in an easier pose, such as Butterfly. If you are struggling to remain in a pose, come out, regardless of whether the timer has sounded.

How Often?

In the yang world, we are advised to rest our muscles for at least a day between workouts. This is to allow the muscles a chance to repair the microscopic damage that occurs during workouts and to allow the metabolic waste products to be removed. To accommodate this rule, we choose to work different groups of muscles on succeeding days: the upper body one day, the lower body the next. In the yin world, things are quite different. The waste products produced in our yang workouts are a result of producing energy in our muscle cells. In our yin practice, the muscles are quiet and we do not metabolize our fuels, so there is less or no waste to get rid of.

During our yin practice, we do cause microscopic damage to our connective tissues, and we do want time to allow them to heal and become stronger, but studies have shown that we do not have to wait days between practices to allow this healing to take place. One particular study that looked at therapeutic stresses of a damaged joint concluded that "the clinician's ideal treatment program for a patient with [non-bony], passive joint limitation should be mild stretching, as much as is practical throughout the 24-hour day, 7 days a week, and to start this program as soon as joint motion is allowed."[16]

It turns out that bed rest is never the best option for any ailment; we need to stress our bodies often.[17] But can we do too much? Of course! We can do too much of anything, including Yin Yoga. However, consider people who wore dental braces when they were younger; perhaps you did. If so, did you take the braces off each night before going to bed? Of course not. You left the braces on, possibly for several years. Braces are a yin stress of the yin tissues (bones) of the jaw. This long-held, constant stress was not the maximum that your jaw could tolerate, but it was significant. Time was more important than intensity, and so too with our Yin Yoga practice. We can do this every day and not need time for recovery, at least for normal, healthy tissues.

If you are injured, damaged or not normal in some way, you may well need to take more frequent breaks from the practice.

Remember the arc of aging mentioned earlier? When we are young, we are in the yang time of life and have lots of mobility; what we need when we are young is stability and yang exercises. As we age, we move into the yin time of life and get stiffer, so we need mobility. The older we get, the more we should be doing Yin Yoga every day.

Pay attention to how you feel, both during the practice and in the days that follow. If you start to experience pain or tingling, think about what you were doing in your yoga practice (whether yin or yang) that may have caused the discomfort, and then modify the practice: don't go so deep, don't hold so long. Again, practice with both intention and attention.

The Portable Yin

The yin practice is very portable—you can take it with you anywhere. You don't need a yoga studio or even a yoga mat. All you need is 4 cubits of space on the floor. That is to say, all you need is enough room to stretch out. You can do these poses while engaging in other activities. Although this may not provide you with the deepest benefits (the meditation you get with a dedicated practice will be absent), you can still affect your tissues physically. Sitting in yin poses while reading or talking on the phone, while eating at the coffee table or watching television, will help open the tightest hips.[18]

One last bit of advice: people love to do things that they love to do. Sounds obvious. Said another way, when you are in balance, you will tend to keep doing things that keep you in balance. However, when you are out of balance, you will tend to continue to do things that keep you out of balance! Active people love to do active yoga. Calmer people (a nice way of saying less active people) love to do calming yoga. Don't always practice what you love; practice what you need! Active people probably need Yin Yoga more than anyone else.

Using Props

Many students and teachers unconsciously equate using a prop with cheating. The inner dialogue goes something like this: "I can do this pose! I don't need props!" This is a very yang attitude, but yinsters know something that yangsters haven't quite grasped yet: the intention of their yoga practice is not to look any particular way, the intention is to feel a particular way. Yinsters don't care if a little extra help is needed to get sensation into the targeted area: if props can help, let's use props!

Benefits of Props

There are several key reasons for using props in our asana practice:

- To increase stress in desired areas
- To decrease stress in undesired areas
- To create length and space
- To make certain positions available and accessible
- To provide support: when the bones feel supported, the muscles can relax
- To increase comfort, which means we can linger longer in the pose

When we take a functional approach to yoga practice, we decide on the area we want to target, then we decide where we want to apply a stress to the body and the nature of the stress (either a stretching kind of stress, called tension, or a squishing form of stress, called compression). If we cannot get the level of stress we desire in the targeted area, then we can either choose a different posture or employ props. Props can help to increase stress where there is too little, or they can assist with decreasing stress if there is too much.

Through applying stress intelligently, props can help to lengthen or open the body, creating more room to move. One example is to use sandbags on an inner thigh in Half Butterfly, which will add a bit more juice to the adductor muscles' and inner thigh's fascial network. With this extra space, it may be easier for a student to then add pelvic flexion and fold forward.

Props may also make certain poses possible. There are a number of reasons why a student may not be able to stay long enough to really marinate in the juiciness of the posture. One is the body's proportions. For example, in Baby Dragon, some students' arms are shorter than their shinbones, and they cannot easily rest their hands on the floor. This means that all the students' upper body weight is supported in the hip sockets, which may be fine, but not if the stress there is too much. For other students, the compression of the top/front of their pelvis onto their thigh is very painful or uncomfortable, and they will not enjoy staying in this position for very long. Their body will tighten up to avoid the discomfort, which is exactly the opposite intention of the pose. We want to be able to relax and bear it, not contract and swear at the teacher. In either case, using blocks under the hands allows the student to back off a bit and reduces the stress of the pose enough so that she can linger longer.

One of the principles in Yin Yoga is that we relax the muscles so that the stress of the posture seeps into the deeper connective tissues. If the muscles are engaged, they will take up the stress, which reduces the stress in the targeted areas. Sarah Powers says it like this: "When the bones feel supported, the muscles can relax." Thus, another benefit to the use of props is that the bones are supported, so the muscles can release tension. Very experienced yogis miss out on this: they feel so open and flexible already that they don't need to use props, but if they were to try placing blocks under their knees in Butterfly, they might be surprised by how much muscular engagement they were employing before. Now, with the bones supported, the muscles relax more completely and the stress of the pose goes deeper into the fascia.

Physiologically, the magic ingredient of Yin Yoga is time: we linger long in the delirious delicacy of the postures. Props can assist in lengthening the lingering. The intention in Yin Yoga is to arrive at an appropriate edge and stay. But if the edge is a bit too strong, we won't be able to stay. Using a prop may take just enough edge off the pose to allow us to marinate more. This is not an excuse to back off so much that you don't feel any stress at all; we need stress, just not too much. Using a prop so we can linger longer is a good trade-off.

The Panoply of Props

In Chapter 3, as we review the various Yin Yoga asanas, examples of some prop uses will be shown.[19] But, there is no definitive description of what can be used as a prop. The table shown here lists standard props that are commonly found in yoga studios and many other things that can be used in uncommon ways. This is not an exhaustive list, but it is sufficient to get us started on looking at how to use props in a wide variety of ways.

Standard Props	Esoteric Props
Cushions	Dowels & towels
Blocks	Balls & walls
Bolsters	Chairs & stairs
Straps	Ropes
Blankets	Books as blocks
Sandbags	Handbags/purses
	Yoga mats
	Furniture
	Partners & pets

Remember your intentions! We want to use the props to help us access the targeted area for the poses or to help us stay in the pose longer. If a prop doesn't help us stay longer or feel the pose where we want to feel it, there is no point in using the prop.

Cushions

The standard use of cushions is to help us gain height. We can sit up taller, which allows a more neutral curve in the lumbar spine. Sitting taller also changes our orientation in the field of gravity when we start to fold forward. When we tilt forward, gravity does the work of drawing us down. If we are constrained by tight hamstrings when sitting and cannot even get to a 90° flexion of our hips, let alone go beyond 90°, then a cushion makes all the difference. The extra height changes our orientation enough that gravity comes into play. Common examples include Butterfly and Caterpillar. Many students cannot flex the pelvis enough to come forward if they are sitting on the floor. They will strain with their abdominal muscles and hip flexors to stay sitting upright. However, sitting up on a cushion changes the orientation enough that the student can now relax and let gravity do the work.

Blocks

Similar to cushions, blocks add height or length to the body, making more poses available and effective. Blocks are generally higher/thicker than cushions, but they are harder and thus less comfortable. Sitting on a cushion may not be enough for someone to reach their "tilting point" where gravity can take over, so placing multiple cushions together or a block on top of the cushion may be required. Sometimes, when we try sitting on our heels (Saddle or Vajrasana), a block or two between our feet makes the pose more accessible.

Blocks are also useful for simple support: you can rest blocks under bent knees in forward folds, like Straddle or Caterpillar, to allow the bones to relax and thus the muscles to soften. Blocks are great, and you may want to have several on hand when you do a Yin Yoga practice.

Bolsters

Similar to blocks, bolsters also help to take stress off bones. Where blocks can add height or length to the body, bolsters are mostly used to relax the body in the postures. Remember, bones don't like to be left hanging: muscles will engage to support them. But we want the muscles to relax, so a bolster under the bones accomplishes this. A good example is the challenging pose of Saddle. For many people who can't quite come all the way to the floor, a bolster under the spine allows them to relax in this pose. Bolsters can be used to prop the body in many ways: the upper body can relax when folding forward onto a bolster, such as in Half Butterfly.

Straps

Straps are great for preventing unwanted movement and, when folded several times, for prying open the body. A good example of the first intention is Wall Straddle, where the legs are allowed to fall widely apart. For many students, this can be too intense. Using a strap or two to limit the abduction of the legs allows the student to come to an appropriate edge, then relax without having to use her muscles to keep her there.

When folded several times, straps can be used to keep two parts of the body separate, such as when we employ a strap behind the knees in Half Butterfly (useful for students who suffer knee pain when the knee is fully flexed), or between the hip and thigh in Dragon Poses (for students who feel a painful or uncomfortable pinching there.)

A final common use of a strap is to create greater reach. For example, in Shoelace (aka Cowface or Gomukhasana), when we want to clasp our hands behind our back but can't quite reach, a strap bridges the gap. (And here, creativity is allowed! If a strap is not available, use a necktie or a towel. Even strong socks can serve—just wash them before offering them to your students.) Straps are used often in Hatha Yoga classes to help students reach the feet in straight-legged seated poses, or in supine backbends where the intention is to reach back for the feet (think Bow Pose). Straps looped around the feet make the feet accessible. In Yin Yoga, we do not have to pull on the straps, just hold with enough intensity to remain where there is the appropriate amount of stress in the targeted area.

Blankets

Blankets can keep us warm. Nothing surprising about that. We use them for Shavasana for that reason. Yin Yoga is a cool practice—we don't warm up the body at all, so we can use blankets to keep us warm and comfortable while we marinate in the postures. Beyond their heat-regulating properties, blankets can be used like cushions (fold them up a couple of times) or like bolsters (roll them up into cylinders), but they can be used as unique foundational supports as well. Many teachers recommend blankets for inversions, such as Shoulder Stand or Plough Pose, to raise the shoulders while the head remains on the floor. This changes the angle of the neck and makes the pose less stressful there. We can use a folded blanket in the same way in the Yin Yoga posture called Snail.

Blankets in Yin Yoga can also be used in place of a regular yoga mat. We don't do standing postures in Yin Yoga, so we don't need a sticky yoga mat, but a nice soft blanket underneath us may make poses like Frog possible. Blankets can cushion the knees and allow them to slide apart. For the same reasons, a blanket under the back knee in Dragon lunges or Swan may make the pose possible for students who suffer kneecap pain.

Sandbags

Sandbags add resistance, stability and weight. Remember, one of the key principles in Yin Yoga is to find the appropriate edge and linger. But many people come into a pose and find no real edge. Sandbags can help make the postures juicier—but remember the Goldilocks Philosophy and don't get too juicy! Sandbags on the inner thighs in Butterfly or Half Butterfly can add that little bit of extra stress you may be craving. Placing a sandbag along the spine in Half Butterfly or Child's Pose can also feel quite lovely.

Sandbags can also create stability and prevent us from slipping out of poses. Bananas can be slippery, but in Bananasana, strategically placing a sandbag beside the feet can help anchor them in place. A sandbag on the bent knee in a Reclining Twist can anchor that knee, even if a bolster underneath the knee already props it up.

Esoteric Props

As long as you remember the intention behind the use of props, you can use many things this way. Instead of a sandbag to restrain your movement, you can use walls or a heavy piece of furniture. (Think again of Bananasana: use a wall or the leg of your sofa to stop your feet from sliding out of the pose.) There are numerous things you can use to support you and help you stay in a pose. Many yoga studios have no props, but they have yoga mats! A yoga mat or two rolled up can be a cushion, block or bolster. Your dog or partner can be a nice bolster under your lower back for a supported Bridge Pose. If you don't have a bolster or small child handy, use a chair or a coffee table to lean on in forward-folding, seated poses such as Caterpillar. You can do the Swan with your front leg on a stair, or a chair, or the kitchen counter. As we will discover at the end of Chapter 4, a wall can be an excellent and fun prop. Get creative, but remember your intentions.

BEGINNING THE PRACTICE

Many students faced with the challenge of practicing yoga at home feel overwhelmed by the possibilities and are not sure how to proceed. Beginning teachers face the same quandary; what do I do to get started well? Before you even start your practice, it is helpful to think about your intention. Once you have that clear in your mind, it's easy to choose the asanas you will do.

Intention

Why are you going to do yoga today? You may never have asked yourself this question, and yet you still feel driven to practice. Why? There are no wrong answers; anything that brings you to your mat is to be respected. But understanding your inner drive will help you to focus on your goal, to pay *attention*.

Reminding yourself of why you are doing yoga throughout your practice will help you achieve your purpose. For some, the intention is to regain or maintain optimal health. If this is your intention, remind yourself to feel your state of health as you practice, feel the healing energies flowing through you. You will heal faster when you remember this intention. For others, the purpose may be to strengthen the body or improve mobility.

Perhaps you are going through a very hectic time in your life and you need to slow down. That will be your goal today: balance. Some people do yoga as part of a meditation practice or because they know they will feel better after they are finished.

These are all perfectly valid reasons for doing yoga. But there can be more—we can set an intention beyond our own benefit. We can make an offering of our practice for the benefit of others. This can be done at the beginning of every practice. Certainly all the other physical, psychological and emotional benefits will still be there, but we can achieve even more. For centuries, prayer has been used in the same manner; we dedicate our efforts to a greater purpose than ourselves.

In the *Yoga Sutra*, this is called *ishvara-pranidhana*—a surrendering of your efforts to something greater than yourself. As you sit or stand at the beginning of your practice, bring to mind someone or something that needs assistance or help right now. Another attitude you can adopt is gratitude. Dedicate your efforts during your practice to that person or thing that you are grateful for, grateful to or want to help. This dedication fills you with a resolve to do the practice with full *attention* along with the *intention*. When a challenging time comes up in the practice (and it usually will), you will find the extra strength you need because of your dedication.

Invocation

Making an intention into a dedication is sending your energy outward. Sometimes, this is not what you need. Sometimes, what you really need is to draw energy inward through an invocation. Invoking resources and support from outside the self is a common way to begin a yoga practice.

Invocations can be as simple as chanting "Om" and allowing the vibration to fill our bodies and then linger. Longer chants can also be nice. Chanting is a wonderful form of breath work. It not only stimulates energy to flow through us but also has a calming, centering effect on the mind. Test them out: some chants are too energizing and distracting—that is not what you need right now. Find and use ones that are centering and calming.

Not all invocations need to be chanted; you can invoke whatever symbols or energies you relate to. Simply ask in your mind for their support, strength, guidance or whatever it is you feel you need right now. Your practice is your payment.

Opening Meditation

Once you are clear about why you are practicing today, you are ready to begin. Most beginnings are gentle. A period of meditation is nice. Sit, lie down, or stand in Mountain Pose and meditate. Spend 3 minutes or more to take inventory and notice from where you are starting.

Here is one option: begin by allowing your awareness to sink into your lower belly. From here, notice the rhythm of your own breath. Feel the rising and falling of each inhalation and exhalation. Do not try to change anything. Notice and accept the breath exactly as it is.

After a few breaths, allow your awareness to broaden. Notice other feelings in your body: feel the earth beneath you … the sky above you … the temperature of the air against your skin … the touch of your clothing … the space and sounds all around you.

After a while, bring your awareness to the heart and check in with the state of your emotions. This can be difficult, but they need not be big, dramatic feelings. Look closely and don't dismiss anything that appears. The emotion may be as small as boredom. Perhaps there is a little bit of irritation. Contentment can also appear from time to time. The key is to notice what is arising, without judging yourself for what is there. Don't criticize yourself for being bored or irritated; don't congratulate yourself for being content. Simply notice what is happening right now.

After another minute or so, allow your awareness to rise to that point right between the eyes. From here, start paying attention to the thoughts arising. Don't try to stop them; just watch each new one arise, notice it and let it float away.

Begin to move your energy. Yin Yoga removes the blockages deep in our connective tissues, allowing the chi or prana to flow unhindered. In a yang practice, we use movement to start this flow of energy, but that engages the muscles, which we generally avoid in the yin practice. In Yin Yoga, we can use other techniques, which will be discussed in Chapter 7.

While you move into, hold and move out of the postures, keep taking inventory. Notice how the practice affects you physically, emotionally and psychologically. Accept whatever you find out and stay curious. There may not be enough time in a short meditation to do all the above practices; don't worry—you will have lots of time during the poses to come back to them.

FLOWING

Depending upon what intentions you set and the areas you are targeting, your choice of asanas will vary. Knowing what you want to do makes it a lot easier to choose postures. For example, let's suppose your intention today is to work your hips. From the list of asanas in Chapter 3, you would choose any of the several postures that target the hips. If one particular pose doesn't work for you, try another one—for any particular area, there are usually several suitable asanas.

Chapter 4 provides several example flows designed with specific themes or intentions in mind. There are flows that work the hips, spine, upper body and legs. There is even one that works the whole body. If your intention is to do some energy work, there are 2 flows you can try; one works the Kidneys and the other works the Liver.[20] If your intention is to have a more mindful, meditative practice, then any of these flows will suffice. For those just starting out and with little experience of Yin Yoga, 3 introductory flows are offered. In time, you will begin to intuitively know which asanas work for you, and you will create your own flows. Until then, it is perfectly fine to use the flows found in Chapter 4.

Beginning Asanas

At the start of our practice we want to ease into the body. Before going deep into a backbend, we'll want to do a gentler backbend to prepare. The same applies to forward bends or twists. Open the body with easier postures before going to the deeper openings.

Unlike in more active practices, in Yin Yoga we are not trying to warm up; we want the muscles to remain relatively cool so they are not taking up all the stress of the postures; when the muscles are cool, the stress can go deeper into the connective tissues. Here are a few beginning asanas that get us under way by starting shallower rather than by warming us up:

- Butterfly: loosens up the hips and spine
- Child's Pose: grounding and soothing
- Caterpillar or Dangling: loosens up the spine for deeper forward bends
- Frog (the Tadpole version): loosens up the hips and upper back
- Sphinx: loosens up the spine for deeper backbends and stimulates the Kidney meridian, which helps to support all the other organs

Each of these postures begins to work specific targeted areas and prepares the body for the deeper postures to come. Consider your intentions and which areas of the body you want to work, then choose your first asana to help you work toward your goals. A very flexible student can start her practice with almost any posture if she remembers the first tattva of Yin Yoga: play your edges appropriately. However, a few asanas definitely need preparation before you attempt them (e.g., even the most flexible students will want to work up to asanas such as Snail, the full Seal and the Winged Dragon). Before the Snail, loosen up the neck. Before the deepest backbend, as in the Seal, do a gentler backbend. Before the deepest hip openers, start with milder versions.

The Butterfly can be a great first pose for almost any practice because it mildly works into the hips and spine; it is a gentle flexion of the spine and hips, a gentle abduction of the thighs and a gentle external rotation of the hips. From here you can go in many directions: deeper hips work, deeper spine work, etc. However, if you practice Yin Yoga in the evening and if you spent your whole day hunched in front of a computer screen, you may wish to start your practice with a gentle backbend such as Sphinx rather than Butterfly. The point is to choose your first pose deliberately, with consideration of where you want to go and with where you have been.

Paying Attention

Memorize this little saying: "Awareness of present experience, with acceptance."[21] This is a great recipe for mindfulness, which is a synonym for meditation. The benefits of a strong mindfulness practice are discussed in Chapter 8, but for now—just do it! Pay attention, on purpose, in a specific way. Notice what you are feeling. If you have chosen a targeted area for the posture you are in, notice what sensations are present in this area. (If you are not feeling anything in the targeted area, then wiggle around a bit until you do, or use a prop. If you still don't get the desired sensation, perhaps choose a different posture that will generate the sensations you seek.)

At first, answering the question "What are you feeling?" may leave you lost and wondering. This is not answering "*How* are you feeling?" but "*What* are you feeling?"

What sensations are arising? We are not used to looking within, so many people can't identify what they are feeling without guidance and practice. It takes attention, intention and persistence.

Once you can identify these sensations, delve deeper. For example, if you feel a physical sensation, where is it exactly? Is it superficial or deep? Is it in one place or spread out? What shape does it have—is it long like a ribbon or spherical or block-like? Does it have a temporal quality to it—does it throb, come and go, or remain constant? Is there a quality of temperature—is it cool, warm, hot or burning? (Don't stay if it is burning!) Is it stretchy (tension) or squishy (compression)? Is it sharp, dully or achy? (Don't stay if it is sharp!) Is it tingling or electrical? (Don't stay if it is!) When the main sensation ebbs away, notice the next most obvious sensation that is occurring and investigate that.

The table below illustrates some of the types of sensations that can arise during a Yin Yoga practice. This is not a complete summary. Unless the sensation is painful, stay and investigate what is happening. Accept the sensation; don't try to change it or mentally run away from it. Remember: awareness of present experience with acceptance.

For beginners, the strongest noticeable sensations will likely be physical ones, but in time, you may also notice emotional, psychological or even energetic sensations. What are they? We can investigate whatever arises. This also applies to our breath: we can investigate it as well.

Sensations of Tension	Sensations of Compression	Sensations of Pain
Superficial	Soft	Achy
Localized	Squishy or bouncy	Burning
Spread out	Pinching or impinging	Scratchy
Stretchy	Hard	Circling
Tugging	Stuck or blocked	Radiating
Tight	Deep	Sharp
Linear or rope-like		Sparkling
Dull		Electrical
Warm		Zingers (shooting)
Hot		Boring
Burning		Risky
Throbbing		

The Ocean Breath

At this point, you are in the flow. You've entered a posture and applied the 3 principles of the practice. Now, let's investigate the very yin-like style of breath mentioned earlier: the "ocean breath."[22]

There are many forms of breath work in yoga (called pranayama). Some are very active and stimulating, and there are times when these pranayamas are beneficial. But to turn on the parasympathetic nervous system, which is our rest-and-digest system, we can use the slow, even pranayama known as ujjayi, which means "victorious breath." A more poetic term for this is "ocean breathing."

Max Strom in his book *A Life Worth Breathing* describes the practice of ocean breathing well:[23] imagine you are trying to fog your sunglasses for cleaning. Try to make this "haahhh" sound on both exhalation and inhalation. At first, do this with your mouth open until you can create the soft sound of the waves coming ashore habitually, without thinking about it. At that point, move to making the same sound with your mouth closed.

Max notes that ocean breathing enlivens and expands the lungs, dynamically pulling in fresh air and expelling stale air and stress. He has discovered that it calms the mind and can be very effective for processing grief. If you experience emotions or even some tears from using the ocean breath, receive it as a healing experience.[24]

In his book *The Heart of Yoga*, the late T.K.V. Desikachar recommends that our attention be focused first on the exhalation. Practice watching your out-breath until you know everything about it. Then allow your awareness to encompass the inhalations. Know everything about the in-breath. Don't worry about the practice of retaining your breath, of holding the breath with lungs full or empty.[25] Instead, allow your ocean breath to slowly lengthen, but don't force it. Surf the breath, and flow with the waves. Desikachar advises that lengthening the breath is okay, but it is not the point. The point is to do whatever it takes to stay focused and present, paying attention to the breath. There definitely are physiological and psychological benefits to an extended breath, which we will investigate in Chapter 7.

It is also worth knowing that in our Yin Yoga practice, we do not have to keep using the ocean breath all the time. Since we are turning off our stressed, fight-or-flight state (called the sympathetic nervous system) and turning on the parasympathetic nervous system, once the switch is made, we do not have to keep using this breath. It is like turning on a light: once you have flipped the switch, you don't have to turn it on more. Similarly, it may only take a couple of minutes of ocean breathing to turn off your sympathetic nervous system and turn on the parasympathetic; once the switch is made, there's no need to keep doing it.

Here's how you might use ocean breathing. When you have arrived at that still point in your first pose, begin to make the sound of the ocean. Start with your mouth open. Allow the breath to slow. Count to 4 as you inhale, pause for 1 count, count to 4 as you exhale, and again pause for 1 count. This totals 10 counts, equivalent to 6 breaths per minute. Next, try it with your mouth closed. Make this into a habit. Whenever you begin your yoga practice, start to surf your ocean breath for a couple of minutes. Eventually, you will be able to use the ocean breath to help you calm down and release stress at other times in your life.

Once you are relaxed, focus your full attention inward. Release the breath and allow it to be whatever it needs to be, but notice what it feels like to breathe. Notice everything about your breath and what happens as you happen to breathe. Explore the yin side of your breath.

Linking Asanas

In the yang world, yogis love to create wonderful flows; as if dancing, we move from one pose into another. There is a rhythm and a logic to these flows: they open the body in stages, prepare us for the more challenging postures, take us to great heights, and allow periods of calm. The yin world is quite different. We hold the poses longer, thus we have less time for many postures in our practice.

We do want to begin the journey with shallower poses before going deeper. Shallow postures naturally precede deeper postures. Examples mentioned already include starting with Sphinx or Bridge Pose if you want to work on backbends or stimulate the Kidneys. After a mild backbend, you will be ready to move into more challenging postures such as the Seal or Saddle, which create more stress in the spine.

Many asanas seem to beg to be paired with each other; Shoelace seems to flow naturally, organically into Swan. Twists easily flow from one side to the other. Straddle folding over one leg easily invites folding over the opposite leg, and then a final fold right down the middle feels very natural, or vice versa.

In the yang styles of yoga, some sort of counterpose to release the tissues follows every deeply held posture. Counterposes move the body in the opposite direction of the previous pose. In the yin style, counterposes are also recommended, but they do not need to occur right away. (In Chapter 6, we will be discussing why counterposes are so necessary, as we meet the reality of "creep"—a natural elongation of tissues when they are subjected to a constant stress.) It is nice to do some gentle yang movements between postures to relieve any incipient stagnation and to get the energy flowing again. However, it is not necessary to do a counterpose immediately after any particular asana. Feel free to do all your forward bends before moving into backbends. Do all your hip work before moving on to the counterposes. But don't overdo this—if you are really craving a counterpose at any time, do one!

Counterposes are very logical. Backbends balance forward bends and vice versa. Right balances left. Internal rotation of the hips balances external rotation. Twists can be used to balance almost any pose involving the spine. Sometimes these counterposes are simple movements, sometimes they are long-held poses of their own.

Some yang poses seem to be made for when we come out of yin poses: Down Dog feels so good after Swan. And if you never really cared for Down Dog before, after 5 minutes of playing with the Dragons, you will quickly learn why the Dog is a yogi's best friend.

By the time you have finished your practice, make sure you have done counterposes for all the deep postures you've held. Some suggested yang counterposes are offered at the end of Chapter 3.

Another option is to let the body rest for a short time between each pose, especially if the pose was very deep. If the sense of fragility is high coming out of a yin posture, take the option of being still and enjoying the echo of the previous pose. Paul Grilley suggests doing a 1-minute Shavasana (which he terms "Pentacle") after every Yin Yoga pose. In the stillness, enjoy the "rebound" feeling—Paul says that is the feeling of chi flowing. Respect the body's wishes, and take your time between the postures.

Finishing Asanas

In the yang styles of yoga, the teacher will allow a significant amount of time at the end to cool the body down. In the yin practice, this is not necessary because we never warmed up! But we still want to find a way back to neutrality and balance. Any of the beginning asanas can work well at the end, but a pose often done is the Reclining Twist. This asana allows the body to fully relax and release. It is one of the most yin-like asanas of all.

The twist in the spine can be directed higher or lower to relieve whatever area was most worked in the practice. Moving the knees higher, toward the armpit, brings the twist more up the spine by curving the spine forward. Pointing the knees straight to the side brings the spine to neutral, allowing the twist to be even along its length. Moving the knees downward arches the spine slightly, bringing the emphasis in the twist to the lumbar/sacrum.

Twisting the spine can be done in many orientations. You can do it sitting up or lying down. It is not the only way to end your practice, but twisting seems to get a lot of the residual kinks out.

Other Considerations

For some students, one side of the body is definitely more open than the other. Many teachers suggest starting your asana on the more open side first. Your closed side will watch with amazement at what is happening and will be inspired to open that much as well. Of course, if you don't know which side is more open, it really doesn't matter. But make sure you don't do the same side twice. One way to make sure that doesn't happen to you is to always start with your right side. That way you will always know that your next side will be the left.[26]

If you are short of time, do fewer postures instead of holding more poses for less time. Those last few breaths give you the most benefit in a pose. It is like that last push-up that strengthens you the most, or that last sugar-filled, creamy doughnut that puts on the most weight. Of course, there are no absolutes, so feel free to do the opposite too; do more poses for shorter holds if you have less time. But shortening the time in the poses moves us away from the real yin nature of the practice. If you have time for only one posture, do either the Butterfly or the Sphinx Pose.

Finally, be aware of how much time you have allowed for your practice. The opening meditation and poses can take up to 15% of this time, and finishing postures, including Shavasana, may be another 15% or so. That leaves you 70% of the time for the key poses you really want to get into. Be aware of the time as you flow. Don't shortchange the ending because you got carried away with the fun postures in the middle of the practice. Shavasana is the most important part of the practice.

ENDING THE PRACTICE

While we do not need to cool down, we do want to restore the body to neutrality. Once we have completed our last pose, it is time for rest and then a transition back to the world we left behind. This rest period is Shavasana.

There are 2 parts to any exercise: stressing the body and resting the body. Most teachers, trainers and students spend a great deal of time learning how to stress the body in a myriad of ways. Equally important is Shavasana, the rest period at the end or our practice where the tissues we just used get the chance to become more usable.[27] Unfortunately, too many students are unaware of the need to balance stress with rest. They may skip their Shavasana or shorten it too much if they are practicing at home or by themselves. But it's better to shorten the other asanas and keep the full amount of time available for Shavasana.

Not all forms of rest are equal. One medical study showed that the effects of stress were reduced in significantly shorter time by Shavasana than by simply sitting quietly or lying down.[28] It is an active form of relaxing, which sounds like an oxymoron. Shavasana has been proven to be a very effective form of rest. Don't skip it!

When we have finished, we should feel completely balanced. After Shavasana, or even just before it, some quiet pranayama or energy work may be nice. Right after Shavasana, you may find yourself in a deep, yin-like, altered state. Performing some guided breath work can balance your yin and yang energies and wake you up again. Nadi shodhana, also called alternate nostril breathing, is a good way to balance yin and yang energies. (These are discussed in Chapter 7.)

Closing Meditation

After relaxing and balancing your energy, you may wish to conclude with a brief meditation. This can mirror your opening meditation; perhaps you'll remind yourself of your intention for the practice and/or conduct an inner inventory. Compare how you feel now with how you felt at the beginning. Note the differences, if any, but do not judge your practice as good or bad. It was what it was.

You may wish to finish with some sort of gesture of completion. Bring your palms together in prayer, leaving a bit of space between the hands to symbolize the space in your heart. Bow down to the floor.

When you rise, you may wish to chant something brief. "Om" will suffice, or you can chant "*Lokah samasta sukhino bhavantu.*"[29] Or simply end by saying "*Namaste*" to all the teachers in your life who have guided you.[30]

For some dedicated yogis, the time after Shavasana is for a full meditation practice. The body is open and strong. Sitting may feel easier. The breath is calm right now. The heart is content. It is a perfect time to train the mind.

Transition to Your Next Activity

When the practice is over and everyday life is waiting for you, don't just jump right back in—savor the quietness for a while. Whatever your next actions are, do them with mindfulness. Allow this heightened awareness to linger throughout the rest of your day. Notice the openness in your body as you move. Smile often and pause frequently. Take time to return to awareness.

Endnotes

1 That is, yoga was not a competitive sport until the early 20th century. Unfortunately, it has recently become just that! There are yoga competitions now—an interesting oxymoron.

2 In the YinYoga.com Forum, other teachers and students offer their own favorite flows. Feel free to check these out and add your favorite ones.

3 Swatmarama, *Hatha Yoga Pradipika*, I-14.

4 Ibid., I-12 and 13. A cubit was considered to be the length of a man's forearm, from the elbow to the tip of the fingers, or about 18 inches. So this would mean you need only about 6 feet of space (500 years ago, apparently, no yogis were over 6 feet tall).

5 It is generally not a good idea to do any significant exercises immediately upon awakening. The vertebral discs swell up during the night due to osmosis, placing greater stress on the restraining ligaments and fascia of the back. If we practice yoga within the first 30 minutes or so after waking up in the morning, we may place too much stress on these tissues. People with back issues, such as herniated, bulging or slipped discs, should be especially cautious of flexion first thing in the morning.

6 Listen to your inner voice, but really listen! Most people tend to do what they like, not what they need.

7 Metal circles distort and interfere with electromagnetic energy flow, which may be one of the forms of chi. In physics, this is known as Lenz's law.

8 It has been adopted by Alcoholics Anonymous and is called the Serenity Prayer. Wikipedia claims that the theologian Reinhold Niebuhr originally wrote it in the 1930s or early 1940s.

9 We have an unfortunate saying in the West: "No pain, no gain." The translation into Sanskrit, the liturgical language of yoga, is: "Bullshitihi!" The East has a better saying: "No pain, no pain!"

10 See Stuart McGill, *Low Back Disorders* (Champaign, IL: Human Kinetics, 2002), 32.

11 This is especially true for women, whose bodies change during their monthly cycles.

12 The ujjayi breath is obtained by slightly constricting the back of the throat, the same way as when you try to fog a mirror or glasses with your breath. With lips closed, a yin ujjayi has a "haahhh" sound on both inhalation and exhalation. The sound may remind you of the wind in the trees or the waves on the shore. A yang ujjayi may sound more like Darth Vader. Cultivate the softer, ocean-sounding breath.

13 Several scientific studies show the benefits of the ocean breath. These will be covered in Chapter 7.

14 The stress that happens when the curves cross can be thought of colloquially as "the straw that breaks the camel's back." It can be a very small stress, such as bending over to pick up your socks off the floor. When we injure ourselves, we like to blame that last movement for causing the injury—also called the *proximal event*. In reality, it was the accumulation of all the stresses we subjected ourselves to that set up the condition for the injury. Sometimes, a student will injure herself in a yoga class and then blame the teacher or the studio. Often, workers' compensation boards will claim that a worker's job was not responsible for an injury because the worker was at home when she picked up that sock and hurt her back. In both cases, it was repetitive strains over time that created the conditions for the injury to happen, not the proximal event.

15 More flexible Yin Yoga students do not need to do more and more difficult poses; they simply need to stay in the poses for longer and longer periods of time.

16 See George R. Hepburn, "Case Studies: Contracture and Stiff Joint Management with Dynasplint," in *Journal of Orthopaedic and Sports Physical Therapy* 8.10 (April 1987): 498–504, doi:10.2519/jospt.1987.8.10.498.

17 See Selina M. Parry and Zudin A. Puthucheary, "The Impact of Extended Bed Rest on the Musculoskeletal System in the Critical Care Environment," in *Extreme Physiology and Medicine* (2015), doi:10.1186/s13728-015-0036-7.

18 Thanks to an insidious invention called the chair, our Western backs are very weak and our hips very tight. We constantly lean against the backs of our chairs and couches, which means our back muscles don't have to do any work. To really strengthen our backs, to preserve the natural curve in our lumbar and to open the hips, we should get out of our chairs, slide off our couches and live on the floor whenever we can.

19 You can view a video of Diana Batts and Bernie Clark illustrating many ways props can be used in Yin Yoga at www.yinyoga.com/newsletter19_using_props.php.

20 Note the capitalization of Kidney and Liver here! I am referring to the Daoist organs now.

21 From Ronald D. Siegel, *The Mindfulness Solution: Everyday Practices for Everyday Problems* (New York: Guilford Press, 2009).

22 A slow ocean breath while you are holding your poses will reduce stress, activate your parasympathetic nervous system, improve your heart and lung function, lower your blood pressure, and lead to a healthier and happier life. That seems like a lot to gain from simply breathing, so we will investigate these claims in detail in Chapter 7.

23 Max Strom, *A Life Worth Breathing: A Yoga Master's Handbook of Strength, Grace, and Healing* (New York: Skyhorse Publishing, 2010), 111.

24 Ibid., 112–113.

25 Desikachar warns: "[M]any people think that they can progress quickly along the yoga path by practicing breath-retention techniques, but in fact problems often arise with this emphasis"; *The Heart of Yoga: Developing a Personal Practice*, 2nd ed. (Rochester, VT: Inner Traditions, 1999), 60.

26 Diana Batts, who co-teaches with me our Yin Yoga teacher training courses, switches every January 1st which side she starts with. She doesn't have to wonder which side she started on, because she knows this is a left-side-starting year or a right-side-starting year.

27 My thanks to Sarah Powers for this lovely turn of phrase.

28 D.D. Kulkarni and T.K. Bera, "Yogic Exercises and Health – A Psycho-Neuro Immunological Approach," *Indian Journal of Physiology and Pharmacology* 53.1 (January 2009): 3–15.

29 This means, "May all beings everywhere be happy."

30 Namaste is an acknowledgment of the divinity in you and in others.

3

YIN YOGA ASANAS

The *Hatha Yoga Pradipika* lists only 15 asanas, and of these, 8 are seated positions. Those postures are meant to be held for a long time. Today, we would call them yin postures. In Paul Grilley's book *Yin Yoga*, he lists 18 yin poses, along with 5 yang poses to be used in between them. If you are planning to hold each pose for 5 minutes, and if you allow a 1-minute rest between postures, a 5-minute meditation at the beginning, and a 10-minute Shavasana at the end, in 90 minutes you will have time for only 12 poses. There will be even fewer if you are doing two sides or other variations in each posture.

There is not a great need for a lot of postures in the Yin Yoga practice! Paul states in his book, *"The more yin you practice, the less variety is needed, and the emphasis is placed on a few basic postures."* He also has a nice saying: "Twenty is plenty!" More simply stated, you do not need a lot of postures to do Yin Yoga!

This chapter will describe 25 individual Yin Yoga asanas and will follow this structure:

- Pictures of the pose, including some common variations
- The intentions of the pose, citing the key targeted areas
- Contraindications (reasons for avoiding the pose)
- How to get into the pose
- Alternatives and options while in the pose
- How to come out of the pose
- Some possible counterposes
- Meridians that may be stimulated and their pertaining Organs
- Suggested hold times
- Other notes of interest, including further benefits of the postures

While the pictures of the asana will provide examples of how the posture might look, please remember that every body is different. The shape is not what's important. To paraphrase David Williams: The real yoga is what you can't see. Remember, what is important is not what a posture looks like but what it feels like.

The intentions and benefits listed in the asana descriptions are not exhaustive but provide guidance to help you choose when to add a particular asana to your practice. If you wish to arrange your practice time around a particular area of the body, the advice here may be useful. Occasionally, several potential benefits claimed by B.K.S. Iyengar will be cited. However, please know that Iyengar's claims are based upon anecdotal evidence, references to other claims by yoga researchers in India in the early 20th century, as well has his own inferences and speculations. Today, the Western medical community would take these claims with many grains of salt, and it must be noted that they have not been verified by modern scientific research.[1] Indeed, all the benefits suggested for each posture are indications of what may be possible, but there is no guarantee that the benefits will be realized for every student. However, anecdotal evidence is still evidence. Will you benefit from these postures? Only you can tell!

Always check out the contraindications before trying a posture for the first time. Included, where available, are contraindications suggested by Dr. Loren Fishman and his co-developers of the website *Yoga Injury Prevention* (YIP).[2] The site includes explanations of why certain postures have been deemed contraindicated for specific conditions, for readers who want to delve deeper.

Know and respect your limits. If a certain pose is not right for you, there are lots of other ways to work the targeted areas. Choose another posture that is more appropriate or accessible from the suggestions offered in the alternatives and options. Or skip this posture completely and choose another pose that is accessible to you.

The recommended times to hold poses are subjective. These are guidelines only, which you should completely ignore if they are not appropriate for you. Some students can remain in the asanas much longer than indicated; others must come out much earlier. Pregnant women, for example, may wish to limit their time in any posture to 3 minutes. Listen to your inner teacher, and respect your body's unique needs.

When coming out of a pose, we may experience a natural sense of fragility—we have been deliberately stressing the body and holding it there. The sense of relief is to be expected. Enjoy your practice! Smile when you come out of the pose! Laugh or even cry. Thank the Buddha, Jesus, Allah, Paul Grilley... Shout, "Om namah Shivaya!"[3] Enjoy the moment.

One of the benefits of Yin Yoga is this experience of coming out of the asana. After a deep, long-held hip opener, you may feel like you'll never be able to walk again—but be assured the fragility will pass. (As long as you didn't experience any pain! Remember, pain is a one-way ticket out of the pose.) Sometimes, a movement in the opposite direction will help to more quickly dissipate the fragility. This is a counterpose, a balancing posture that brings us back to neutral. Short descriptions of the offered counterposes are provided at the end of this chapter. Another option after coming out of a pose is to remain completely still, in a Shavasana position, and monitor the rebound effect for a minute or two.

Many of these asanas will be familiar to experienced yoga students. However, the names may be different in the yin tradition, and this is deliberate. For example, the yin pose of Swan looks identical to the yang pose of Pigeon, but in the yin practice, we relax the muscles; our intention is to soak deeply into the joints and the deep tissues wrapping them, not the more superficial tissues of the muscles. There is no consensus in the world of yoga on naming asanas; different names abound. The ones shown here are the names more commonly used in the Yin Yoga tradition, but they are not universal, and there may be other names for these postures.

THE ASANAS

This selection will suffice to work all the areas of the body normally targeted in a Yin Yoga practice: from the navel to the knees, which generally means the hips and lower spine.

53

1. Anahatasana (aka Melting Heart)
2. Ankle Stretch
3. Bananasana
4. Bridge (aka Supported Bridge)
5. Butterfly
6. Half Butterfly
7. Cat Pulling Its Tail
8. Caterpillar
9. Child's Pose
10. Dangling
11. Deer
12. Dragon
13. Frog
14. Happy Baby
15. Reclining Twists
16. Saddle
17. Shavasana
18. Shoelace
19. Snail
20. Sphinx and Seal
21. Square
22. Squat
23. Straddle (aka Dragonfly)
24. Swan and Sleeping Swan
25. Toe Squat
26. Yin Postures for the Upper Body

ANAHATASANA
(MELTING HEART)

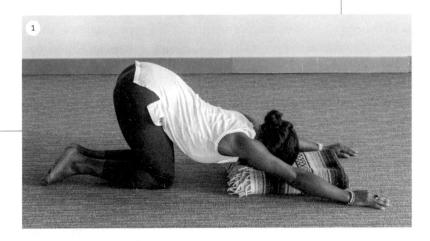

INTENTIONS AND TARGETED AREAS

- Primary targeted areas: middle and upper back (extension).
- Secondary targeted areas: neck (extension) and arms/shoulders (flexion).

CONTRAINDICATIONS

- If you have a bad neck, take care, as the looking-forward option could strain it too much or cause sensations of lightheadedness.
- Be aware of any tingling in the hands or fingers! This is often a sign that a nerve is being compressed, and if you continue to compress it, you may permanently damage it. If you feel tingling, adjust the arm and hand positions (fig. 2) or skip the pose entirely.

GETTING INTO THE POSE

From your hands and knees, walk your hands forward, allowing your chest to drop toward the floor (fig. 1). Keep your hips above your knees. Find the neutral position for your arm width (which may or may not be shoulder-width apart).

ALTERNATIVES AND OPTIONS

- If shoulder pain or tingling prevents the arms from going overhead, move them further apart or rest your forehead on your forearms (fig. 2).
- You may also stretch out just one arm at a time (fig. 3), resting the head upon the other forearm.

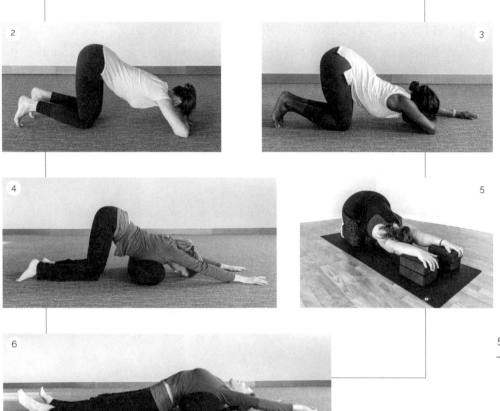

- If you're very flexible, you can bring the chin to the floor and look ahead, but this could strain the neck.
- If your knees are uncomfortable here, place a blanket underneath them.
- Toes can be tucked under (fig. 2).
- The chest can rest on a bolster, allowing the body to relax (fig. 4).
- Another option is to rest your outstretched hands on blocks (fig. 5).
- If this pose just doesn't work for you, another way to get the extension in the upper back is to recline over a bolster, as shown in fig. 6.

COMING OUT OF THE POSE
Either move back into Child's Pose or slide forward onto your belly.

COUNTERPOSES
Lying on your abdomen or in Child's Pose can be nice here. Since this posture is a backbend (extension), Child's Pose is a good choice for a counterpose because it is a mild forward fold (flexion) of the spine.

MERIDIANS AND ORGANS AFFECTED

○ Sensations (compression) along the middle and upper spine may stimulate the Urinary Bladder meridians.

○ Stress in the chest may stimulate your Stomach and Spleen meridians.

○ This posture may juice up the arm meridians through the shoulders, especially the Heart and Lung meridians.

RECOMMENDED HOLD TIME

○ Three to 5 minutes.

○ If resting your chin on floor, the hold may need to be shorter. Carefully watch the sensations in the neck.

OTHER NOTES

○ Other common names for this pose are Half Down Dog and Puppy Dog.

○ Mildly extends and compresses the lower spine.

○ The head and neck also extend if the student looks forward, bringing the chin to the floor.

○ If you are worried about the cleanliness of your yoga mat, use a towel or blanket under your forehead, as shown in fig. 1.

○ Extension of the upper back may be good for hyperkyphosis.

○ We spend a lot of time flexing our upper spine throughout the day (sitting at desks, etc.). This pose is a great way to create some balance for the upper back.

○ If the knees spread apart, this becomes Frog Pose!

○ Can be used as a precursor for deeper backbends.

○ If you feel pinching in the back of the shoulders, you may be reaching a compression point. Abducting the arms (moving them farther apart) may allow you to go around this point.

ANKLE STRETCH

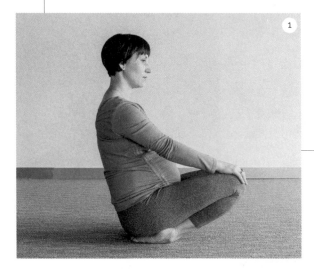

INTENTIONS AND TARGETED AREAS

- Primary targeted area: the ankles (plantarflexion).
- Secondary targeted areas: the knees (full flexion).

CONTRAINDICATIONS

- If there is any sharp pain in the ankles, back off.
- This can be painful on a hard floor, so try placing a blanket or towel under the feet to cushion them.
- Knee issues (knee replacement, ligament or cartilage damage, chronic inflammation) may prevent sitting on the heels; sitting on a cushion may be helpful. You can also try placing a rolled-up towel behind the knees or a cushion between the thighs and calves.
- If your ankles or knees still complain, this may not be the pose for you. Skip it and try Swan or Dragon Pose (where the back leg's foot will also be plantarflexed but with much less stress).

GETTING INTO THE POSE

Begin by sitting on the heels (fig. 3). If sitting on the heels is too challenging, sit with blocks or cushions between your feet. This may be enough for the ankles! Check in with how it feels before trying other options. If it is too intense, lean back on the hands (fig. 2) and check in again.

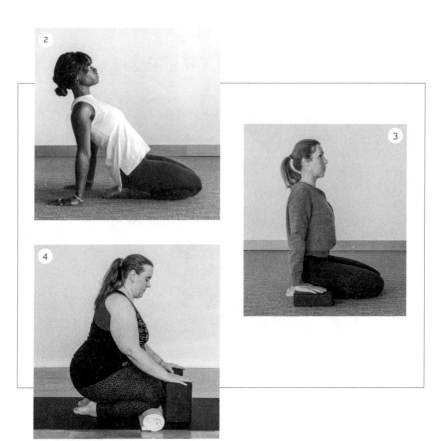

ALTERNATIVES AND OPTIONS

- Leaning back on the hands (fig. 2) is the easiest, least stressful position, but beware of collapsing backward. Keep the heart forward, and imagine you are trying to do a backbend.

- After a few moments, bring the hands to the floor or to blocks beside your legs (fig. 3).

- Padding under the knees may make the pose more accessible (fig. 4).

- Most challenging is holding the knees and gently pulling them upward (fig. 1).

COMING OUT OF THE POSE

Lean forward and bring your hands to the floor beside the knees. Slowly step one foot at a time back to a push-up position or just lie on your belly.

COUNTERPOSES

- Push-up, Plank on elbows or any posture that straightens the legs and tucks the toes under.
- Dangling or squatting.

MERIDIANS AND ORGANS AFFECTED

Sensations along the top of the foot may stimulate the Stomach meridians, while sensations along the back of the calves and thighs may stimulate the Urinary Bladder meridians. Any sensations of stress along the top of the thigh may indicate stimulation of the Stomach and Spleen meridians.

RECOMMENDED HOLD TIME

One to 3 minutes, especially if the sensations are relatively intense. You may eventually be able to sit like this for a very long time.

OTHER NOTES

- This is a nice counterpose for many postures that dorsiflex the feet, such as Toe Squat, Down Dog, Squat and some cross-legged seated meditations. For some people, it can even be therapeutic for the knees.
- Sitting on the heels is known as Seiza (a Japanese meditation position) but B.K.S. Iyengar calls this Virasana. He doesn't suggest lifting up the knees. His version involves sitting between the feet if possible. (Other teachers call sitting on the feet Vajrasana, but Iyengar calls that a variation of Virasana.) He recommends holding this pose for 1 minute initially, and then working up to 5 minutes. He claims it can help strengthen the arches of the feet, fix flat feet, relieve gout, improve circulation in the feet, relieve heel spurs, knee pain and knee inflammation, and even correct herniated discs.[4] These claims have not been verified.

BANANASANA

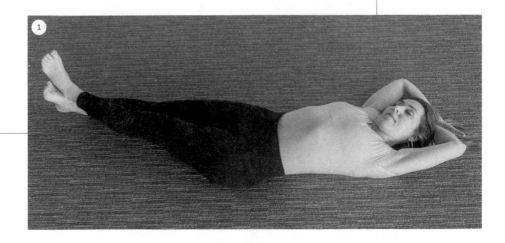

INTENTIONS AND TARGETED AREAS

- Primary targeted area: the lateral side of the torso, neck and hips (side flexion).
- Secondary targeted area: the armpits (abduction).

CONTRAINDICATIONS

- If you are prone to tingling in the hands when extending your arms overhead, you may need to place a bolster under the arm or simply bring the hands down.
- If you have low back issues, you may wish to not go too deep in this pose.

GETTING INTO THE POSE

Lying on your back with your legs together and straight on the floor, reach the arms overhead and clasp your hands or elbows. With your buttocks firmly glued to the earth, move your upper body to the right. When you have gone as far as you can, move the legs (fig. 2). (Note the order! It is easier to move the legs, so move those last.) Arch like a nice, ripe banana. Be careful not to twist or roll your hips off the floor. Find your first edge. When your body opens more, move both feet further to the right and pull your upper body further to the right as well.

ALTERNATIVES AND OPTIONS

- After marinating for a while, try crossing the ankles (fig. 1). Most students feel the greatest stress by crossing the outside ankle over the inner ankle, but some feel more "locked in" with the other ankle on top. Experiment.
- If you feel any tingling in the hands, support the arms with a bolster or rest them on the forehead. If tingling persists, lower the arms.

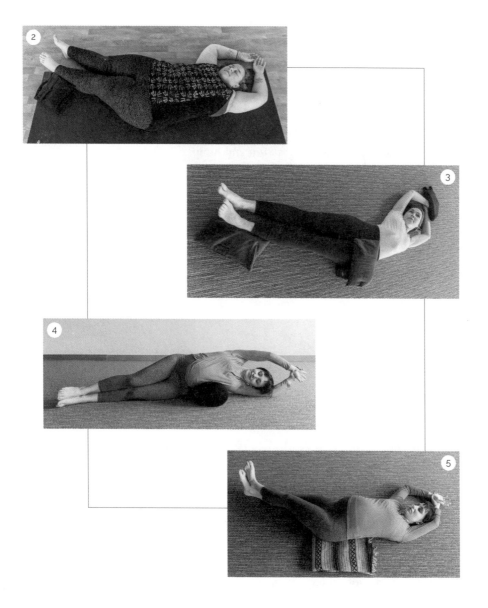

- If your hips tend to roll up, a sandbag or heavy bolster here may be helpful. If it tends to slide off the hip, use a block beside the hip to support it. Sandbags beside the outer foot can also be used to hold the feet in place. Or they can be placed on the hands if the arms are straight overhead (fig. 3).
- Pregnant women who are uncomfortable on their backs can try a side bend over a bolster. Have the bolster under the lower ribcage and side belly to maximize the arch as shown in fig. 4.
- Another option for pregnant women is to have support under one hip (fig. 5).

COMING OUT OF THE POSE

Move your legs back to a straight position and bring your arms down. Be still and enjoy the echo of the posture. (Don't forget to do the other side.)

COUNTERPOSES

- Hug the knees to the chest to release the back in a gentle forward fold.
- Circle the knees to massage the sacrum and lumbar.
- Spontaneously erupt into any pose that feels organic.

MERIDIANS AND ORGANS AFFECTED

- Sensations along the side of the hips and torso may stimulate the Gall Bladder meridian.
- Stress closer to the spine may stimulate the Urinary Bladder meridians.
- Stress along the arms and into the shoulders while they are overhead may stimulate the Heart and Lung meridians.

RECOMMENDED HOLD TIME

Can be held for 3 to 5 minutes.

OTHER NOTES

- This is a lying down version of Half Moon or Blown Palm.
- This is a delicious way to stress the whole side of the body. It works the spine in a lateral flexion (side bend) from the iliotibial (IT) band to the top of the side rib-cage. It stretches the oblique abdominal muscles and the side intercostal muscles between the ribs. If you feel tugging at the outside of the hip (the greater trochanter), then you may be working your tensor fascia latae (this is not a drink from Starbucks but the muscle that connects the IT band to the iliac crest) or gluteus maximus, both of which attach to the IT band.
- Don't forget to do both sides; however, you may wish to hold one side longer than the other if you have significant asymmetry in the spine, such as scoliosis. In this case, stress the tight side longer than the open side or skip the open side entirely and do the tight side twice.

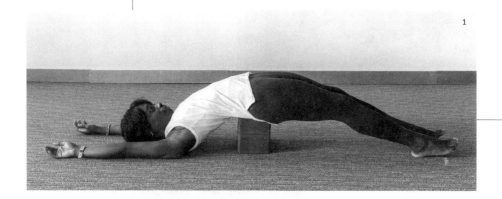

BRIDGE
(SUPPORTED BRIDGE)

1

INTENTIONS AND TARGETED AREAS

- Primary targeted area: the sacrum/low back (extension).
- Secondary targeted areas: the arms/shoulders (flexion) when arms are overhead. For many students, having the arms overhead also creates a nice stress in the lower belly. Tension may also arise through the hip flexors.

CONTRAINDICATIONS

- Students with arthritic hips, hip replacements and low back issues may find the stress here too much. Either modify the pose to be lower or skip this entirely.
- If any tingling occurs in the hands when your arms are overhead, rest your forearms on your forehead or a block. If that doesn't resolve the tingling, lower the arms completely.
- This is not ideal for pregnant women, who may prefer to do Sphinx Pose with bolsters under the thighs and elbows.
- Contraindications from YIP: anterior total hip replacement, anterolisthesis, arthritis hip, gastroesophageal reflux disease, hernia (abdominal), herniated cervical disc, Lasik surgery, lumbar spinal stenosis, nosebleed.

GETTING INTO THE POSE

Start lying on your back with knees bent. Lift the hips high enough to slide a block or bolster under the pelvis. Make sure the support is under the pelvis/sacrum and NOT under the low back (fig. 2). We want the lumbar spine to be unsupported. Do

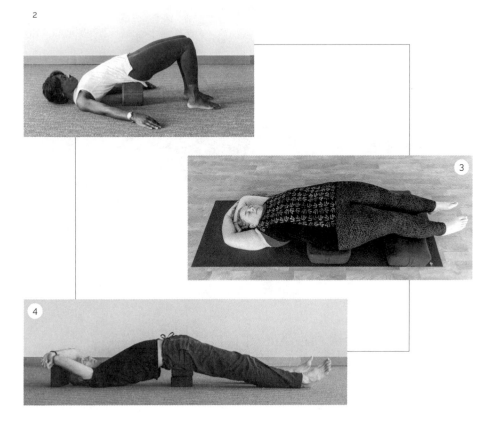

NOT put a block on its thin edge, as that is potentially unstable and could tip while you're in the pose; only put blocks on their widest sides. If more height is needed, add more blocks.

ALTERNATIVES AND OPTIONS

- Once the pelvis is supported, walk the feet away, thus straightening the legs. Legs fully straight (fig. 1) create the deepest stress into the low back, sacrum and hip flexors.

- Not quite as deep is resting your legs on another bolster (fig. 3). This should still create a sense of compression in the low back.

- After a few minutes, more flexible students may increase the height of the support, perhaps by adding more blocks.

- Raising the arms overhead (fig. 1) increases the tension in the lower abdomen and hip flexors. If this creates any tingling or electrical feeling in the hands, there are 2 options to reduce this: rest the arms on a block (fig. 4) or on your forehead.

COMING OUT OF THE POSE

This is a surprisingly juicy pose, so come out slowly, gingerly. Start by bending the knees again and walking the feet toward you. Engage your core muscles and then lift your hips just an inch, just enough to allow you to slide the support away. Slowly lower your hips to the floor and pause there in awe.

COUNTERPOSES

Give yourself a minute or so before moving. Since we were extending the spine, a little flexion is nice: hug your knees to your chest.

MERIDIANS AND ORGANS AFFECTED

- Sensations along the sacrum and lower spine may stimulate the Kidney and Urinary Bladder meridians.
- Stress along the thighs or lower belly may stimulate the Spleen and Stomach meridians as well as the Kidney meridians.
- Stress along the arms and into the shoulders while they are overhead may stimulate the Heart and Lung meridians.

RECOMMENDED HOLD TIME

We can marinate in the pose for a fairly long time, but 3 to 5 minutes should be plenty to start.

OTHER NOTES

- This is very similar to Setubandha Sarvangasana, but instead of using our arms to hold the hips up, we use props. This makes it possible to stay in the pose passively for a long time.
- Bridge is great preparation for deeper backbends but also a juicy "work-in" to the low back all on its own.
- In B.K.S. Iyengar's version, a bench is used to support the lower body. He recommends holding this pose for 3 minutes initially, and then working up to 5 to 8 minutes. He claims it can help relieve backache and neck strain, prevent varicose veins, improve digestion, relieve headaches and improve blood circulation.[5] These claims have not been verified.

BUTTERFLY

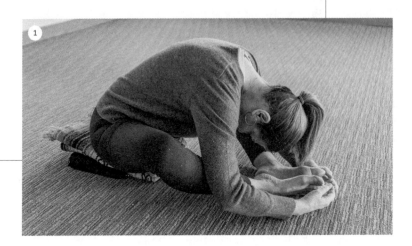

INTENTIONS AND TARGETED AREAS

- Primary targeted areas: the whole spine (flexion) and hips (flexion, external rotation, abduction).
- Secondary targeted areas: the inner thighs/adductors (tension) and the hamstrings (tension).

CONTRAINDICATIONS

- Can aggravate sciatica. If you have piriformis sciatica, elevate the hips by sitting on a cushion so the knees are below the hips. If you have discogenic sciatica, avoid rounding the spine. In either case, if this pose makes the symptoms worse, avoid it entirely.
- Many knees do not like this pose. If your knees complain, have the feet further away, support the thighs with blocks or cushions (fig. 2) or skip this pose.
- If you have any low back disorders that do not allow flexion of the spine, then do not allow the spine to round: keep the back as neutral as you can. You could choose the reclining version (fig. 3), which many pregnant students prefer, or Wall Butterfly (fig. 4).
- If you have had a hip replaced, check with your surgeon before trying this pose.
- Avoid dropping the head down if you have neck issues.
- Contraindications from YIP: arthritis hip, arthritis knee, chondromalacia patellae, herniated lumbar disc, osteoporosis, posterior total hip replacement, retinal tear, retrolisthesis, sacroiliac joint derangement, spinal fracture (vertebral body), compression fracture, total knee replacement.

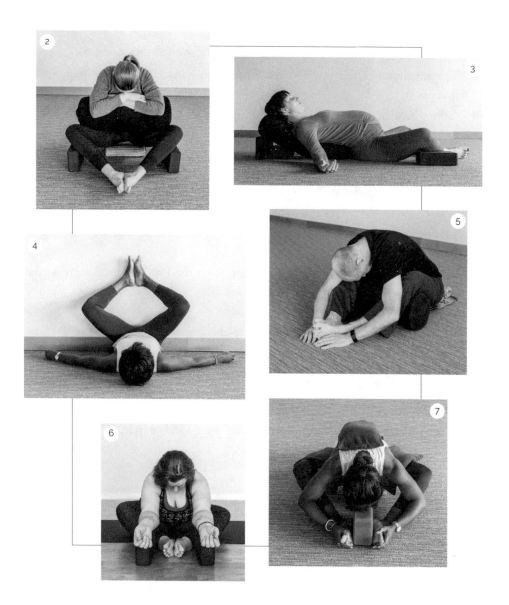

GETTING INTO THE POSE

Sitting on a cushion, bring the soles of your feet together and then slide them away from you. Consider this to be a "long-legged Butterfly"! Allowing your back to round, fold forward, lightly resting your hands on your feet or on the floor in front of you. Your head can hang down toward your heels (fig. 1).

ALTERNATIVES AND OPTIONS

- Elevating the hips with a bolster or cushion will help tilt you forward.
- If your neck is too stressed, support your head in your hands, resting your elbows on your thighs or a block, or support your head with a bolster.

- You can rest your chest on a bolster positioned across the thighs (fig. 2).
- For complaining knees, support the thighs with blocks (fig. 2) or with a bolster under both legs (fig. 5).
- Various hand/arm positions are possible: hold your feet, place your hands on the floor in front of you or relax your arms behind the body. Another option is to place blocks under the hands (fig. 6).
- If the back doesn't like this pose, do the reclining variation: lie down, keeping your legs in Butterfly. You may lie on a bolster for support (fig. 3) or rest against a wall.
- Another option is the Wall Butterfly, with legs up the wall (fig. 4), which again spares the spine.
- Sandbags on the inner thighs, on the feet or on the low back may increase the sensations without you having to go lower (fig. 7). You can even combine the sandbags with blocks under the knees.
- Placing a block between the feet increases the amount of abduction in the legs, changing the level of stress in the hips (fig. 7).

COMING OUT OF THE POSE

- Use your hands to push the floor away and slowly roll up.
- Before straightening your legs, lean back on your hands to release the hips. Then slowly straighten each leg.

COUNTERPOSES

- This was a flexion for the spine so spinal extension is nice. Do a gentle sitting backbend or lie on the belly. You could also do Cat's Breath or flow into Tabletop (aka Hammock).
- Seated twist is another way to release the spine.
- This was also an external rotation for the hips, so some internal rotation, like Windshield Wipers, may feel nice.

MERIDIANS AND ORGANS AFFECTED

- Sensations along the outside of the hips may stimulate the Gall Bladder meridians.
- Sensations through the inner knees, thighs and groin may stimulate the Liver and Kidney meridians.
- Sensations along the spine may stimulate the Urinary Bladder meridians.

RECOMMENDED HOLD TIME

Three to 5 minutes or much longer if desired.

OTHER NOTES

- A nice way to stress the low back without requiring loose hamstrings.
- If the legs are straighter and the feet further away from the groin, the hamstrings will get more stress. If the feet are in closer to the groin, the adductor muscles get more stress.
- Sarah Powers suggests that if you only have time for one pose, do Butterfly. It also is a nice way to start a Yin Yoga practice, as it is a gentle way to work into the spine and hips.
- If the feet are closer in, tightness in the adductors or low back may prevent you from folding forward. Move the feet farther away. (It is not wrong to do this pose with the feet in close: that will stress the adductor muscles more, but it also prevents many people from flexing at the hips. With the feet further away, more hip flexion is possible, which allows more spinal flexion too.)
- This pose is nice for pregnant women because the legs are abducted, providing space for the belly.
- B.K.S. Iyengar calls this Baddhakonasana (although he suggests having the feet in close to the groin and keeping the spine neutral) and claims it is good for the kidneys and prostate gland, treats urinary problems, prevents hernias, removes heaviness in the testicles, regulates periods, helps ovaries function properly, and makes childbirth easier.[6] These claims have not been verified.

HALF BUTTERFLY

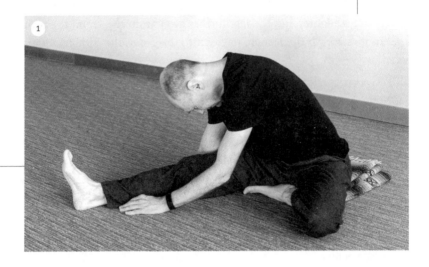

INTENTIONS AND TARGETED AREAS

- Primary targeted areas: the whole spine (flexion and lateral flexion) and hips (flexion, external rotation, abduction).
- Secondary targeted areas: the hamstrings (tension). Depending upon how far apart the legs are abducted, there may be some tension in the inner thighs and the inner knee.

CONTRAINDICATIONS

- Can aggravate sciatica. If you have piriformis sciatica, elevate the hips by sitting on a cushion so the knees are below the hips. If you have discogenic sciatica, avoid rounding the spine. In either case, if symptoms are made worse, avoid this pose entirely.
- If you have any low back disorders that do not allow flexion of the spine, then do not allow the spine to round: keep the back as neutral as you can.
- Beware of any sharp pain in the knees if the legs are wide apart. If you have issues in this area, bring the legs closer together.
- If the bent knee complains, place support under that thigh (fig. 2) or move that foot away from the groin. Some students find relief by placing a folded strap or rolled-up towel at the back of the bent knee.
- If the hamstrings protest, bend the straight knee and support the thigh with a blanket or block (fig. 2).

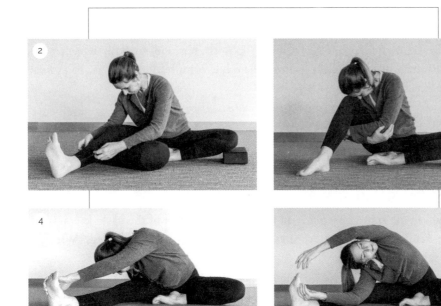

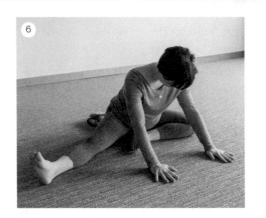

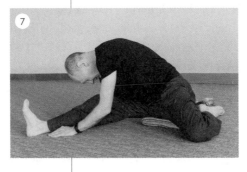

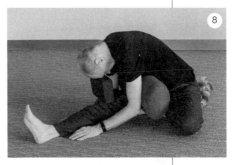

- Contraindications from YIP: anterior cruciate ligament tear, arthritis hip, arthritis knee, chondromalacia patellae, herniated lumbar disc, ischial bursitis, lateral meniscal tear, medial meniscal tear, osteoporosis, posterior total hip replacement, retrolisthesis, spinal fracture (vertebral body), compression fracture, total knee replacement.

GETTING INTO THE POSE

From a seated position, draw one foot in toward you and stretch the other leg straight out to the side. Allowing your back to round, fold over the straight leg (fig. 1).

ALTERNATIVES AND OPTIONS

- Rounding the spine may place more stress in the fascia of the back; keeping the spine neutral may place more stress on the hips and back of the legs. Which is your targeted area?
- If the hamstrings are tight, folding forward may be restricted. Very tight students may bend the knee so much that the foot is on the floor (fig. 3), in which case, they can wrap their arms under the thigh and over time let the leg become a bit straighter.
- Reach the opposite hand to the extended foot and/or lower that shoulder to emphasize the side of the spine (fig. 4).
- Add a twisting side bend to the spine by resting the elbow on the thigh and the head in that hand (or for more flexible students, by placing the arm alongside the straight leg) and placing the other arm behind the back or over the head. Rotate the chest toward the sky (fig. 5). This deepens the emphasis along the side of the ribs and spine.
- Folding down the middle (fig. 6) can change where you feel the stress. Maybe it is more into the adductors/inner groin? You decide whether this is better. This may be a preferred option for pregnant students.
- For the Half Frog option, place the foot of the bent knee in Virasana (fig. 7), but only if the knee doesn't complain. This is one of the few chances we get in yoga to internally rotate at the hip.
- For more flexible students who easily bring their chest to their thigh, try placing a bolster under the chest to encourage more spinal flexion (fig. 8).

COMING OUT OF THE POSE

Slowly roll up, pushing the floor away with your hands. Before straightening the opposite leg, lean back on your hands to release the hips. Then slowly straighten the leg. (Don't forget to do the other side.)

COUNTERPOSES

- This was a flexion for the spine, so spinal extension is nice. Do a gentle sitting backbend or lie on the belly. You could also do Cat's Breath or flow into Tabletop (aka Hammock).
- Seated twist is another way to release the spine.
- This was also an external rotation for the hips, so some internal rotation, like Windshield Wipers, may feel nice.

MERIDIANS AND ORGANS AFFECTED

- Sensations along the spine and the back of the straight leg may stimulate the Urinary Bladder meridians.
- If you are feeling sensations along the outside of the hips or through the sides of the ribs, this pose may stimulate the Gall Bladder meridians.
- Sensations through the inner knees, thighs and groin may stimulate the Liver and Kidney meridians.

RECOMMENDED HOLD TIME

- Can be held up to 5 minutes, with variations added after 2 or 3 minutes.

OTHER NOTES

- This can be great for pregnant women because the legs are abducted, providing space for the belly.
- B.K.S. Iyengar calls this pose Janusirsasana, but in our version, we are allowing the back to round. He claims that this pose will relieve headaches, improve bladder control, prevent enlarging of the prostate (only in men) and reduce menstrual cramps (only in women), along with relieving vaginal dryness and itching.[7] These claims have not been verified.

CAT PULLING ITS TAIL

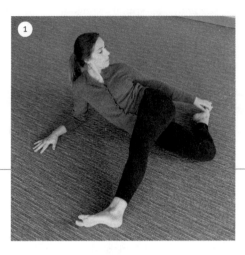

INTENTIONS AND TARGETED AREAS

- Primary targeted area: the quadriceps and iliopsoas (tension).
- Secondary targeted areas: twisting of the spine and perhaps a mild extension of the hips and lumbar.

CONTRAINDICATIONS

- If you have low back issues, go gently. You may not be able to pull the foot away at all.
- This pose is not recommended for most pregnant women.

GETTING INTO THE POSE

- Start by sitting with both legs out in front of you. Twist to the right and recline onto your right elbow. Keeping your bottom (right) leg straight, bring your top (left) leg forward and to the side. Bend the bottom leg, bringing that heel toward your buttock. Reach back with your top (left) hand and grab the bottom foot. Pull the foot away from you (fig. 1).
- You may begin lying down. From here, roll onto your right side. Keeping your bottom (right) leg straight, bring your top (left) leg forward (to the side). Bend the bottom leg, bringing that heel toward your buttock. Reach back with your top (left) hand and grab the bottom foot. Pull the foot away from you (fig. 2).

ALTERNATIVES AND OPTIONS

- It's easiest to be propped up on one arm (fig. 1).
- If the foot is not reachable, try using a strap (fig. 3).
- A bolster under the top leg may also make the pose more accessible (fig. 3).

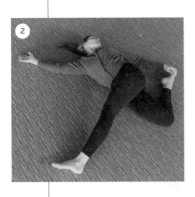 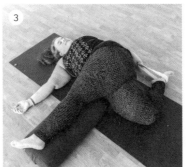 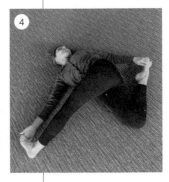

- It's more challenging to recline and look over the shoulder to the bottom foot (fig. 2). This becomes a reclining twist with a backbend. Try pulling the foot away from the buttock; most students will not be able to pull the foot too far, and that's okay!
- A deeper option is to hold both feet (fig. 4).

COMING OUT OF THE POSE

Release the bottom foot and roll onto your abdomen. Straighten the bottom leg. Optionally, roll onto your back.

COUNTERPOSES

Hug the knees to the chest to release the low back in a gentle forward fold. Do this either while lying on your back or in Child's Pose.

MERIDIANS AND ORGANS AFFECTED

- Sensations along the top of the thigh may stimulate the Stomach and Spleen meridians.
- Sensations along the low back may stimulate the Urinary Bladder and Kidney meridians.
- If you feel a twist through the side of the ribcage, this may stimulate the Gall Bladder meridians.

RECOMMENDED HOLD TIME

- One minute if done as a counterpose to a forward bend.
- Can hold for 3 to 5 minutes as a reclining twist.

OTHER NOTES

- A nice counterpose to strong forward bends (such as the Snail or Caterpillar).
- If you are actively pulling the foot away, the pose becomes yang-like in nature. In this case, you may shorten the time or release the pressure after 1 minute.

CATERPILLAR

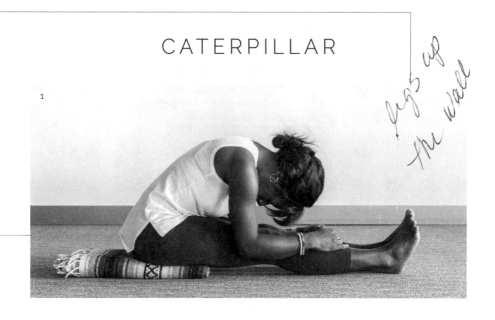

1

legs up the wall

INTENTIONS AND TARGETED AREAS

- Primary targeted areas: the spine and hips (flexion) and the hamstrings (tension).
- Secondary targeted areas: the calves (ankle dorsiflexion).

CONTRAINDICATIONS

- Can aggravate sciatica. If you have piriformis sciatica, elevate the hips by sitting on a cushion so the knees are below the hips. If you have discogenic sciatica, avoid rounding the spine. In either case, if symptoms are made worse, avoid this pose entirely.
- If the hamstrings are very tight, the knees should be bent and supported by a bolster (fig. 2), which allows the hips to flex more.
- If you have any low back disorders that do not allow flexion of the spine, then do not allow the spine to round: keep the back as neutral as you can (fig. 3) or do the legs-up-the-wall version (fig. 6).
- This pose may hyperextend the knees if the legs are straight, but that may be quite good for them. All joints need stress, including the knees, and they are designed to hyperextend a bit. However, if hyperextension is painful for you, keep a little bend there, perhaps with a rolled-up blanket under them.
- Most pregnant women should be able to do this pose if they separate their legs enough for their belly to go between them. In this case, it becomes a mini version of the Straddle Pose.
- Contraindications from YIP: arthritis hip, gastroesophageal reflux disease, herniated lumbar disc, ischial bursitis, osteoporosis, posterior total hip replacement, retrolisthesis, spinal fracture (vertebral body), compression fracture, torn hamstring.

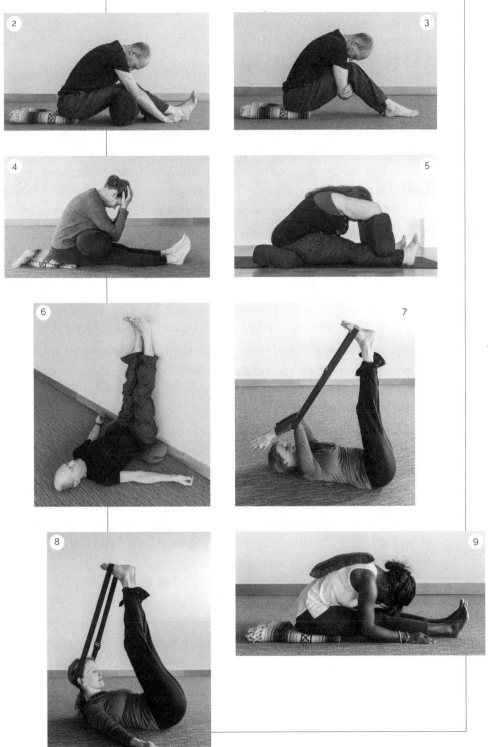

GETTING INTO THE POSE

Sit on a cushion with both legs straight out in front of you. Fold forward over the legs, allowing your back to round (fig. 1).

ALTERNATIVES AND OPTIONS

- Most students have to choose to bend the knees or not. If the hamstrings are tight, the hips won't flex much, which can be okay, as this will create more stress in the targeted areas. But if you are very tight in the hamstrings, you may not be able to flex the hips enough to come past vertical with your torso: in this case, bend the knees enough to allow gravity to draw your spine into flexion rather than using your abdominal muscles. You can use a bolster under the knees for support (fig. 2) or wrap your arms under them (fig. 3). Also try sitting up on additional cushions to tilt the pelvis more.
- Similarly, drawing the chin to the chest, deepening the flexion at the neck, will also increase the stress along the fascial chains of the back body.
- If your neck feels strained by the weight of the head, support your head in your hands, resting your elbows on the legs or a bolster (fig. 4).
- You can rest your chest on a bolster (fig. 4) to help relax into the pose.
- Experiment with hand positions. Rest your elbows on your thighs, bolster (fig. 5) or the floor, or loosely hold the toes with your hands. No need to pull: holding the feet in dorsiflexion will make the tension stronger along the back of the body.
- For students who would prefer not to flex the spine at all but still want a lovely hamstring stress, there are a couple of other options: lie on the back with your legs on the wall and a bolster under the pelvis (fig. 6), which is very nice for people who stand all day. Another option here is to place a sandbag on the feet while they are in the air against the wall; or have your legs in the air and hold the feet with a strap (fig. 7); or, more exciting, use a strap looped between the feet and the back of the head (fig. 8). Note: not the back of the neck! Ouch! This is not as challenging at it looks.
- In most variations, sandbags along the spine can add a bit of juice if more is desired (fig. 9).
- To feel a stress if you're very flexible and can easily rest your chest on your thighs, you may want to separate your legs just enough that your chest fits between the legs. Need more? Sit on a block and have blocks under the calves, building a platform.

COMING OUT OF THE POSE

- Use your hands to push the floor away and slowly roll up.
- Once you are up, lean back on your hands to release the hips and extend the spine.

COUNTERPOSES

- This was a flexion for the spine, so spinal extension is nice. Do a gentle sitting backbend or lie on the belly. You could also do Cat's Breath or flow into Tabletop (aka Hammock).
- Seated twist is another way to release the spine.

MERIDIANS AND ORGANS AFFECTED

- Sensations along the back side of the body may stimulate the Urinary Bladder meridians.
- Sensations through the low back may stimulate the Kidney line meridian.

RECOMMENDED HOLD TIME

Three to 5 minutes, but in time even more.

OTHER NOTES

- Paul Grilley says this pose is excellent for balancing chi flow and preparing the body for meditation.
- Keep muscles relaxed, especially in the legs and abdomen.
- Make sure the tops of the hips are tilted forward. If the hips are rotating backward, sit on higher cushions and bend the knees more. Let gravity have you! Surrendering is yin.
- B.K.S. Iyengar calls this pose Paschimottanasana. He claims it cools the brain, normalizes blood pressure, relieves chronic headaches, soothes the heart, massages the adrenal glands and kidneys, tones the bladder and pancreas, treats the entire reproductive system in women, and treats impotence and builds sex control in men.[8] These claims have not been verified.

CHILD'S POSE

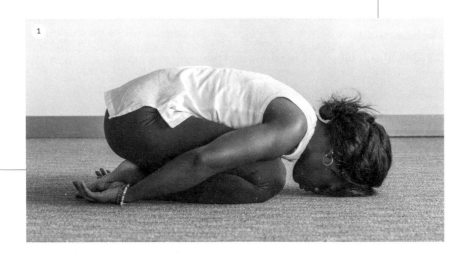

INTENTIONS AND TARGETED AREAS

- Primary targeted area: the spine and hips (flexion).
- Secondary targeted areas: the knees (flexion) and ankles (plantarflexion).

CONTRAINDICATIONS

- If you have diarrhea, are pregnant or have just eaten, either spread the legs apart (fig. 4) or skip this pose.
- If you have hip or knee issues, you may need to place a towel or blanket between thighs and calves or avoid the pose altogether.
- You may need a blanket or other padding under the ankles to reduce discomfort on the top of the feet.
- Contraindications from YIP: anterior cruciate ligament tear, arthritis hip, arthritis knee, bunion, chondromalacia patellae, gastroesophageal reflux disease, herniated lumbar disc, herniated thoracic disc, posterior total hip replacement, retrolisthesis, spinal fracture (vertebral body), compression fracture, total knee replacement.

GETTING INTO THE POSE

Begin by sitting on your heels and then slowly fold forward, bringing your chest to your thighs and your forehead to the earth. Hands go back beside the feet, allowing elbows to bend out to the sides (fig. 1).

alternative is happy baby.

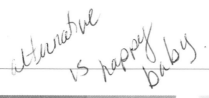

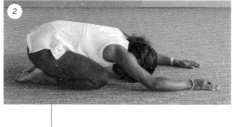
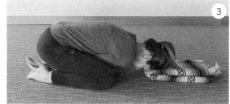

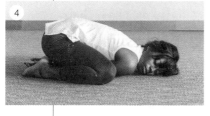

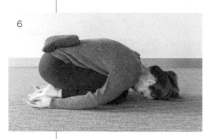
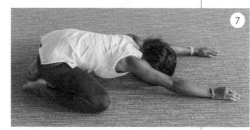

81

add thread the needle twist.

ALTERNATIVES AND OPTIONS

- Can be done with arms stretched forward, which may avoid placing too much pressure on the neck (fig. 2). This may, however, increase shoulder tension.

- Another favorite option is to thread the arms between the legs (fig. 3).

- If you prefer not to have your forehead on the floor or mat, place a towel or blanket under your head (fig. 3) or turn your head to one side (fig. 4).

- Allow the knees to be as close together as is comfortable, but they do not have to touch. If there is any uncomfortable pinching at the front hips or if there is too much compression in the chest or belly, separate the knees more (fig. 4).

- If you cannot get your buttocks to your heels, or if the head or neck feels too much stress, place a bolster under the chest (fig. 5). This is a nice option for pregnant students.

- If you crave a bit more stress, sandbags along the spine can feel nice (fig. 6).

- You can do this as a preparation for the Frog by spreading the knees wide apart halfway through the pose while continuing to sit on the heels. Optionally, have an arm overhead (fig. 7); we call this the Tadpole.

COMING OUT OF THE POSE

Use your hands to push the floor away and slowly roll up.

COUNTERPOSES

A counterpose is not normally needed after this pose. Just sit tall or lie down for a moment.

MERIDIANS AND ORGANS AFFECTED

- Sensations along the spine may stimulate the Urinary Bladder meridians.
- Sensations along the front body (thighs and belly) may stimulate the Stomach and Spleen meridians.

RECOMMENDED HOLD TIME

- If used as a counterpose, hold for up to 1 minute.
- If used as a yin pose on its own, hold for 3 to 5 minutes. Some people can stay forever! (That may be a bit too long.) If you cannot get your head to the floor, 5 minutes may be too long.

OTHER NOTES

- A healing, restful pose—useful any time a break is needed.
- Gentle compression of the abdomen and chest may benefit the organs of digestion.
- Psychologically soothing when feeling cold, anxious or vulnerable.
- Might relieve back and neck pain when the head is supported.
- If the knees are fairly close together, rocking gently side to side may stimulate the flow of blood and lymph fluids in the upper chest and breast tissues.
- This pose can be used as a preparation for deeper spinal flexion postures such as Straddle, Caterpillar or Snail.
- This is sometimes called Balasana or Garbhasana. However, B.K.S. Iyengar has called this pose Adhomukha Virasana. He claims it can relieve headaches, dizziness, fatigue and breathlessness, reduce high blood pressure and flatulence, and relieve menstrual pain as well as associated depression.[9] These claims have not been verified.

DANGLING

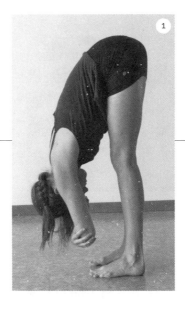

INTENTIONS AND TARGETED AREAS

- Primary targeted areas: stressing the spine (flexion in the lumbar) and the hamstrings (tension) when the legs are straight (fig. 1). The cervical and upper thoracic spine may experience a lovely traction.

- Secondary targeted areas: strengthening the quadriceps when the knees are bent (fig. 2).

CONTRAINDICATIONS

- Avoid if you have high blood pressure. (Poses where the head is below the heart can increase blood pressure.) Related conditions that are a problem when blood pressure is increased include diabetes and glaucoma and other eye issues. If you have these conditions, you may wish to avoid this pose and do Caterpillar instead.

- If you have low blood pressure, to come out of the pose roll up to standing slowly or go into Squat to avoid dizziness.

- If you have bad knees, it may be better to keep the legs straight.

- If your knees are okay but you have a bad back, bend your knees a lot to allow more flexion to occur around the hips, keeping the spine more neutral. You can also rest your elbows on the thighs (fig. 3).

- If you have any low back disorders that do not allow any flexion of the spine, this is not the pose for you.

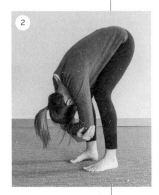

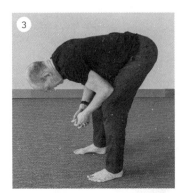

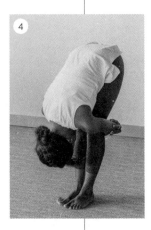

- This is not ideal for pregnant women, who may prefer to do a narrow version of Straddle Pose.
- Contraindications from YIP: arthritis hip, gastroesophageal reflux disease, herniated lumbar disc, herniated thoracic disc, Lasik surgery, nosebleed, orthostatic hypotension, osteoporosis, plantar fasciitis, posterior total hip replacement, pregnancy (second and third trimesters), retinal tear, retrolisthesis, spinal fracture (vertebral body), compression fracture, torn hamstring.

GETTING INTO THE POSE
Stand up with the feet comfortably apart. Bend your knees and fold forward. You can clasp your elbows (fig. 1 and 2) or rest the elbows on the knees (fig. 3).

ALTERNATIVES AND OPTIONS
- Another back-sparing option is to rest your elbows on a table or chair.
- Eventually, allow the hands to dangle to the floor.
- More flexible students can clasp the elbows behind the knees with legs straight (fig. 4).
- If you do this pose more than once, try it with legs bent the first time and straight the second time.

COMING OUT OF THE POSE
- Bend your knees and release your hands to the floor. Slowly roll up. This is often called Rag Doll.

- You can place your hands onto your shins and come up halfway, then fold back down. Do this a couple of times, and when you feel ready, come all the way up with as neutral a spine as possible.
- If you feel dizzy or lightheaded after coming up, one option is to stay up and raise your arms overhead with knees bent a little until the dizziness passes. If that doesn't work, fold back down and try again a breath or two later.
- Another option is to come out by going directly into Squat Pose.

COUNTERPOSES
- Squat is a lovely counterpose for the legs after Dangling.
- This was a flexion for the spine, so spinal extension is nice. Do a gentle sitting backbend or lie on the belly. You could also do Cat's Breath or flow into Tabletop (aka Hammock).
- Seated twist is another way to release the spine.

MERIDIANS AND ORGANS AFFECTED
- Sensations along the back side of the body may stimulate the Urinary Bladder meridians.
- Sensations through the low back may stimulate the Kidney line meridian.

RECOMMENDED HOLD TIME
Three minutes can be intense; 2 minutes may be enough at one time, but the pose can be repeated. One option is to do 2 or more sessions of 2 minutes each, separated by 2 minutes of Squat.

OTHER NOTES
- Balance the weight between toes and heels. You can gently sway or wobble, but avoid bouncing.
- B.K.S. Iyengar calls this pose Uttanasana, but in the Yin Yoga version, the emphasis is not to stretch the hamstrings a lot but rather to release the low back. If the legs are straight, it is a nice stress for the hamstrings. If the knees are bent, it is a great strengthener for the quadriceps and allows the back to release more fully. Iyengar claims it slows the heart rate, regulates blood pressure, tones the liver, spleen and kidneys, relieves abdominal and back pain during menstruation, relieves stomach aches and headaches and cures insomnia.[10] These claims have not been verified.

DEER

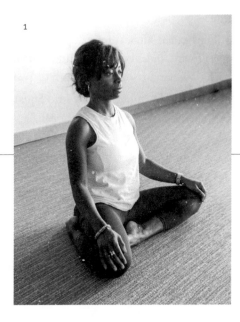

1

INTENTIONS AND TARGETED AREAS

- Primary targeted areas: external rotation, abduction and flexion of front leg's hip; internal rotation, abduction and flexion of back leg's hip.
- Secondary targeted areas: side of torso may twist and flex in several options.

CONTRAINDICATIONS

If any knee issues exist, be careful of deep internal or external rotations of the hip. Tightness in the hip sockets tends to show up in increased stress in the knees. The more the knee is bent, however, the less stress will arise, so one option is to keep the feet in closer to the groin or buttocks, as shown in fig. 1. You could support the front knee with a bolster or folded blanket and/or sit up higher on a cushion or block.

GETTING INTO THE POSE

Start by sitting in Butterfly on the floor, then swing your right leg back behind you, bringing that foot behind your hip. Position the front leg by moving the foot away from you. There is no need to move the foot more forward if the front knee is well off the floor. Move the back foot away from your hip until you start to feel like you are tipping away from that foot. If possible, keep both sitting bones firmly rooted to the ground. Sitting up on a cushion may help.

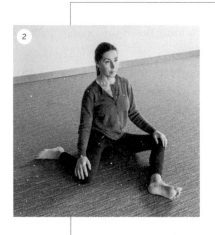

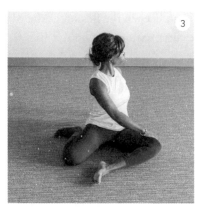

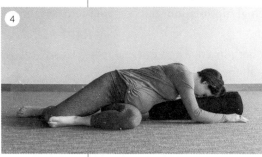

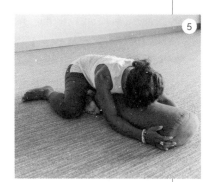

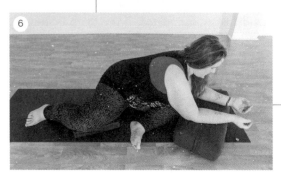

ALTERNATIVES AND OPTIONS

- The tendency here is to tilt away from the internally rotating hip of the back leg; make sure both sitting bones are firmly on the floor. You may need to move both feet more inwards, toward the core of the body.

- If you're very flexible and your knees don't complain, you can begin to move your feet away from the hips (fig. 2).

- To get a nice stress in the side of your torso and the back thigh, twist away from the legs (fig. 3). You can lower down to the floor and rest on your elbow(s) here, or you can rest your chest on a bolster, which is a nice supported option for pregnant students (fig. 4).

- We can deepen the flexion in the hips by folding down the middle, perhaps with the chest resting on a bolster (fig. 5).
- Deer meets Swan: Another option in Deer is to fold over the front leg (fig. 6). This makes the pose into a modified version of Swan for those who tilt too much or don't like to have their back leg straight in Swan.

COMING OUT OF THE POSE

Lean away from the back foot and bring that leg forward, coming back to Butterfly. You are ready to do the second side.

COUNTERPOSES

- Since this is an external and internal hip rotation, the best counterpose is to do the other side.
- Windshield Wipers also includes both internal and external rotations and can be done lying down, sitting up or reclining on the elbows.

MERIDIANS AND ORGANS AFFECTED

- If the front leg is firmly on the floor, creating stress along the outside of the leg or hip, or if you are twisting and feel stress along the sides of the ribcage, then the Gall Bladder meridians may be stimulated. Any inner groin sensations could indicate that the Liver and Kidney meridians are stimulated. If the thigh is stressed, the Stomach and Spleen meridians may be activated.

RECOMMENDED HOLD TIME

- One to 3 minutes should be enough because most people cannot move their feet too far away to really get deep rotations in the hip sockets. The supported versions (fig. 4, 5 and 6) can be held longer, from 3 to 5 minutes.

OTHER NOTES

- This is a combination of Virasana (Hero Pose) for the back leg and Baddhakonasana (Butterfly) for the front leg.
- Useful after long-held external hip rotations such as Shoelace, Swan or Winged Dragon.
- Most students won't easily understand what the pose is about; they won't move their feet far enough away from the groin or hips, or they will tilt too much, allowing the internally rotated hip to rise off the floor. Teachers will have to inspect their students and offer guidance to ensure sensations are felt in the targeted areas.

DRAGON

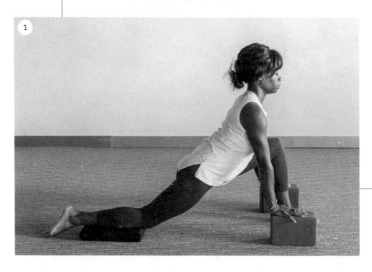

INTENTIONS AND TARGETED AREAS

- Primary targeted area: the quadriceps and hip flexors of the back leg (tension), hip socket of the front leg (flexion but also external rotation and abduction in some options).
- Secondary targeted areas: some options provide minor flexion, extension or twisting of the spine. One option also works into the ankle (dorsiflexion).

CONTRAINDICATIONS

- Can be uncomfortable for the kneecap or ankle of the straight leg. There are several options to reduce kneecap pain: pad the back of the knee with a blanket; place support under the shin, allowing the knee to be off the floor (fig. 1); or keep the knee bent with the foot raised off the floor (fig. 7).[11] If the ankle is uncomfortable, place a blanket underneath it or lift the leg by putting support under the shin.
- Due to asymmetric stresses in the sacroiliac joints, pregnant women may wish to avoid these poses, or not go so low (fig. 2 and 5).
- If you experience discomfort or a painful pinching at the front hip (from compression into the thigh), point the toes and knee outward, allowing you to go around that point of compression.

GETTING INTO THE POSE

Begin either on hands and knees or in Down Dog. Step one foot between the hands. Walk the front foot forward until the knee is over the heel. Slide the back knee backward as far as you can. Keep the hands on either side of the front foot. This first

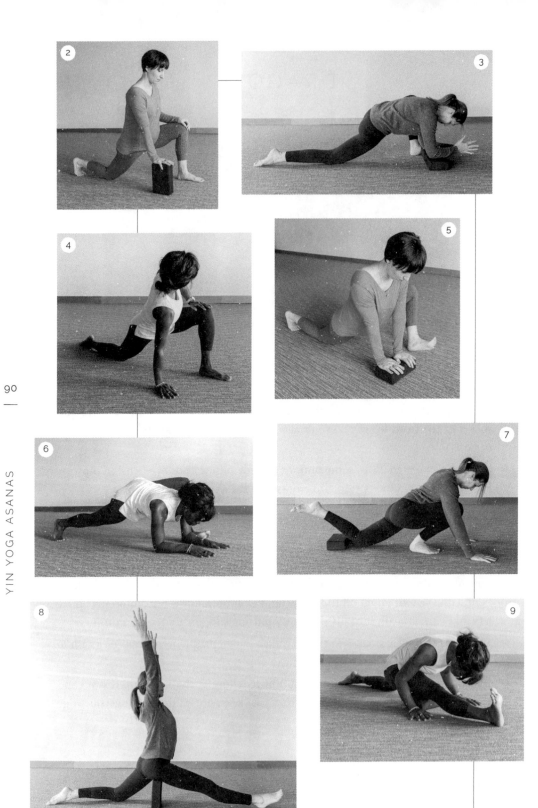

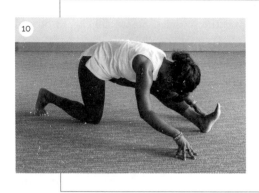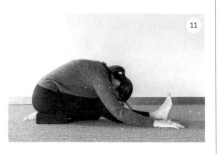

version of the pose is a simple low lunge called Baby Dragon (fig. 1). To help you easily reach the floor, you can rest your hands on blocks.

ALTERNATIVES AND OPTIONS

○ For the High-Flying Dragon, rest the arms or hands on the front thigh and lift the chest. Alternately, you can rest one or both hands on a block or two (fig. 2). Having the chest higher increases the stress in the front hip. Make sure you don't move your hips backward, which reduces the desired stress in the hips and quadriceps and may increase stress on the back knee.

○ For the Low-Flying Dragon (fig. 3), place both hands inside the front foot, move the foot a few inches toward the edge of the mat (so you are no longer blocked by the front thigh) and walk hands forward, lowering the hips. For more depth, come down on the elbows or rest them on a bolster or block.

○ In Twisted Dragon (fig. 4), one hand holds the front knee, while the chest rotates to the sky.

○ In Winged Dragon (fig. 5), with hands on the floor, wing out the knee a few times, rolling onto the outside edge of that foot, and then stay there with the knee low. You could come down on the elbows or rest them on a block or bolster.

○ For the Fire-Breathing Dragon (fig. 6), in any of the above variations, tuck the back toe under and lift the knee off the floor, lengthening the leg. This puts more weight into the hips, increasing the stress. This is much more yang-like, so don't hold this position too long.

○ Overstepping Dragon (fig. 7) stresses the ankle. From Baby Dragon, allow the front knee to come far forward and/or slide the heel backward until the heel is just about to lift off the ground. The sensations we are seeking are at the back of the front leg's calf (tension) or the front of the ankle (compression). It helps to allow the back leg to come forward a lot.

○ Dragon Splits offers the deepest stress in the hip flexors. Straighten both legs into the splits. Support the front hip with a block or bolster under the buttock for balance and to release weight; this relaxes the muscles. Sit up tall (fig. 8) or fold forward (fig. 9) for different sensations.

- Bowing Dragon (fig. 10) is a half-splits version. Keep the front leg straight while moving the hips backward. Fold forward over the front leg. Feel the hamstrings. Another version (fig. 11) is to sit on the floor beside the back foot, which makes this pose into a version of Half Saddle.

COMING OUT OF THE POSE

Move your paws to Down Dog position, move the back knee forward a bit, tuck the back toes under, and with a nice groan, step back to Down Dog. Many students may prefer to go straight to Child's Pose.

COUNTERPOSES

- A short Down Dog is delicious. Bend one knee, lifting that heel and pushing the opposite heel down, and then switch sides repeatedly (this is called Walking the Dog).
- Child's Pose feels really good after Down Dog and before switching to the other side of the Dragon.

MERIDIANS AND ORGANS AFFECTED

This is one posture than can stimulate all 6 lower body meridians! Sensations along the top of the back leg may indicate that the Stomach and Spleen meridians are being stimulated. Sensation in the inner groin may stimulate the Liver and Kidney meridians. Sensations along the spine may stimulate the Urinary Bladder and Kidney meridians. Sensations along the sides of the ribs (in the Twisting Dragon) or outside of the hips may stimulate the Gall Bladder meridian.

RECOMMENDED HOLD TIME

- Hold each variation for 1 to 2 minutes and cycle through 2 or 3 variations.
- Or hold just 1 variation for 3 to 5 minutes.

OTHER NOTES

- This is sometimes referred to as the low lunge (Anjaneyasana).
- You may not feel anything in the outer hip joint. If your hip flexors or quadriceps are tight, these areas will take all the stress. This is still a good pose, but to work your hips, other poses will be needed.
- B.K.S. Iyengar claims that Dragon Splits (which he calls Hanumanasana) can cure sciatica.[12] This claim has not been verified.

FROG

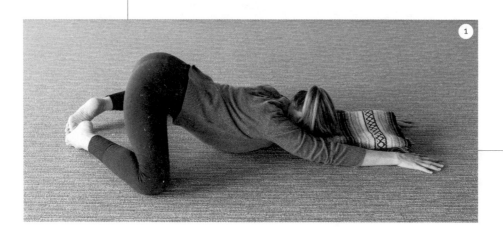

INTENTIONS AND TARGETED AREAS

- Primary targeted area: the inner groin (adductors—tension) and hip sockets (flexion and adduction).
- Secondary targeted areas: the spine may experience extension (backbend) stresses in less flexible students or when the hips remain high; the hips may externally rotate if the feet are together or internally rotate if the feet are wider than the knees.

CONTRAINDICATIONS

- If you have a bad back, compression in the low back may be too much.
- If the knees complain, use padding underneath them.
- If the neck complains when you try to look forward, try resting the forehead on the floor, not the chin, or place a bolster under the chest.
- If you are prone to tingling in the hands or discomfort in the shoulders when you extend the arms overhead, you may need to move the hands wider apart or closer together. If that doesn't help, do one arm at a time.

GETTING INTO THE POSE

To begin, start in Child's Pose and slide both hands forward, separate the knees, but remain sitting on the heels. This is also known as the Tadpole (fig. 2).

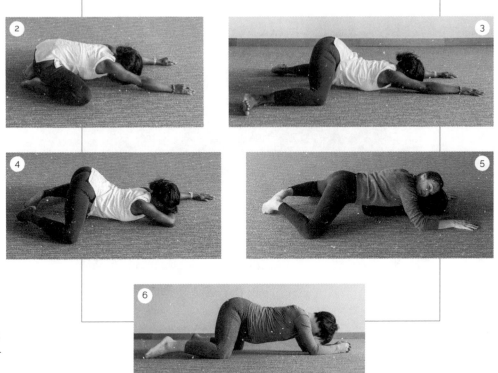

ALTERNATIVES AND OPTIONS

○ Half Frog (fig. 1): Move the hips forward until they are in line with the knees. Keep feet together. It is okay to allow the hips to be high, at least at first. Eventually, the knees widen and the hips may lower.

○ Full Frog (fig. 3): Try separating the feet wider apart. If knees complain, don't!

○ For students with shoulder issues or tingling in the hands, reach only one arm forward at a time (fig. 4). The other arm can be bent with the head resting on that forearm. Alternately, experiment with hand positions (closer or further apart).

○ If stress in the groin or hips is too severe, allow the hips to come forward of the knees (fig. 5) or keep the toes together and allow the hips to be behind the knees (fig. 2).

○ To reduce the amount of backbend and support the upper body, rest the chest on a bolster (fig. 5). Pregnant students may prefer this option, or to rest onto their elbows (fig. 6).

COMING OUT OF THE POSE

Either bring the knees together coming onto your forearms and then sit back into Child's Pose, or slide forward onto your belly, bringing your legs together.

COUNTERPOSES

- Child's Pose.
- Lying down Windshield Wipers to adduct and internally rotate the legs at the hips.
- Lying on your back, hug your knees to your chest and rock side to side or move the knees in circles.

MERIDIANS AND ORGANS AFFECTED

- Sensation along the front of the belly may stimulate the Spleen and Stomach meridians.
- Sensation through the inner groin may stimulate the Liver and Kidney meridians.
- Sensation along the spine, especially in the low back, may stimulate the Kidney and Urinary Bladder meridians.
- The arms stretched forward may stimulate the Heart, Lungs, and Small and Large Intestines meridians.

RECOMMENDED HOLD TIME

Three to 5 minutes.

OTHER NOTES

- This is also called Mandukasana or Bhekasana.
- When the hips are in line with the knees, gravity has maximum effect. However, often students will move hips forward to avoid painful compression in the hips—that is okay. Allowing the hips to move a bit may move the stress from the hips and low back to the inner thighs.
- If the knees are kept together, this becomes Anahatasana (Melting Heart Pose)!
- If doing this right after eating, rest on the elbows and don't let the abdomen rest on the floor. Allow it to hang, which is nice for digestion.
- To advance in this posture, don't go deeper, stay longer! But don't go overboard; 5 minutes of being a frog should be enough for most princes.
- You could do the first half of the pose in Tadpole and then move to Full Frog for the second half.

HAPPY BABY

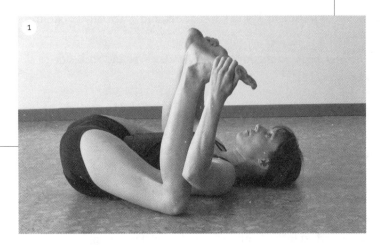

INTENTIONS AND TARGETED AREAS

- Primary targeted area: abduction, flexion and possibly external rotation in the hip sockets.
- Secondary targeted areas: can create flexion stress in the low back and tension in the hamstrings and adductor muscles.

CONTRAINDICATIONS

- If the hips roll up off the floor, this can become a mild inversion and a mild flexion of the spine. If you have any low back disorders that do not allow flexion of the spine, then do not allow the spine to round: keep the back as neutral as you can. Do not allow the hips to roll off the floor.
- Women during menstruation may also choose not to allow their hips to roll off the floor.
- This is not ideal for pregnant women, who may prefer to do Squat, Child's Pose or Frog instead.

GETTING INTO THE POSE

Lying on your back, hug the knees to your chest. Grab the soles of the feet, the ankles or the back of the legs. Move the feet apart so they are above the knees, and pull the knees toward the floor, alongside your chest (fig. 1). Relax your head and shoulders down to the floor.

if people cant squat - happy baby alternative.

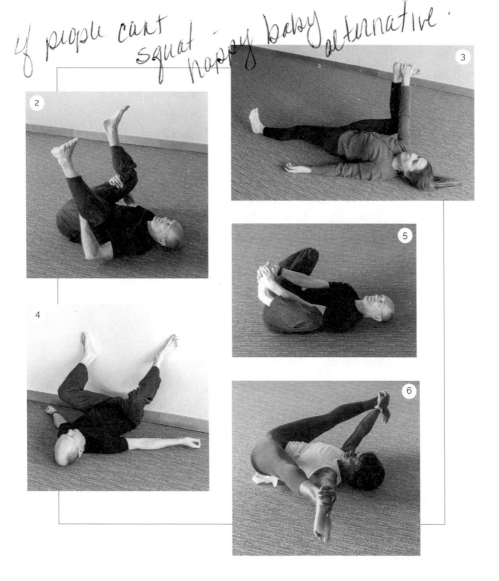

ALTERNATIVES AND OPTIONS

- If the feet are too far away, hold the backs of the thighs (fig. 2) or use belts or straps to hold the feet.

- Half Happy Baby (like an upside-down Baby Dragon), holding one foot at a time (fig. 3). The free leg can be either straight along the floor, or bend the knee and rest the foot on the floor.

- After a few minutes of active pulling with the arms, relax and let the weight of the arms and legs draw the knees down to the floor.

- Another easy alternative is to do this against a wall, called the Wall Squat (fig. 4).

- The Happy Baby Butterfly version can be a good starting option. Keep your feet together for an initial stage, holding them near the groin (fig. 5); for a deeper version, bring the toes to your nose like babies can do. Eventually, feet go behind the head! (Eventually, but not necessarily in this lifetime.)

- One option to create more stress in the hamstrings, adductors and hips is to gradually straighten the legs while still pulling the feet down and wider apart (fig. 6). In this option, do not allow your hips to lift off the floor.
- If you feel you have had enough but other students want to stay longer, come into a reclining Butterfly (feet together, knees bent, feet on the floor) and wait there for everyone else to come out. Reclining Butterfly can be very juicy too!
- Where should the hips be? There are two schools of thought:
  1. Allow the tailbone to curve up in the air. This creates more flexion in the spine.
  2. Keep the tailbone low to the ground. This reduces spinal flexion but may increase stress in the legs and hips. Which one works better for you? What is your intention?

COMING OUT OF THE POSE

Release the feet, placing them on the floor, with the knees bent. Walk the feet away from each other, keeping the knees together. Pause for a moment.

COUNTERPOSES

- Gentle backbends (lying on abdomen) or, while on the back, a mild spinal lift, coming up only halfway.
- Windshield Wipers moves the hips into both external and internal rotations. Lying down with your knees bent and your feet on the floor as wide apart as the mat, drop the knees from side to side.

MERIDIANS AND ORGANS AFFECTED

- Sensations along the back of the legs or along the spine may stimulate the Urinary Bladder meridians.
- Sensations along the inner groin (adductors) may stimulate the Liver and Kidney meridians.

RECOMMENDED HOLD TIME

Two minutes if you are actively pulling with the arms, but if you relax the arms, you can linger up to 5 minutes.

OTHER NOTES

- This pose is sometimes called Ananda Balasana but is also known as Window Pose, and in Los Angeles as Dead Bug Pose. Sarah Powers call this Stirrup Pose.
- This is one of the few postures in yoga where one can strengthen the bicep muscles in the arms if you use the hands rather than gravity to pull the feet or legs down.
- It can be a nice preparation posture for Squats or deep external hip rotation poses.

RECLINING TWISTS

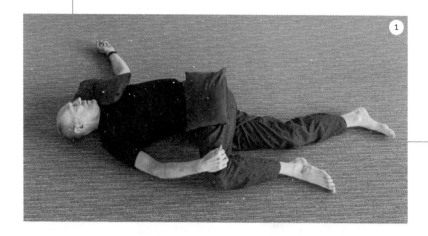

INTENTIONS AND TARGETED AREAS

- Primary targeted area: rotation along the spine and torso.
- Secondary targeted areas: can create tension along the outer hip and the legs and in the arms and shoulders.

CONTRAINDICATIONS

- Students with back issues may find too much stress along the spine.
- Similarly, students with instability in the sacroiliac (SI) joints may want to pin the hips first and move from the shoulders, which can reduce stress in the pelvic area (fig. 3).
- For shoulder issues (such as rotator cuff injuries) or if tingling arises in the hands when the arms are out to the side or overhead, don't raise your arms. Instead, lower the arms or support them with bolsters or blankets. If tingling persists, rest the hands on the chest. Do not tolerate tingling, because this could be a sign that you are damaging a nerve.
- Contraindications from YIP: gastroesophageal reflux disease, herniated lumbar disc, herniated thoracic disc, posterior total hip replacement, pregnancy (second and third trimesters), spinal fracture (vertebral body), compression fracture, torn hamstring, trochanteric bursitis.

GETTING INTO THE POSE

- To initiate the twist from the hips, pin the shoulders first: lying on your back, draw one or both knees into your chest. Open your arms to the side like wings

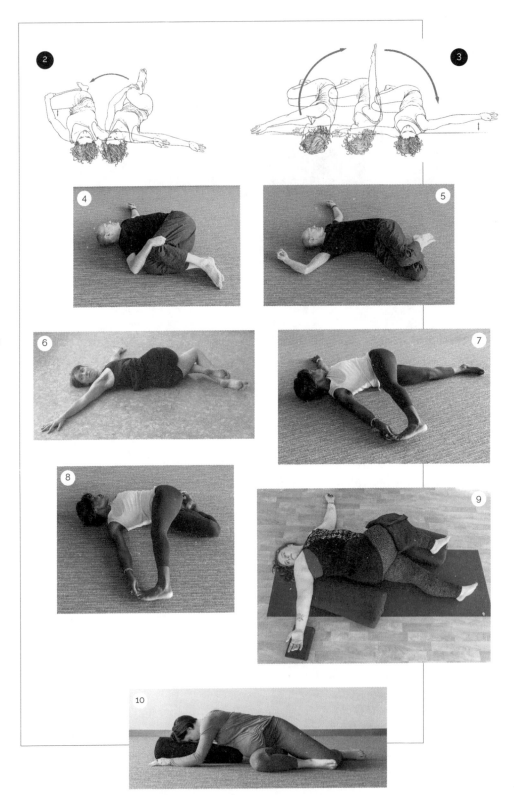

and then drop the knee(s) to one side (fig. 2). This may generate more stress in the lower spine and pelvis than in the upper spine.

o To initiate the twist from the shoulders, pin the hips first: lying on your back, draw the knees into the chest and roll over onto your side (in a fetal-like position). Keep the knees on the ground, raise the top arm up in the air and allow gravity to draw it to the floor behind you (fig. 3). This may generate more stress in the upper spine than the lower spine and pelvis.

ALTERNATIVES AND OPTIONS

o Directing the knees lower or higher may affect where in the spine the stress is felt. If the knees are higher (fig. 4), stress may be more obvious in the upper back, which is more flexed/rounded; lowering the knees (fig. 5) may make the stress more obvious in the low back, which is more extended.

o For the deeper one-knee twist, draw one knee into the chest and, holding that knee with the opposite hand, draw it across the body (fig. 1).

o For the Twisted Roots option (fig. 6), cross the legs as in Eagle Pose (Garudasana) and if available, hook the toes under the opposite calf. Dropping the knees to the opposite side of the top leg creates the greatest spinal twist, but going to the same side as the top leg (called the Twisted-Twisted Roots Pose) may create more stress along the outside of the hips. It is more challenging to keep the foot hooked in this latter position.

o If a shoulder is floating uncomfortably, place a blanket under it or a bolster under the bent knee(s).

o Experiment with turning your head to either side and notice how the sensations change. If lightheadedness or dizziness arises, do not keep the head turned.

o The extended arms can be resting on the floor or on a bolster.

o If the legs are floating, place support under the legs or between them (fig. 9).

o Sandbags on the top thigh or shoulders may help you stay in the pose or may create more stress in the targeted areas (fig. 1 and 9).

o Placing the top leg straight out to the side applies the most leverage, which helps to keep the hips fully turned. For some, it's less of a twist and more stress in the outside of the leg and hip; this can be great for the iliotibial band. The deepest version of this option is to hold the foot with the opposite hand (fig. 7), which may increase stress along the hamstrings as well. Another option is to also hold the bottom foot and pull it away, much like the Cat Pulling Its Tail Pose (fig. 8).

o For students who feel they are rolling out of the twist (usually larger-bodied students), a bolster placed along the spine may be supportive and keep them in the pose (fig. 9).

o For pregnant women who prefer not to lie on their backs, seated twists or the folding forward version of Deer Pose (fig. 10) may be a better option.

COMING OUT OF THE POSE

Slowly roll onto your back and hug the knees into the chest to release the sacrum and lumbar. (Don't forget to do the other side.)

COUNTERPOSES

- Hug the knees and rock on your back from side to side.
- Windshield Wipers while lying back can be a nice release. Lying down with your knees bent and your feet on the floor as wide apart as the mat, drop the knees from side to side.

MERIDIANS AND ORGANS AFFECTED

- Sensations along the sides of the ribcage or the outside of the hips may stimulate the Gall Bladder meridians.
- Sensations along the spine may stimulate the Urinary Bladder meridians.
- One or both arms overhead may stimulate the Heart, Lung, Small Intestines and Large Intestines meridians.
- Twists can physically compress the abdomen and massage the internal organs.

RECOMMENDED HOLD TIME

- Three to 5 minutes.
- As a teacher, this a nice "contingency posture" to end the class with: you can shorten the amount of time spent in the twist if the class is overrunning the clock, or you can lengthen the amount of time the students marinate in the pose if you have extra time left in the class.

OTHER NOTES

- Another name for this pose is Jatharaparivartanasana. It is much easier to say "Reclining Twist."
- An excellent final pose of the practice because it removes kinks and tension along the spine. You can slide right from this pose into Shavasana.
- Twisted Roots is a great way to internally rotate the hips after a lot of external hip rotation work, such as Shoelace, Swan, Square or Winged Dragon poses.
- Don't force the twist; relax and let gravity do the work.
- When the twist is initiated from the upper body first (with hips pinned), more stress may be generated in the shoulders and upper spine.
- When the twist is initiated from the lower body first (with shoulders pinned), more stress may be generated in the lower spine, hips and SI joints.[13]

SADDLE

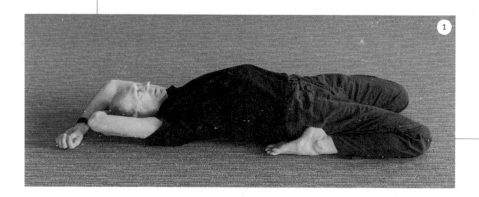

INTENTIONS AND TARGETED AREAS

- Primary targeted areas: extension along the spine and counternutation in the sacroiliac joints.
- Secondary targeted areas: Many! This pose can create stress in the ankles (dorsiflexion) and knees (flexion), tension in the hip flexors (quadriceps, iliacus and psoas), sacroiliac joints (SIJ—counternutation) and lumbar (extension), and tension in the lower belly if the arms are raised overhead, which may also stress the shoulders. If sitting between the feet, internal rotation happens in the hip sockets.

CONTRAINDICATIONS

- If you have a bad back or tight SI joints, choose another pose.
- Knees can be tested too much here, in which case, sit higher on more support.
- Ankles can protest, in which case, place padding (blankets or towels) under them.
- Tingling may arise in the hands if the arms are overhead, in which case, lower the arms.
- If any sharp or burning pain occurs anywhere, you must come out of the pose!
- Pregnant women may like this pose, but they probably won't go all the way to the floor and will rest on an angled bolster (fig. 4).
- Contraindications from YIP: anterior cruciate ligament tear, arthritis hip, arthritis knee, arthritis shoulder, chondromalacia patellae, gastroesophageal reflux disease, lateral meniscal tear, lumbar spinal stenosis, medial meniscal tear, posterior cruciate ligament tear, posterior total hip replacement, sacroiliac joint derangement, sprained ankle, total knee replacement.

GETTING INTO THE POSE

o There are several options for coming into this pose. Start with sitting on the heels and noticing how this feels. If there's pain in the knees, sit higher on cushions or skip this pose and choose another one that works your primary targeted area. If your ankles are complaining, try a blanket under them or skip the pose. Lean back on your hands, creating a little arch in the low back (fig. 2). Check in with how this feels. This may be it for you today! If you can go further, come down onto your elbows. If that is easy, lie down all the way to the floor (fig. 1).

o Some students find this pose challenging not because they cannot do the pose but because they cannot get into the pose from sitting on their heels.[14] For these students it is better to come into the pose from Windshield Wipers (fig. 9): lying on your back, bend your knees with the feet on the floor but as wide apart as possible (as wide as or wider than the mat) and drop both knees to one side; now you are in a version of Half Saddle! To make it deeper, pull the foot close to your hip even higher and move that knee wider, past the edge of the mat.

ALTERNATIVES AND OPTIONS

o If this is too deep for any of the many reasons cited above, choose Sphinx Pose, which also affects the main targeted area.

o Play with sitting on the heels and between the heels; the first emphasizes the lumbar extension, and the second works the quads and hip flexors more. Lifting the hips higher by placing a block between the feet and under the buttocks increases extension in the spine.

o Resting the top of the head on the floor opens the throat, but it may be too much of a deep neck extension.

o Arms overhead can open the shoulders and intensify the stress in the hip flexors. If tingling arises, try resting the arms on your forehead or a bolster. If that doesn't resolve the tingling, lower your arms.

o If you can only go as far back as your elbows, rest on a bolster to relax here (fig. 3). There are various ways you may use bolsters—crossways under the shoulders or lengthwise under the spine. If you can't quite rest on the bolster, try making a higher wedge out of it by placing blocks under the end of it (fig. 4).

o For many students, it is better to do one leg at a time, called Half Saddle. There are many versions. You can straighten one leg, keeping one knee bent (fig. 5), or you can bend the straight leg and place the foot on the floor (fig. 6). Alternatively, that bent leg's foot can rest on a block or against a wall. A deeper variation is to hug the top knee toward the chest (fig. 7). That can get quite juicy, but if you want even more juice, straighten that leg up in the air and hold it with your hands or a strap.

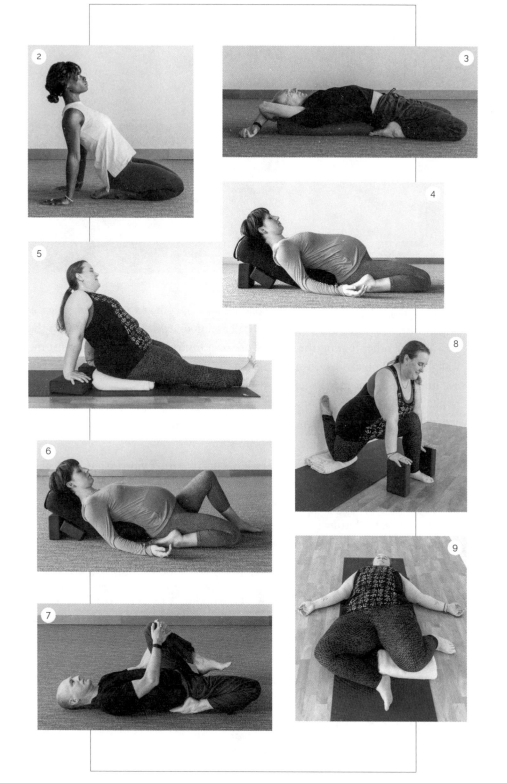

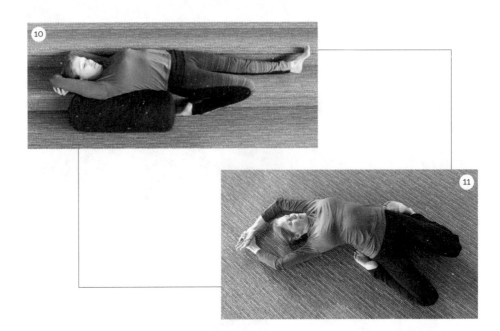

- For the King Arthur version of Half Saddle (fig. 8), come to a wall and have the targeted leg's knee at the corner of the wall and floor, with its shin up against the wall and the other foot on the floor. Work over time to get your back against the wall. Initially, you can have your hands on the floor or on blocks for balance, but eventually, the arms may be raised up against the wall.

- If the targeted area is your upper thigh (quadriceps stretch), a side-lying thigh stretch may be a good alternative. Lying on your side, reach down and grab the top foot (or use a strap) and pull it away from your pelvis.

- An exotic version of Half Saddle uses wide stairs (fig. 10). Lying on a middle stair, allow your bent leg to rest on the lower stair.

- It is possible to add a side bend if you can lie all the way down, called Banana in the Saddle (fig. 11). Sitting between the feet, if possible, clasp your elbows overhead and arch your upper body far to one side.

COMING OUT OF THE POSE

- There are several ways to end this pose. One option is to come back up the way you went down, propping yourself up on your elbows and then onto the hands. Then lie down on your belly, straightening your legs slowly to allow the knees to release.

- If that doesn't work or you are stuck, rent a crane, hire a forklift or call for help. If they are not available, trying rolling to one side and slowly straighten the opposite leg. Before rolling onto your back, you may want to wait a bit or hold your sacrum with your free hand and ease down to your back.

- If you're flexible, you can just lift both knees up and pop your feet out, or free one leg at a time.

COUNTERPOSES

- After coming out, lie quietly on your back for a few breaths with the legs straight, tightening and releasing the kneecaps. When you are ready, hug the backs of the thighs and pull the knees to the chest to release the low back.
- Child's Pose: Move into it slowly. You may need to rest your head on your palms before coming into a full Child's Pose.
- Plank on elbows (Crocodile) engages the knees and tones the core of the body.
- Windshield Wipers works well for many students.

MERIDIANS AND ORGANS AFFECTED

- Sensations along the top of the thighs and through the belly may stimulate the Stomach and Spleen meridians.
- Sensations along the spine, especially the low back, may stimulate the Kidney and Urinary Bladder meridians.
- If your arms are overhead, you may also stimulate the Heart and Lung meridians.

RECOMMENDED HOLD TIME

- One to 5 minutes.
- Iyengar says up to 15 minutes![15]

OTHER NOTES

- This is not a deep backbend for experienced yogis who are already very open in the low back; however, this pose does work many areas at once: ankles, knees, quadriceps, iliacus, psoas, sacrum, lumbar and shoulders.
- There is space for the belly to expand, so this pose can be done soon after eating, and many pregnant women like this pose when they are supported on a bolster.
- If your job requires you to stand all day and you do this pose at night before bed, your legs may feel rested in the morning.
- Tucking the tailbone (posterior tilt of the pelvis) may increase sensations in the hip flexors, but it decreases extension in the spine. Anterior tilting of the pelvis deepens the backbend extension but reduces stress in the hip flexors. Which option you choose to do depends upon your intention for the pose.
- B.K.S. Iyengar calls this pose Supta Virasana and, as mentioned, suggests it should be held for as long as you can, even up to 10–15 minutes! This shows that the Yin Yoga style is not new, even though he never uses this terminology. Holding postures for a long time has been around since the beginning of Hatha Yoga. He also claims it massages the heart and thereby improves blood flow, improves resistance to infections, relieves indigestion and flatulence, corrects a prolapsed uterus and flat feet, reduces menstrual and ovarian disorders, and reduces pain in the feet, legs and knees.[16] These claims have not been verified.

SHOELACE

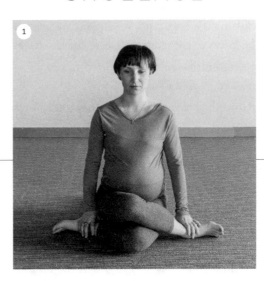

INTENTIONS AND TARGETED AREAS

- Primary targeted areas: the hips (flexion, external rotation, adduction).
- Secondary targeted areas: when folding forward the whole spine (flexion); for the Half Shoelace, tension in the hamstrings (due to hip flexion).

CONTRAINDICATIONS

- Many knees do not like this pose because of the external rotation at the hips. If your knees complain, raise the knees higher with supports (fig. 2) or try another option. If knee pain persists in all variations, skip this pose.
- Can aggravate sciatica. If you have piriformis sciatica, elevate the hips by sitting on a cushion so the knees are below the hips (reducing hip flexion). If you have discogenic sciatica, avoid rounding forward (reducing spinal flexion). In either case, if symptoms are made worse, avoid this pose entirely.
- If you have any low back disorders that do not allow flexion of the spine, then do not allow the spine to round: stay sitting up and keep the back as neutral as you can.
- Pregnant women will probably not be able to fold forward after the first trimester. They may also prefer to twist away from the top leg (fig. 5) or side-bend away from the top leg (fig. 7). Another option for pregnant students is the Sitting Swan (Eye-of-the-Needle) pose (fig. 11).

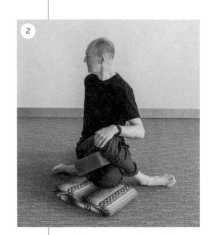

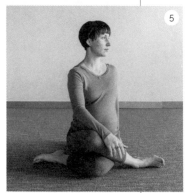

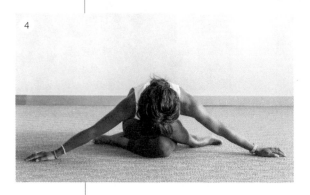

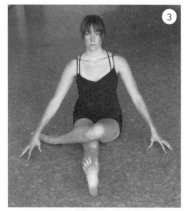

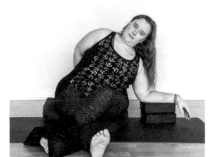

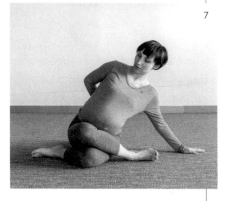

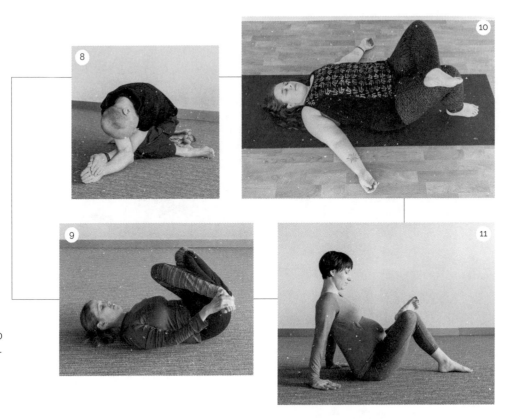

- Contraindications from YIP: anterior cruciate ligament tear, arthritis hip, arthritis knee, ischial bursitis, posterior total hip replacement, sprained ankle, torn abductors, total knee replacement.

GETTING INTO THE POSE

- There are several options for coming into this pose. One method is to begin by sitting on your heels, slide onto one buttock and bring the opposite foot toward its opposite hip. A second approach is to begin by sitting cross-legged and then draw one foot under the opposite thigh and the other foot over toward its opposite hip.

- A riskier approach (for the knees) is to begin by kneeling on all fours, then placing one knee behind the other and sitting back between the heels. (For some students, this approach involves a free-fall into sitting, and if their hips are not sufficiently open, too much stress can suddenly be placed onto the knees.)

ALTERNATIVES AND OPTIONS

- If this is not available due to pain or discomfort, sit cross-legged and fold forward.

- Try not to sit on the feet, but slide them as far forward as they can go, anchoring both sitting bones to the ground (fig. 1).

- If hips are tight, sit on a bolster to reduce the amount of hip flexion occurring. However, more flexible students may prefer to sit on the floor, increasing hip flexion, which may paradoxically reduce stress in the knees.[17]

- If the bottom knee complains, place a prop under the bottom knee (fig. 2) or do the pose with the bottom leg straight. This is the Half Saddle (fig. 3). Folding forward now makes the hamstrings feel really juicy.

- If the top knee complains, place a bolster or blanket under that knee or slide its foot more forward, increasing flexion at that hip. Some students may need to prop both knees (fig. 2).

- Folding forward over the legs (fig. 4) increases flexion in the hips and spine. If this is too challenging, support the chest on a bolster or rest the head in your hands. The further forward you fold, the more you can externally rotate the hips, and thus you may be able to move the feet further apart. Sensations may also increase in the buttocks.

- If you choose to remain sitting upright, your hands can be to your side or you can stretch the arms back behind the body and add a backbend (spinal extension). This may create more stress in the knees, however.

- Twists, side bends or Eagle Arms can be added. For the side bends, bending to the side of the top leg may feel more stable (fig. 6) but some people prefer bending away from the top leg (fig. 7). Similarly, you can twist toward the top knee (fig. 2), which pins the hips more, or twist away from it, which compresses the belly less (fig. 5). While in Eagle Arms, you may add a forward fold (fig. 8).

- Many students love to do this pose lying down: a reclining Shoelace, holding the feet of the crossed legs (fig. 9).

- Other alternatives include Eye-of-the-Needle Pose, either lying down (fig. 10) or sitting (fig. 11), Square Pose or Swan.

- Very flexible students can bring their feet more forward, until their shins are parallel to the front of their mat, with their knees still on top of each other. This in effect makes the pose into a version of Square Pose.

COMING OUT OF THE POSE

Lean back to release the hips, and slowly straighten the legs. (Don't forget to do the other side.)

111

COUNTERPOSES

- Windshield Wipers lying down or sitting (to provide an internal rotation of the hip).
- Deer Pose (which again provides internal rotation at the back hip).
- Tabletop (aka Hammock) to release the spine.

MERIDIANS AND ORGANS AFFECTED

- Sensations along the outside of the hips may stimulate the Gall Bladder meridians.
- Sensations through the inner knees, thighs and groin may stimulate the Liver and Kidney meridians.
- Sensations along the spine or the back of the legs may stimulate the Urinary Bladder meridians.
- Variations that include upper-body stresses through the arms and shoulders may stimulate the Heart and Lung meridians.

RECOMMENDED HOLD TIME

Three to 5 minutes per side.

OTHER NOTES

- This pose is also known as Cowface (Gomukhasana); if you can see a cow here, you have a good imagination!
- It is nice to follow this with Swan or Sleeping Swan before doing the other side.
- Start with the more open hip (whichever hip is more open, place that knee on top).
- Keep your weight back into the sitting bones when you come forward, preventing the weight from moving into the knees.
- Keep the hips even. There is a tendency for the top hip to be pulled forward.
- While you are lingering in this pose, try some poses targeting the shoulders or wrists. Check the upcoming section on the upper body for some suggestions.
- You could do the first half of the time in a variation like side bend or twist and then fold forward for the remaining time.

SNAIL

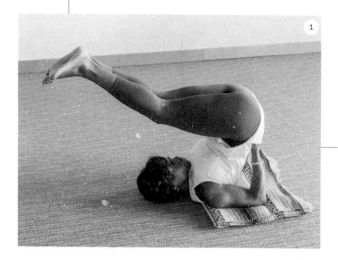

INTENTIONS AND TARGETED AREAS

- Primary targeted area: the whole length of the spine (flexion).
- Secondary targeted areas: can create tension in the hamstrings.

CONTRAINDICATIONS

- This pose may put a lot of pressure on the neck, so be cautious! Avoid if you have any neck problems.
- Not recommended for anyone with high blood pressure, upper-body infection, vertigo, glaucoma or a cold. Women who are menstruating may also find it better not to do this pose.
- If you have any low back disorder that does not allow flexion of the spine, this may not be a great pose for you.
- Do not do this posture if you have recently eaten or are pregnant.
- Contraindications from YIP: arthritis hip, congestive heart failure, coronary arterial disease, gastroesophageal reflux disease, glaucoma, herniated lumbar disc, Lasik surgery, menstruation, nosebleed, osteoporosis, posterior total hip replacement, retinal tear, retrolisthesis, spinal fracture (vertebral body), compression fracture, torn hamstring.

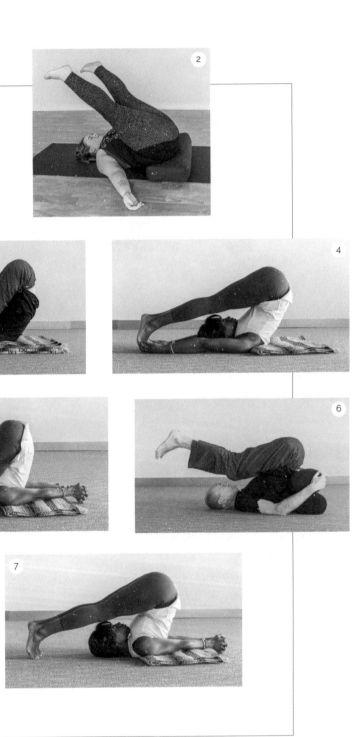

GETTING INTO THE POSE

Lie down, lift your hips and support them with your hands. Allow your back to round (unlike the Plough Pose, Halasana, in which we strive to keep the spine and legs straight). Let your feet fall over your head toward the floor (fig. 1). Position the weight of your body onto your shoulders; note how much weight is on your neck—some is okay, but not too much!

ALTERNATIVES AND OPTIONS

- For beginners or those not wishing to invert, replace this pose with a seated straight leg, a forward fold (such as Caterpillar) or a legs-up-the-wall pose.
- An option for less flexible students is the mini version of Snail, with the hips lifted just enough for them to rest on bolsters (fig. 2).
- There are many variations that can increase stress:

    1. Support the back with the palms (fig. 1).
    2. More challenging is to place the palms under the feet and lower the feet to the floor, or rest the feet on a bolster (fig. 3) or a chair, or even press them against a wall.
    3. Deeper is to have the legs straight and feet on the floor (fig. 4). However, this version has less rounding of the spine, more flexion in the hips and more stress in the hamstrings. It may also create the deepest flexion of the neck, so blankets under the shoulders may be required.
    4. Most challenging is to bend the knees toward the floor (fig. 5), which may create the deepest stress along the spine.

- Unlike in Plough Pose (Halasana), we want the spine to round. A deeper stress in the mid and upper back may be created if you back off from the desire to have your feet on the floor and hips over the head. Instead, move your hips back, as shown in fig. 6. Hips can be supported in the hands, on bolsters or even against a wall. This position may be better for the neck, as there is much less neck flexion occurring now.
- If the legs are straight and the feet are touching the floor, the hands can come to the floor behind the back. Your hands can be apart (easier) or together (if there are no shoulder problems), but be careful; bringing the hands together can aggravate rotator cuff problems. This is more like the classical Plough Pose (fig. 7).

COMING OUT OF THE POSE

- The simplest way to come out is to keep the knees bent and hold your hips, allowing yourself to slowly roll down. Your head will likely lift up as you come down and that is okay.

- More challenging is to come out with the legs straight and holding the feet. Slowly roll down, holding the feet as a way to slow your descent.

COUNTERPOSES
- After coming out, lie down for a few breaths with the knees bent and feet on the floor.
- Do Windshield Wipers, then a gentle backbend, such as by lying on the abdomen, or a mild spinal lift. Come up only halfway.
- Upward Facing Cat.
- Child's Pose.

MERIDIANS AND ORGANS AFFECTED
- Sensations along the spine and back of the legs may stimulate the Urinary Bladder meridians.
- The internal organs are physically compressed, and each breath adds to the massage.

RECOMMENDED HOLD TIME

Three to 5 minutes.

OTHER NOTES
- This is a very deep flexion for the spine, so it is not a pose to start your practice with. First prepare the spine with gentler flexions, such as Butterfly or Caterpillar.
- Indeed, many students do not need to do this pose at all and can simply linger longer in Caterpillar. However, for more flexible students who do not feel much in the easier postures, Snail may be perfect. Even so, don't start with Snail. Spend a couple of minutes in Caterpillar and then roll onto your back for Snail.
- Allow the spine to fully round. Unlike Halasana, do not try to keep the spine straight.
- B.K.S. Iyengar claims Halasana controls blood pressure, improves digestion, can assist with treating hemorrhoids, reduces fatigue, insomnia and anxiety, alleviates symptoms of asthma, bronchitis and congestion, relieves heart palpitations and breathlessness, and improves the function of the thyroid and parathyroid glands.[18] These claims have not been verified.

SPHINX AND SEAL

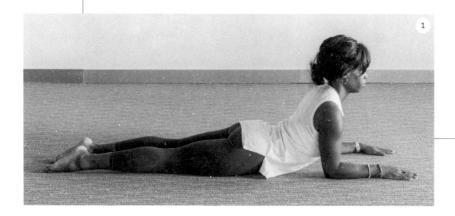

INTENTIONS AND TARGETED AREAS

- Primary targeted area: the sacral-lumbar spine (compression).
- Secondary targeted areas: the front torso (tension).

CONTRAINDICATIONS

- If you have low back problems or sacral instabilities, this pose may not be for you.
- If any sharp pains arise, you must come out!
- Avoid lifting the head in Sphinx if you have a headache or if it causes a headache.
- Contraindications from YIP: anterior total hip replacement, anterolisthesis, carpal tunnel syndrome (Seal), cervical spinal stenosis, Dupuytren's contracture, facet syndrome, lumbar spinal stenosis, tennis elbow (Seal).

GETTING INTO THE POSE

Lie down on your belly. Move the elbows just ahead of your shoulders, propping yourself up (fig. 1). Notice how this feels in your low back. If the sensations are too strong, move your elbows further ahead, lowering your chest closer to the floor. Even lying flat on the floor may be enough stress for the low back (fig. 2).

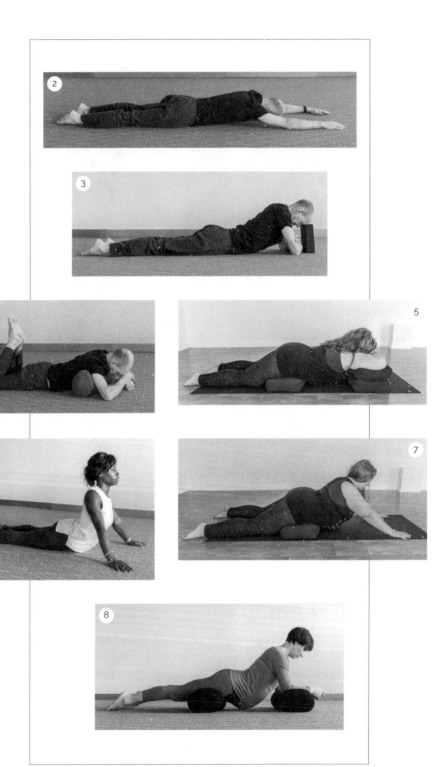

ALTERNATIVES AND OPTIONS

- Hands can hold the elbows (fig. 3), be clasped together or be flat on the floor.

- If your head gets too heavy for your neck, try resting your head in your hands or on a block (fig. 3), or your chin on your fists.

- If there is too much discomfort in the shoulders or upper chest, try a bolster or two under the armpits (fig. 4).

- If after a few minutes in the pose there is not enough stress in the low back, try bending the knees (fig. 4) and/or propping the elbows higher on blocks (fig. 5).

- How far apart the knees should be is variable. Which position feels best for you? (Where do you get the appropriate amount of stress in the targeted areas?)

- If the stress in the low back is still not enough, Seal Pose may be required. To come into Seal, turn your hands outward, straighten the arms (locking the elbows) and walk the hands toward you (fig. 6). It is okay if the elbows hyperextend here, because they are not bearing much weight. Indeed, this may be a good time to stress the elbow joints.

- You may feel the greatest amount of compression in the low back in Seal Pose if your hands are not right under the shoulders but slightly forward.

- Rather than coming into Seal with the arms in front, have the hands and arms straight out to the side, and walk them in toward you.[19]

- You can place a bolster or blanket under the pubic bone or thighs to reduce uncomfortable pressure (fig. 5 and 7).

- Pregnant women may enjoy this pose if they place a bolster under both the thighs and elbows; there is no pressure at all in the belly (fig. 8).

- Tightening the buttocks is okay within reason. Sagging the shoulders is also okay. These actions will not affect the stress in the targeted areas.

- To arch the neck and stimulate the cervical spine, lengthen the neck, drop the head back, lift the chin and open the throat. This is for Seal only; it is not a good idea to do this in Sphinx, as it involves too much neck extension, which can cause headaches or lightheadedness.

- If you're very flexible, try these postures with the legs in Lotus.

COMING OUT OF THE POSE

- To come out, slowly lower your chest to the floor. Turn your head to one side and rest your cheek on your palms. You may wish to decompress the low back more by sliding one knee alongside you on the floor.

COUNTERPOSES

- Child's Pose is a nice, gentle forward fold; move into it slowly. You may need to rest your head on your palms.
- On your way to Child's Pose, you may crave Cat's Breath: flow from the Upward Facing Cat to the Downward Facing Cat (aka Cat/Cow) but flow gently, in time with the breath. Don't make these your deepest Cats ever.

MERIDIANS AND ORGANS AFFECTED

- Sensations along the spine and low back may stimulate the Urinary Bladder and Kidney meridians.
- Sensations along the front of the body may stimulate the Stomach and Spleen meridians.
- There is a physical compression of the kidneys as well.

RECOMMENDED HOLD TIME

- Sphinx can be held for a long time: 5–10 minutes for most people. Or do the pose twice with each set lasting 3–5 minutes.
- For Seal, start with one-minute holds, come down, rest, and repeat 2–3 times.
- Eventually Seal can be held for 5 minutes or more.
- Eventually Sphinx can be held up to 20 minutes!

OTHER NOTES

- If tingling arises in the hands in Seal Pose, this is not good. Probably nerves are being compressed or blood flow is restricted. Come back to Sphinx.
- Seal Pose is a deeper backbend than Saddle and thus can be done after Saddle. Sphinx, however, is not as deep as Saddle, so it may be done before Saddle.
- This is a great pose for watching television or reading on the floor.
- People with bulging or herniated discs may find this very therapeutic.[20]
- According to Daoists, between the L2 and L3 vertebrae is found the "Door of Life," where jing energy is housed. You may feel a lot of stress right there.
- In Seal, if the neck is dropped back, the thyroid and parathyroid glands may be physically stimulated.
- B.K.S. Iyengar calls this Bhujangasana (Cobra), but his version requires a lot of muscular engagement. He claims it is a panacea for injured spines.[21] This claim has not been verified.

SQUARE

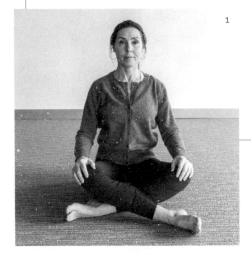

1

INTENTIONS AND TARGETED AREAS

- Primary targeted areas: the hips (flexion and external rotation).
- Secondary targeted areas: when folding forward, the whole spine (flexion).

CONTRAINDICATIONS

- Watch the pressure on the knees; if the hips are too tight, the stress will go to the knees. If you feel any pain or burning sensations in the knees, modify the pose or skip it.
- This pose can aggravate sciatica. If you have piriformis sciatica, elevate the hips by sitting on a cushion so the knees are below the hips (reducing hip flexion). If you have discogenic sciatica, avoid rounding forward (reducing spinal flexion). In either case, if symptoms are made worse, avoid this pose entirely.
- If you have any low back disorders that do not allow flexion of the spine, then do not allow the spine to round: keep the back as neutral as you can.
- Pregnant women should be okay doing this pose, but skip the folding forward options.

GETTING INTO THE POSE

This can be a tricky one to get into. The key is to go where you feel some juiciness in the outer hips, never in the knees. Start by sitting with legs crossed. Move your feet forward until your shins are parallel to the front edge of your mat (your legs are "square" to it). (Notice which leg is in front because when you do the other side, you will want to bring the other leg in front.)

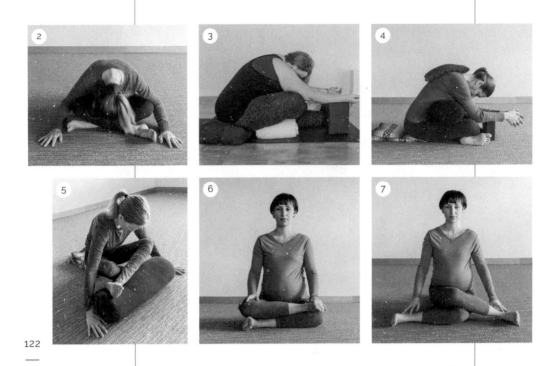

- Try to move your knees closer together without allowing your feet to come back closer to you (fig. 1).
- Ideally, the thighs are parallel to each other and the shins are parallel to each other. But who cares about ideals! That alignment is not available to every body, so do what works for you.

ALTERNATIVES AND OPTIONS

- If this is not available due to pain or discomfort, try sitting cross-legged and folding forward.
- Folding forward stretches the low back and can intensify the stress in the buttocks (fig. 2). However, folding forward (deepening the hip flexion) may reduce stress in the knees, allowing you to move your feet further away from you or to stack the legs on top of each other.
- If you're tight or experience discomfort in the knees, or if the knees are high off the floor, you can place blankets or some form of support under the knees (fig. 3).
- If you can't come forward, sit higher on cushions. It is also okay to support the upper body with a bolster (fig. 4) and/or rest your head in your hands or on a block.
- If you crave a little more stress, a sandbag along the spine may be delicious (fig. 4).
- If you remain sitting up, you can add twists, side bends and other arm/shoulder work.

- A deeper option is to place the front leg on a bolster (fig. 5) or come into the version of the pose where one ankle is over the opposite knee and the other ankle under its opposite knee (fig. 6). If the top knee is very high in the air, you are not ready for this variation! Bring that foot to the floor in front of its opposite knee.
- If you're very flexible, try to slide the knees closer together, allowing the feet to go further apart (fig. 7). This is where Square meets the deeper version of Shoelace.
- If none of these options works for you, other alternatives for working into the hips include Eye-of-the-Needle, Shoelace, Butterfly and Swan.

COMING OUT OF THE POSE

Lean back and slowly straighten the legs out in front of you. Remember to do both sides!

COUNTERPOSES

- Bounce out the legs and tighten/release the knees a few times.
- This was a fairly deep external rotation of the hips, so we want to move the hips in the opposite direction. Some nice internal rotations of the hips are Deer or Windshield Wipers.
- If you're craving a backbend, perform Tabletop or lie down and do some Spinal Lifts.

MERIDIANS AND ORGANS AFFECTED

- Sensations along the outside of the hips may stimulate the Gall Bladder meridians.
- Sensations through the inner knees, thighs and groin may stimulate the Liver and Kidney meridians.
- Sensations along the spine or the back of the legs may stimulate the Urinary Bladder meridians.

RECOMMENDED HOLD TIME : Three to 5 minutes per side.

OTHER NOTES

- If you're a beginner, you may tend to bring your feet very close to the groin. That may be okay! Even a simple cross-legged sitting posture may be enough for your body. If you are feeling it, you are doing it! Be there and enjoy.
- Square Pose is in the middle of a continuum between Butterfly (legs abducted) and Shoelace (legs adducted). All 3 postures include external rotation and flexion at the hips. If one of these poses doesn't work for you, the others might.
- Other names for Square are Double Pigeon, Boxcar, 90-90 and Fire Log.
- B.K.S. Iyengar calls cross-legged sitting (the easy version of Square Pose) Swastikasana. He claims it rests tired legs and feet, reduces inflammation in the knees and the veins of the legs, strengthens knee cartilage and makes the hips supple.[22] These claims have not been verified.

SQUAT

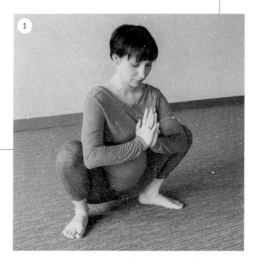

INTENTIONS AND TARGETED AREAS

- Primary targeted areas: dorsiflexion of ankles, flexion of knees and hips.
- Secondary targeted areas: flexion of the lumbar spine can feel like a decompression; for some students, those with feet wider apart, this also creates abduction and a little bit of external rotation in the hip sockets.

CONTRAINDICATIONS

- If hips are too tight, this might overly stress the knees.
- If you have knee issues and cannot fully flex your knees, avoid this pose.
- For students with tight ankles who have to have their heels in the air, so be it! Just because your ankles are tight doesn't mean you can't do this pose.
- Contraindications from YIP: anterior cruciate ligament tear, arthritis hip, arthritis knee, chondromalacia patellae, herniated thoracic disc, medial meniscal tear, orthostatic hypotension, osteoporosis, plantar fasciitis, posterior cruciate ligament tear, posterior total hip replacement, pregnancy (second and third trimesters), sprained ankle, total knee replacement.

GETTING INTO THE POSE

Start by standing with the feet hip-width apart, feet turned slightly outward. Squat down with your arms in front of you for counterbalance (fig. 1). When all the way down, your hands can be in prayer, with the elbows pulling lightly against the knees or shins.

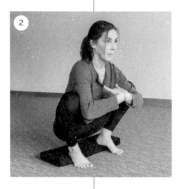
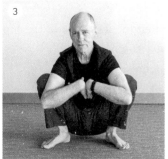
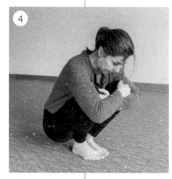

ALTERNATIVES AND OPTIONS

- Many students cannot easily do this posture due to tightness in the hips, knees and/or ankles. If your heels are off the floor, there are several options to try: use a folded blanket or bolster under the heels (fig. 2); widen the distance between the feet; or turn the feet more outward (fig. 3).

- Find the place where you can relax in this pose. But if that is not going to happen at all, try the Wall Squat or Happy Baby, which are similarly shaped postures. Child's Pose with legs apart also shares similar movements at the joints (except the ankles) with less stress.

- In a classroom setting, if the pose gets tiring, switch to Butterfly while everyone else remains in Squat.

- When the feet are wide apart (hip width or more), you may feel more stress in the hips.

- When the feet are close together (perhaps even touching—fig. 4), you may feel more stress in the ankles.

- You can try other hand variations, such as reverse prayer, where the backs of the hands are together (palmar flexion—fig. 2 and 3). This can be a nice counterpose after a lot of wrist extension from Down Dog or Sun Salutations.

- Another option is to place your hands behind your head and gently draw the chin to the chest; this adds stress to the back of the neck.

COMING OUT OF THE POSE

- An easy exit is to just sit down and then slowly straighten the legs out in front of you.

- A more challenging exit is to come to Dangling by straightening the legs and folding forward. As you straighten the legs, your feet may change their alignment as well.

COUNTERPOSES

- Postures that straighten the legs, extend the hips and spine, and plantarflex the ankles, such as Sphinx Pose.
- For the knees—Dangling or Caterpillar.
- For the ankles—Ankle Stretch, Vajrasana (sitting on the heels) or Virasana (sitting between the feet).

MERIDIANS AND ORGANS AFFECTED

- Sensations through the inner groin may stimulate the Liver and Kidney meridians.
- Sensations along the thighs and lower belly may stimulate the Spleen and Stomach meridians.
- Sensations along the lower spine may stimulate the Urinary Bladder and Kidney meridians.
- If you feel this all around your ankles, you may stimulate the Stomach, Spleen, Gall Bladder and Urinary Bladder meridians.

RECOMMENDED HOLD TIME

- Two to 3 minutes at one time is plenty for most people, but you can revisit this pose a couple of times during the practice.

OTHER NOTES

- The challenge for many people is getting into the pose, not the end posture itself. Coming down into Squat requires the knees to move in front of the toes to counterbalance the hips going backward; this is one reason for the arms coming forward as you descend. If your range of dorsiflexion in the ankles is restricted, you may not be able to descend easily; if so, having your feet wider or lifting your heels may make the pose doable. If this doesn't work, try coming into Squat from sitting on the floor.
- Approximately two-thirds of the world's population goes to the bathroom this way every day! It is a natural position for humans. If you find it challenging, this may be a sign that you need to do this pose more.
- A nice sequence is to go from Dangling to Squat, back to Dangling, back to Squat, over and over again, holding each position for 1 to 2 minutes.
- Elbows in front of knees can be used as levers to pull the chest forward, allowing the tailbone to drop lower.
- A common yoga belief claims that this can be a great pose to prepare for childbirth.
- This is sometimes called Malasana. B.K.S. Iyengar claims that this posture offers relief to women suffering severe low back pain due to their menstrual cycle and strengthens the abdominal organs.[23] These claims have not been verified.

STRADDLE

(DRAGONFLY)

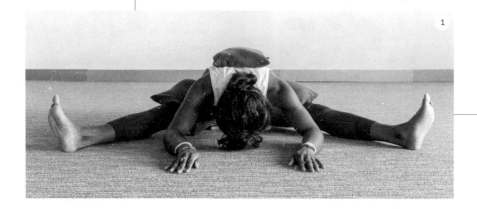

INTENTIONS AND TARGETED AREAS

- Primary targeted areas: the hips (flexion, external rotation, abduction) and the inner thighs/adductors (tension).
- Secondary targeted area: the whole spine (flexion), the hamstrings (tension) and the inner knees (tension).

CONTRAINDICATIONS

- This pose can aggravate sciatica. If you have piriformis sciatica, elevate the hips by sitting on a cushion so the knees are below the hips. If you have discogenic sciatica, avoid rounding the spine. In either case, if symptoms are made worse, avoid this pose entirely.
- If you have any low back disorders that do not allow flexion of the spine, then do not allow the spine to round: keep the back as neutral as you can.
- If you have any inner knee trauma or issues and if this pose creates any burning pain there, bring the legs closer together.
- Contraindications from YIP: anterior total hip replacement, arthritis hip, cervical spinal stenosis, gastroesophageal reflux disease, herniated lumbar disc, ischial bursitis, osteoporosis, posterior total hip replacement, pregnancy (second and third trimesters), retinal tear, retrolisthesis, sacroiliac joint derangement, spinal fracture (vertebral body), compression fracture, torn adductor, torn hamstring.

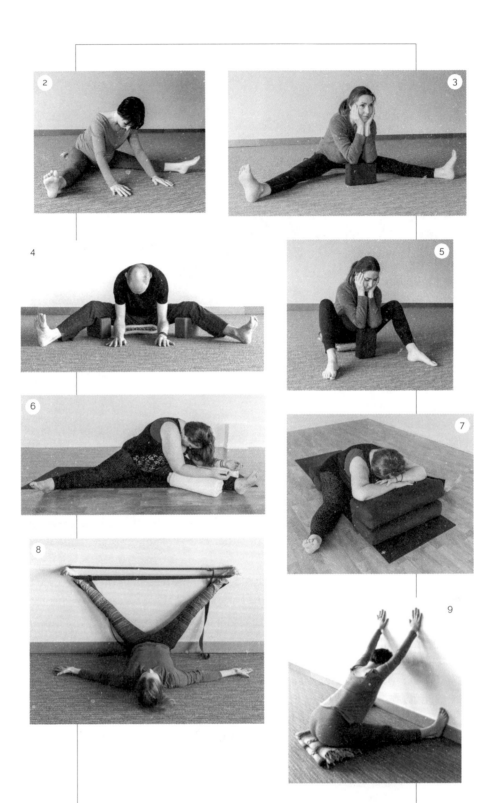

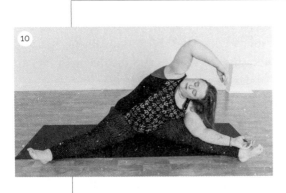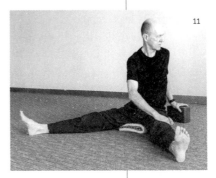

GETTING INTO THE POSE

From a sitting position, spread your legs apart until they won't go any further. Sitting on a cushion will help tilt your hips. Fold forward, resting your weight into your hands (fig. 2) with your arms locked straight, or rest your elbows on a block (fig. 3).

ALTERNATIVES AND OPTIONS

- Use a bolster to raise the hips; this makes it easier to come forward.
- You can keep the hands behind the back, which may make it easier to keep the spine straight if desired.
- Another option is to do Half Butterfly over one leg, then the other leg, then to do the full Straddle down the middle.
- Legs can be 90° apart for stiffer students to 120° for flexible students. The full split of 180° is not necessary, but if you can do it, go for it.
- If you're more flexible, fold right down onto your abdomen. To increase sensations, sandbags along the upper spine or on the thighs can help (fig. 1).
- If your head is too heavy for your neck, support it in your hands (fig. 3).
- If the hamstrings feel too tight, bend the knees and place blocks under the thighs (fig. 4).
- If you are very stiff, bend the knees a lot (fig. 5)! It is also okay to place the feet flat on the floor. When the knees are bent, and while sitting on a cushion, you can bend forward more easily and allow gravity to do the work.
- Fold over just one leg (fig. 6) instead of down the middle. Notice the differences in sensations along the spine and hamstrings.
- Use a bolster under the chest or arms if you are close to the floor (fig. 6 and 7).
- Using straps to hold onto the feet is okay, as long as you are not actively pulling.

- Using the wall can also be great, especially if you don't want to flex the spine at all. If the legs feel too stressed by gravity pulling them apart, you can place bolsters or blocks under the thighs or wrap a strap or 2 around the feet (fig. 8). You can also use the wall by folding toward it, allowing the wall to keep the feet apart (fig. 9). This is a nice option for pregnant students.

- You can also side-bend toward one leg and rotate the chest skyward (fig. 10). If you are very flexible, hold the foot with both hands.

- You can also do a sitting-up twist (fig. 11), which may help to stimulate the upper body meridians.

- Pregnant women can do this pose, but if they get too close to the floor, they may want to rest on a bolster.

- Very flexible students may not feel much here, and that's okay. They are still getting benefits.[24] But if they insist on going further, they can place blocks under their hips and calves to create a platform.

COMING OUT OF THE POSE

- Use your hands to push the floor away, and slowly roll up.

- Once you are up, lean back on your hands to release the hips, tighten the leg muscles, and drag or lift your legs to bring them together. Bounce or shake out the legs. Groaning is allowed![25]

COUNTERPOSES

- This was a flexion for the spine and hips, so spinal extension is nice. Do a gentle sitting backbend or lie on the belly. You can also do Cat's Breath or flow into Tabletop (aka Hammock).

- Seated twist is another way to release the spine.

- This was also an external rotation and abduction for the hips, so some internal rotation and adduction, such as Windshield Wipers, may feel nice. Twisted Roots is another option.

MERIDIANS AND ORGANS AFFECTED

- Sensations through the inner knees, thighs and groin may stimulate the Liver and Kidney meridians.

- Sensations along the spine and/or back of the legs may stimulate the Urinary Bladder meridians.

- If you are feeling sensations along the outside of the hips or through the ribcage when you add a twist, you may stimulate the Gall Bladder meridians.

RECOMMENDED HOLD TIME
Three to 10 minutes.

OTHER NOTES

- Straddle provides a gentle stress on the inner knees, which may be very therapeutic for people suffering trauma there, as long as the sensations generated are not painful.
- This can be very frustrating for beginners: the adductor muscles tug on the sitting bones, as do the hamstrings, which causes the top of the hips to tilt backward, making forward folding difficult. Persistence (and bent knees!) is required. Sitting on a bolster helps.
- You can sequence this into a 3-pose flow—first folding over one leg, then the other, then down the middle, holding each position for 3–5 minutes. Or start down the middle and then do each leg. While folding over a leg, you may want to add a twist for the last half of the time.
- B.K.S. Iyengar calls this pose Upavista Konasana. He claims it relieves sciatic pain, prevents and treats hernia, massages the reproductive organs, relieves menstrual disorders, and corrects a prolapsed bladder or uterus.[26] These claims have not been verified.

SWAN AND SLEEPING SWAN

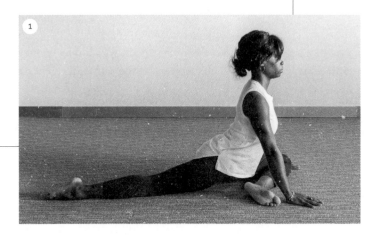

INTENTIONS AND TARGETED AREAS

- Primary targeted areas: the front leg's hip is in flexion, external rotation and perhaps abduction, while the back leg's hip is extended.
- Secondary targeted areas: in the full Swan, the spine is extended; in Sleeping Swan, tension may also be created in the glutes and along the iliotibial band.

CONTRAINDICATIONS

- Many knees do not like this pose. If your knees complain, have the front foot closer in, perhaps sitting on it (fig. 4), or skip this pose and do Eye-of-the-Needle Pose (fig. 11) or another hip opener.
- If the back kneecap feels uncomfortable due to pressure against the floor, there are several options: pad the back knee with a blanket; or place support under the shin (fig. 8 and 9), allowing the knee to be off the floor; or keep the knee bent with the foot raised off the floor.[27]
- Due to asymmetric stresses in the sacroiliac joints, pregnant women may wish to avoid this pose.
- Contraindications from YIP for the full Swan: anterior cruciate ligament tear, anterior total hip replacement, anterolisthesis, arthritis hip, arthritis knee, chondromalacia patellae, facet syndrome, lateral meniscal tear, lumbar spinal stenosis, medial meniscal tear, posterior cruciate, ligament tear, posterior total hip replacement, sprained ankle, total knee replacement.

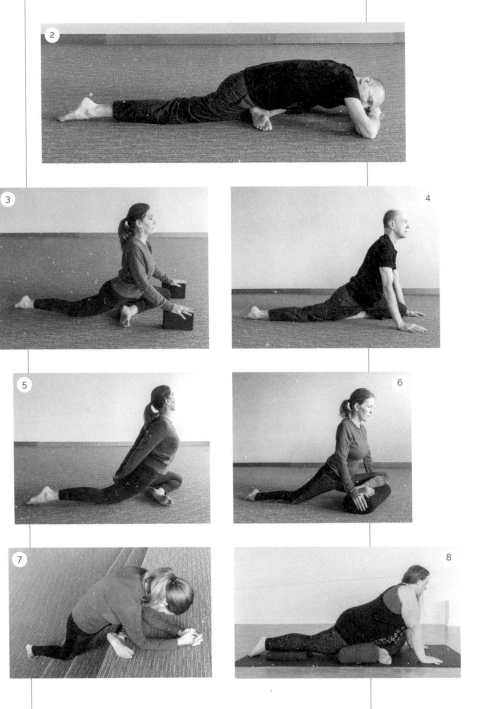

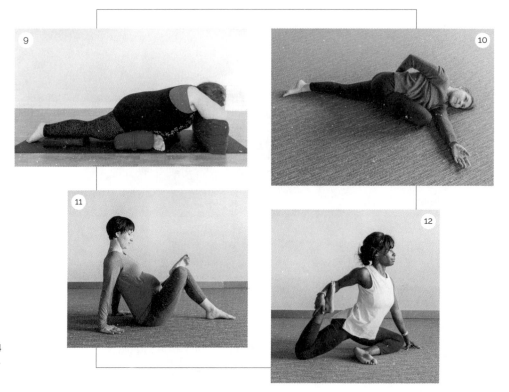

GETTING INTO THE POSE

You can come into this pose from Down Dog, Deer or hands and knees. Slide a knee between your hands, lean a bit to that side and check in with how your knee feels. If the knee is fine, flex the front foot and move it forward (fig. 1); if the knee feels stressed, bring the foot closer in toward the hip (fig. 3). You may even sit right on the foot (fig. 4). Center yourself so your weight is even. Try tucking the back toes under and sliding the back knee away. Do this a few times until your front leg's buttock is on the floor or as low as it is going to get.

ALTERNATIVES AND OPTIONS FOR THE FULL SWAN—STAYING UPRIGHT (FIG. 1)

- To protect the front knee, keep the front foot flexed; this engages the fascia all around the knee, stiffening it.
- Less flexible students may rest their hands on blocks in front of them (fig. 3). Moving the hands closer to the hips increases the weight over the front hip (fig. 1). Very flexible students may clasp hands behind their low backs (fig. 5).
- If you are leaning to the bent leg side, that may be perfectly okay for you. Indeed, another version of Swan is the Deer, where you have considerable weight on that

front hip. If, however, you want to be more centered, place a support, such as a folded blanket, under the bent knee's hip.

- If you're really externally rotated at the hip, try to bring your front foot forward, parallel to the front of your mat, and slide that knee more to the side. Deeper options include placing a bolster under the front shin (fig. 6) or resting that leg onto a chair, counter top, desk or stair (fig. 7).

- Many students prefer to have a bolster under both hips so they can relax more and thus stay longer in the pose (fig. 8).

ALTERNATIVES AND OPTIONS FOR THE SLEEPING SWAN—THE FOLDED FORWARD VERSION (FIG. 2)

- To come into this version, keep the weight back into the hips as you walk your hands forward, lowering down in stages. If you come down too fast, all the weight goes into the front knee; so walk hands forward, but snuggle the hips back; walk forward, snuggle back; eventually, come onto the elbows or all the way down.

- You can lie on a bolster placed lengthwise under the chest, or support your upper body on blocks (fig. 9). This may be ideal for pregnant women, but if that doesn't work for them, they could stay in full Swan or do Deer Pose.

- If you're really flexible, try to bring the front foot forward, pull the bent knee more to the side, and lay your chest on top of the shin.

- You may want to rest your chest on your thigh, if that is better/juicier, or to walk your chest away from the front thigh. Which version works better for you?

- You may want to add a twist by threading the opposite arm from the front leg under your head and turning your chest to look up. You can raise the free arm up and behind your back (fig. 10).

- Another option to the full Swan is the sitting Eye-of-the-Needle Pose (fig. 11), which maintains the back extension with the hip work. Other options include the reclining Eye-of-the-Needle Pose, Deer, Shoelace or Square.

- If the targeted area is your upper thigh (quadriceps stretch), Screaming Swan is a really yang version that can be fun if tried at the end of the pose (fig. 12). Bend the back leg, reach the hand of the same side to that heel, and pull the heel to the buttocks. (Or until the screaming starts.)

COMING OUT OF THE POSE

Use your hands to push the floor away and slowly come up. Tuck the back toes under, plant your front paws in Down Dog position, and with a nice groan, step back to the Downward Facing Puppy. If you never liked Down Dog before, you will love it now!

COUNTERPOSES

- A short Down Dog is delicious. Bend one knee, lifting that heel and pushing the opposite heel down, and then switch sides repeatedly (this is sometimes called Walking the Dog). Many students also love to lift one leg up, stretching it, and then switch sides.
- Child's Pose feels really good after Down Dog and before switching to the other side of Swan.
- If you were strongly externally rotating at the hips, internal rotations such as Windshield Wipers or Twisted Roots may be ideal.

MERIDIANS AND ORGANS AFFECTED

- The full Swan is one posture than can stimulate all 6 lower body meridians! Sensations along the top of the back leg may indicate that the Stomach and Spleen meridians are being stimulated.
- Sensation in the inner groin may stimulate the Liver and Kidney meridians.
- Sensations along the spine may stimulate the Urinary Bladder and Kidney meridians.
- Sensations along the outside of the hips or the sides of the ribs (in the Twisting Swan) may stimulate the Gall Bladder meridian.

RECOMMENDED HOLD TIME

The full Swan is a moderately yang posture when the chest is raised: hold 1 to 3 minutes. After a couple of minutes, switch to Sleeping Swan for another 1 to 3 minutes.

OTHER NOTES

- Full Swan is a deeper hip opener than Sleeping Swan because more weight is placed right above the front hip.
- If you are feeling it, you are doing it! If you have lost the feeling in the targeted areas, wiggle around until you find it again. Sometimes a subtle adjustment of the legs can increase the sensation in the front hip but reduce the stress in the quadriceps of the back leg. You can decide where your priority is today.
- This is also called Rajakapotasana. B.K.S. Iyengar claims it can control sexual desires due to increased blood flowing through the pubic region and can improve the health of the urinary system.[28] These claims have not been verified.

TOE SQUAT

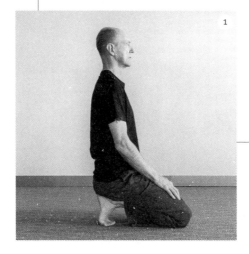

INTENTIONS AND TARGETED AREAS

- Primary targeted area: flexes the toes and dorsiflexes the ankles.
- Secondary targeted areas: deep flexion for the knees, mild flexion for the hips; the plantar fascia at the bottom of the foot may get a lovely stress (tension).

CONTRAINDICATIONS

- If the knees complain from the deep flexion, sit up higher on blocks (fig. 2).
- If ankles or toe joints are very tight, don't stay here long.

GETTING INTO THE POSE

Begin by sitting on your heels with the feet together. Tuck the toes under and try to be on the balls of the feet, not the tippy-toes (fig. 1 and 4). Reach down and tuck the little toes under—let them join the party.

ALTERNATIVES AND OPTIONS

- If the pose becomes too challenging, stand up on the knees, relieving most of the pressure on the toe joints (fig. 3). When you feel you can handle it again, sit back down on the heels.
- Don't stay if in pain!
- If you need a bit more juice, allow your knees to slide more forward, deepening the flexion and stress in the toes (fig. 4).
- You can combine this posture with shoulder exercises such as Eagle Arms or Cowface Arms.

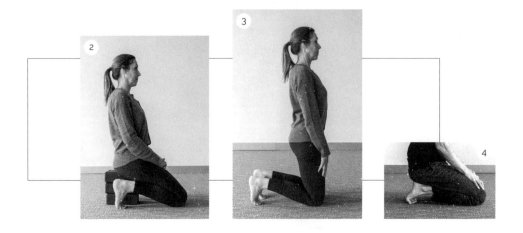

- If the knees are uncomfortable, place a blanket under them or a cushion between the hips and heels. You may enjoy a rolled-up towel behind the knees, which helps to release the knee joints.

COMING OUT OF THE POSE

This one can be quite juicy, so come out slowly, enjoying every single moment! Lean forward onto your hands, lift your hips forward and release your feet. Point the feet backward and sit on your heels again. Sigh! Om.

COUNTERPOSES : Ankle Stretch, Child's Pose or any posture that plantarflexes the ankles, such as Saddle.

MERIDIANS AND ORGANS AFFECTED

- All the meridians of the lower body may be stimulated due to the stresses in the toes.
- The front of the ankles also become stressed, which may help to stimulate the Stomach meridians.

RECOMMENDED HOLD TIME : Two to 3 minutes.

OTHER NOTES

- Our feet are the furthest things from our minds, literally! Most of us imprison our toes all day long in shoes, and then when we are in our 70s and 80s, our toes stop working and we fall down. There is an old Daoist saying; "A person with open toes has an open mind." Open your toes now!
- This pose can become quite intense for most people fairly quickly. Monitor the level of intensity. It is better not to stay in the pose if you are in pain. Come out, rest a bit, then try again.
- If doing shoulder work while holding the pose, take a break between sides. Do an Ankle Stretch, and then come back into Toe Stretch and resume the shoulder work on the other side.

SHAVASANA

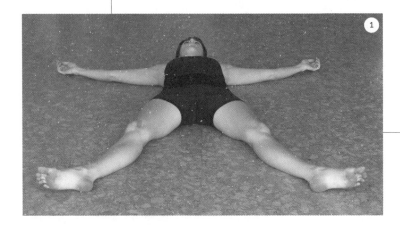

Time to relax. Time to rest the body, to become younger, stronger, healthier, whole. Time for the little death of *Shavasana* (which literally means the "dead posture"). Shavasana symbolizes the end of your practice—a natural completion to the journey you have been on.

If you are practicing on your own, you may want to set a timer for your Shavasana. It is not uncommon for students to fall asleep. Falling asleep is okay, but most teachers prefer that you remain alert and aware while the body is relaxed. A timer will help rouse you at the end of the Shavasana. Decide how much time you need to relax. For an active yang practice, a good rule of thumb is to allow yourself 10–15% of your practice time. For the yin style, since the muscles were not used, a shorter period may be okay—maybe 5% or 8% will suffice. However, check in with your inner guide and see how much time would be right today. Most of us can benefit from a longer Shavasana regardless of what we have been doing.

Shavasana is not just a time to relax the body; in this quiet time, the mind should remain alert yet relaxed and aware of the body relaxing. Pay attention to the energies flowing. This is an ideal time to develop your ability to feel your energies. It may be difficult to do this when you are in the postures. Practicing watching the energies during your Shavasana will help you feel energy flowing at other times. As you actively relax, watch the flow of chi or prana into and out of the areas you worked in the asana practice. At first, you may have to pretend or imagine you can feel these energies. Pretending will help you look closely at these areas. In time, you will more easily notice the energy flow.

There are many ways to perform Shavasana, and many teachers have their own unique and favorite methods. Collect several ways of relaxing by taking classes with several teachers. With a larger repertoire, you can choose which way is best for any given day. The following suggestion is just one of the many possible options, and for some students, Shavasana is better done while sitting, or with legs up the wall, or while lying on their side (especially for pregnant students).

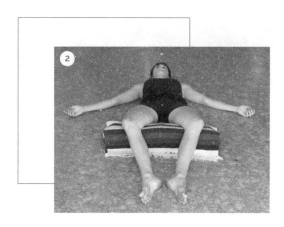

Preparing to Relax

In a yoga studio, your teacher will make sure the surroundings are suitable for relaxation. If you are practicing by yourself, make your environment quiet: disconnect phones; turn off noises; open the windows to allow fresh air in, but stay warm; put any pets into another room; turn lights down but not off completely—a completely dark room may encourage you to sleep. For the same reason, you may want to avoid doing Shavasana in bed.

Begin by letting the body become open: take off glasses and watches; let your hair down; remove anything that may constrict the flow of energy. Also experiment with removing any metallic circles you have on—things like rings, bracelets and body piercings can interfere with the flow of energy.[29] Notice any differences.

Ensure you will stay warm—put on socks and a sweater, and/or cover yourself with a blanket. If you are doing Shavasana after a sweaty yang practice, you may need to change your shirt to avoid getting too cold, but don't wipe off any sweat; allowing sweat to dry on the body is one of the yogic healing techniques.

Make yourself comfortable as you lie down on the floor. Arms and legs can be out to the sides (fig. 1). Bending the knees a little may allow the low back to release to the floor. If you do bend the knees, place a folded blanket or bolster under them so that the legs can relax (fig. 2). Allow the feet to fall inward or outward, whichever feels more relaxed. To allow the sacrum to lie flat, slide your tailbone away from you. Next, with your arms lying beside you, turn the palms face up. This will allow your shoulder blades to lie flat; snuggle them into the floor. Lengthen the neck slightly by pointing the chin toward your feet. You can even roll your head from side to side a few times until you find a comfortable position in the center. A shallow pillow for the head is

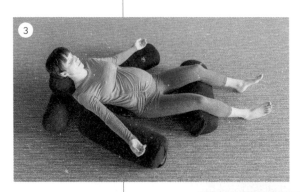

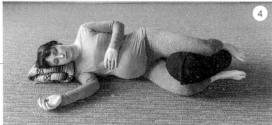

nice. If many bolsters are available, you can use up to 5 to support the limbs and torso, as shown in fig. 3. Pregnant women may prefer to rest on their left side (fig. 4).

Get all of your fidgeting over with, then become still. Often, one or two deep breaths here with a loud sigh are delicious. Release your bones, let go completely—you are ready. Now close your eyes; time to relax.

Relaxing Completely

Scan your body slowly. Start with your toes and feet—allow your feet to relax. Feel them becoming heavy on the floor. Allow your awareness to rise up to the ankles, calves and shins. Feel them melting into the earth; no effort is needed. Feel the space in the knee joints. Move slowly higher. Relax the thighs. Feel them become heavy, warm, soft. Notice your buttocks, hips and groin relaxing; they too become soft and warm. If you have done a lot of hip work in your practice, linger here for a while, feeling the openness, the flow of energy through the hips.

Now allow your awareness to come to the tailbone; feel your sacrum and low back release into the floor. Feel your low back and abdominal muscles relax. Allow this sensation to rise up the spine. Feel each vertebra, the space between the vertebrae and their alignment. Allow the upper back muscles and the shoulder blades to sink into the floor. Relax your chest and all the muscles between the ribs. Come now to the shoulders, where we carry so much tension in our bodies. Let the shoulders release completely. Spend an extra moment here, and really soften. Relax your shoulders! Feel the weight of the shoulders sink into the earth. Allow this sensation of softness to flow down the arms. Relax the upper arms, the elbows and the fore-arms. Feel the space in the wrist joints. Feel the space around each finger and the energy in the palm of each hand.

Bring your awareness to your neck and throat, and release all tension there. Relax your jaw, lips and tongue; relax your cheeks and eyes and all the muscles around the eyes and deep in the eye sockets; relax your forehead and your scalp. Allow your head to rest heavily on the floor.

Now relax your inner organs. Bring your awareness to the reproductive organs, and either feel or imagine them relaxing. Relax your intestines and kidneys. Imagine your liver, stomach and spleen being filled with healing energies. Soften your diaphragm and lungs. Relax your heart. Let your heart become open ... vast ... undefended and ... smiling.

Release the breath totally: let it be whatever it wants to be. Notice it—become aware of the short pauses between each breath. Relax your mind... Notice that the moment between each breath is the moment between thoughts. Enjoy those moments of complete silence and peace; feel this sense of peace growing deeper. Let this feeling of peace fill you; let it fill the space around you; let peace fill the room and beyond, touching everyone and everything.

At a deep, unconscious level, you are becoming healthier, younger, stronger, whole. While this healing will continue throughout the days ahead, all you will remember is the feeling of stillness growing within you. Enjoy this! Enjoy being relaxed—and for the days to come, enjoy being.

Coming out

When the time has arrived—the teacher is calling you, or your timer has beckoned—begin to return to life by allowing your breath to be deeper, longer. Bring some movement to your fingers and toes while you roll your head from side to side. Take a moment to move your wrists and ankles in circles: circle in both directions to stimulate energy flow again. (There is an old Daoist saying that if you roll your ankles in circles every day, you will never die of a heart attack.) When you are ready, hug your knees to your chest in preparation for making the body small and round. Take a deep inhalation, and on the exhalation, bring your head and knees together and squeeze. Make yourself as small and as round as you can—as small as a 10-pound turkey. Release.

Wake up by stretching out the whole body. This is a natural energizer, one that many people forget to do when they wake up in the morning. Move any supports away, stretch your legs along the floor and stretch your arms over your head. Interlock your fingers and turn the palms away from you. Press your low back down; flex your toes toward your nose. Now take a huge inhalation, fill your lungs—and stretch. Make yourself as long as possible; contract all your facial muscles, and make your face as small as possible. Push and pull yourself longer. Then release with a loud, sighing "haaah."

Once more, flex the toes, flatten your low back, and take a big inhalation. Stretch your body. This time, open your face, mouth and eyes as wide as you can; stick your tongue out; touch your chin. Stretch! Reach! Exhale, and relax with a sigh.

Hug your knees once more into your chest, and roll to your left side;[30] pause there a moment, and let the energy settle. Stretch out your bottom arm under your head, and use it as a pillow; enjoy how this feels.

Don't linger too long here. Coming back to life is like being reincarnated. Don't stay in the bardo state between Shavasana (your little death) and rebirth too long, or you may decide to stay there forever. When you are ready, spiral up to sitting and prepare for your final meditation or pranayama practice. If you still feel that you are not quite back to normal, you may want to end your practice with nadi shodhana breathing to fully balance your energies (which is described in detail in Chapter 7).

Adverse Reactions to Shavasana—A Warning!

Several studies of the relaxation response have shown that occasionally, relaxation can have adverse effects. These effects range from a feeling of being dissociated from your body or from reality, to feelings of anxiety or panic. Sometimes deeply repressed emotions start to surface. If these start to trouble you, remain calm and resolve to watch whatever unfolds with the same dispassion with which you were watching the breath during your practice. If conditions persist, seek assistance.

For some students, physiological reactions can occur; blood pressure can drop after deep relaxation, and a temporary hypoglycemic state can occur. If you are on medication, deep relaxation may intensify the effect of the drugs. Caution is advised for students taking insulin, sedatives or cardiovascular medications. If you are on medication, check with your health-care professional before beginning a yoga practice. These occurrences are rare, but it is good to be aware that adverse reactions can happen. Don't be alarmed. If the situation warrants help, seek it. It is okay to call 911 if you feel the situation demands it.

The practice of Yin Yoga involves stressing the yin tissues of the body safely (which means no pain), for long periods of time, while staying relaxed. Note that this definition does not specify where the tissues must be. We know that the yin tissues we are targeting are the denser, deeper, more plastic and less elastic tissues, such as the ligaments, joint capsules, cartilage, bones and fascial networks, but these tissues are found in the upper body as well as the lower body. We can apply the principles of Yin Yoga all over the body, though so far we have focused on the lower body because as we age, this area tightens up the most. From the navel down, as we get older our mobility decreases, and injuries and pathologies increase. We can, indeed, do Yin Yoga for the shoulders, neck and arms. However, in general, since these upper-body joints are not as big or stiff as those in the lower body, the recommended hold times for the postures are shorter; 1 to 3 minutes may be plenty. Pay attention, and come out of the pose if you feel anything that doesn't feel safe or wise.

THE NECK

We carry a lot of stress in the neck and shoulder areas, especially when we spend great swaths of time typing or working with our hands. Tight neck and shoulder muscles can lead to headaches and shallow breathing. Chronically tight necks can lead to shortened ligaments and a very restricted range of motion. A very common movement pattern can be seen in the elderly. If you call a young child's name from behind her, she may just turn her head to look at you. As an adult, she may have to turn her whole torso, from the hips. If you call an elderly person from behind, he will likely turn his whole body, moving his feet, in order to look at you. There is a saying in yoga: "You are only as young as your spine!" That includes the cervical spine.

We can work the neck in 6 main directions while we linger in Yin Yoga postures. Most of the options offered for the upper body can be done while sitting in Shoelace, Square, Straddle or Toe Squat, or while sitting with the legs comfortably crossed. Try the poses listed below while in the basic seated positions. If you have any neck issues, don't try these until you have checked with your health-care provider. If you experience any lightheadedness, dizziness, nausea or neck pain—don't do these poses!

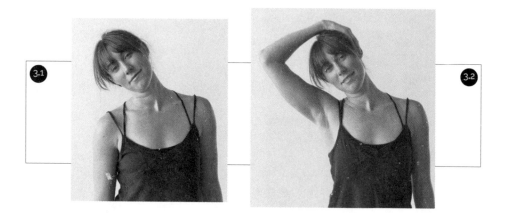

Lateral (Side) Flexion

Sit on a cushion in Shoelace or cross-legged. Keep the spine nice and long, including the neck. Drop your right ear to the right shoulder (figure 3.1). The 3 principles of the practice still apply: find a nice edge so that you feel some stress on the side of the neck away from the shoulder you are leaning toward. Become still, and stay for 1 or 2 minutes. If the edge moves, allow your ear to drop lower. Be cautious that you are not simply tilting your whole body, or worse, collapsing your spine. Keep sitting tall. If you would like a bit more stress, gently rest your right hand above your left ear to add a bit more weight (figure 3.2). Don't pull; just let the hand relax there. When you have had enough, use your right hand to push your head back to center, and pause for a few breaths to allow the sensations to ebb away. Then try the other side.

Another option for increasing the stress of this lateral, right flexion to the cervical spine is to bring your left hand behind your back and try to wiggle the hand up between the shoulder blades as high as it can go. Drop the left shoulder down as you relax the shoulder. As the left shoulder drops, the sensation along the left side of the neck may intensify.

Forward Flexion

Most people tend to have their head hanging forward, with their ears in front of their shoulders. This is because most people spend a lot of time at a computer or watching TV: they slouch back into their chairs or couches, requiring their head to come forward in order to see the screen. Despite this chronic position, it can be healthy to take the head and neck into a deeper flexed position than is done when sitting at a desk all day. Here is your chance!

Once again, come into a seated posture such as Shoelace and sit up nice and tall. Take a deep inhalation, and deliberately try to lengthen the neck by pushing the crown of your head to the sky; this will create the space you need to move the head

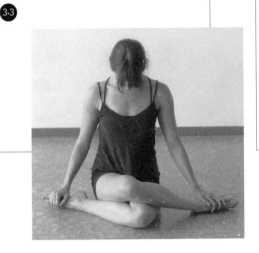
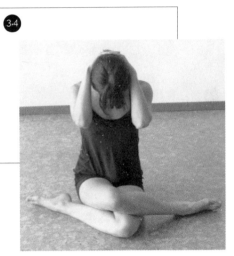

forward. Now stick your chin out, and as you slowly exhale, lower your chin toward your chest (figure 3.3). To help you sit up tall, bring your chest up to your chin with each inhale. Find that first edge, and give yourself time to open up. Again, just a couple of minutes here may be all you need. When you are ready to come out, use your hands to push your head back to neutral. Rest for a few breaths, relaxing the tissues you just worked.

While the chin is lowered to the chest, try some variations. If you turn your head a little to the right you may find the stress has moved a bit diagonally to the right side of the neck. No longer are you only feeling the back of the neck, nor are you feeling the side of the neck as in the lateral flexions. Now you are targeting the tissues between the side and back of the neck. If you feel you are not at your full edge, interlace the fingers of both hands and gently rest your hands on the back of your head (figure 3.4). Again, don't pull; the weight of your hands and arms will be enough to bring you deeper.

You may never get to a place where you feel a deep stretch here; if you have been doing yoga for a long time, you may have already stretched out those tissues enough so that what is stopping you now is compression—your chin is hitting your chest! You have reached your ultimate limit, so there is no point pulling harder with your hands. Sometimes, compression is reached even before the chin hits the chest: the bones at the base of the skull may contact the front of the vertebrae in the neck, or two or more vertebrae may be compressing into each other. Or your chin is compressing the organs at the front of the neck, such as the vocal cords. If you feel that you are stuck due to sensations in the throat area, don't force further. Just chill where you are.

One final comment about flexion of the neck: there are many poses in Yin Yoga where you are naturally flexing the neck. In Butterfly, Caterpillar and the variations of Straddle, your head will be hanging down, thus the neck will be in flexion. There may be no need for you to add a specific flexion exercise for your neck, because you will be in flexion so often already. Instead, you may want to work the neck in the other directions.

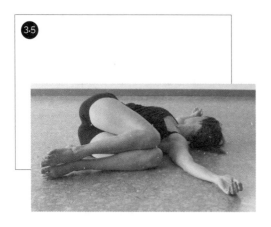

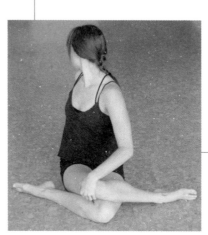

Twists

We can twist our neck any time we are twisting the spine as a whole. Reclining Twists provide a nice chance to twist the neck, as do many of the seated postures. In holding twists for the neck, we are not overly working the ligaments along the spine, but more often we are affecting the fascial bags that envelop the muscles.

In the Reclining Twist, as you move your legs to one side, roll your head to the other (figure 3.5). You may find you can turn the head more if you first lift your head off the floor, turn it while it is in the air, and then lower your cheek to the floor. If you feel lightheaded at all, dizzy, faint or nauseous, don't turn your head! Or simply experiment with turning your head to other side.

In Shoelace or other seated twists, the same philosophy applies. Turn the head by allowing the chin to glide over the shoulder (figure 3.6). Find that first edge. Remember: if you are feeling it, you are doing it. No need to strain and make this a really muscular effort. Just hang out where you feel it. Time is more important than intensity. To come out, turn the head first back to neutral, and then allow the rest of your body to unwind.

Backward Extension

Earlier we noted that most people chronically position their head in front of their shoulders. This has become known as "text neck," but it has been around a lot longer than smart phones. One consequence of this head-forward position is a closing off of the front of the neck, the throat. Moving the neck backward, called extension, can help open the throat and massage the various glands located there, such as the thyroid gland, the 4 parathyroid glands and the many salivary glands.

The way to extend the neck backward is quite simple, but caution is needed. Four major arteries bring blood to the brain: two of these are the carotid arteries, which run up the front side of the neck, and two are the vertebral arteries, which, as the name implies, run through the cervical vertebrae. When some people move their heads backward, their vertebrae compress the vertebral arteries and reduce the flow of blood to the brain, resulting in feelings of dizziness and lightheadedness. This is not good. If it happens to you, don't do those movements.

Please note carefully the sensations you experience when you exercise your neck in any direction, but pay particular attention when you extend the neck!

Begin by sitting up nice and tall in whatever Yin Yoga pose works for you, and lengthen your neck as you inhale. This will create more space to drop the head back. As you exhale, release the weight of your head. You will probably find that you stop quite quickly: this is your edge. Be content and hang out there. Some people will stop due to compression: if you have a lot of flexibility in your neck, you may find that the back of your head will rest upon your upper back. Others may feel compression in the vertebrae of the neck. If you are stopped due to compression, be content that this is as far as you are going to go—don't try to go further. If you do not feel these points of compression, you will probably be stopped by tension in the throat. Let that just soak in for 1 or 2 minutes. To come out, simply bring your head back to neutral and pause for a few breaths.

Often, when we work with the neck, we think we are curving the cervical spine, but actually all we are doing is tilting the head. People with little neck flexibility disguise their lack of movement in the neck by turning, twisting or tilting their skulls on the first two cervical vertebrae. As you do any of the above movements, try to feel the full length of the neck arching or twisting, rather than just the head moving. (You can even try placing your fingers along the neck's spinous processes to see whether you can sense individual movements there.) The lower the vertebrae, the less range of motion it will have, so feel like you are moving your neck right from its lowest base. When you focus on the neck instead of the head, you may find that you are spreading out the intensity over more tissues: it should feel deeper. Increases in flexibility in this region will not come quickly, so be patient with the practice. Do not try to do too much too fast.

THE SHOULDERS

The shoulder is one of the most mobile and complicated joints in the body, capable of a large variety of movements. One reason is because what we refer to as shoulder movement is really 2 separate movements: that of the arm and that of the scapula. The arm has 6 degrees of freedom,[31] while the scapula can move in 8 directions.[32] If we were to analyze all the possible combinations, we would have to look at 48 combined movements. Fortunately, we don't need to have that many postures to keep our shoulders in optimum condition. There are a couple of classic positions for the arms that will work the shoulders quite nicely.

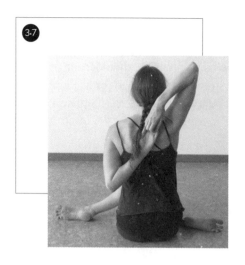

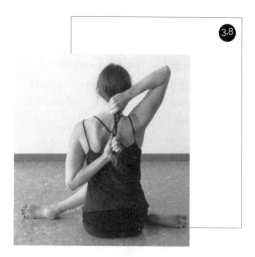

Cowface Arms

From sitting tall we can work the shoulders in several ways. In the classical Cowface arm position, bring your right hand up from the side, raising the hand as high as you can so the arm is beside the ear (this is full abduction at the shoulder), bend the elbow (which is flexion at the elbow), pointing the elbow forward (this is external rotation at the shoulder), and pat yourself on the back. Raise your left hand out to the side with the palm facing down, and try to rotate the palm to the back of the room

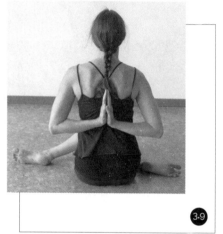

or even up to the ceiling (this is internal rotation at the shoulder), then move the arm backward (extension) and slide your hand up your back (adduction). If you have the range of motion, clasp your hands (figure 3.7); if you cannot do that, use a strap or belt and hold it with both hands. If a strap is not handy, use your ponytail (figure 3.8). Find a place where you feel a lovely stress, and let this soak in for 2 or 3 minutes. You are externally rotating, abducting and flexing the upper arm and internally rotating, adducting and extending the lower arm. The scapulae are mostly neutral.

A final variation is placing your hands in reverse prayer, sometimes called *Paschima Namaskara* (figure 3.9). This is a very juicy position for both shoulders at the same time. You can do it throughout the day: when you are walking around the house, place your arms in this position—your shoulders may loosen up quickly.

When you decide to come out of these postures, you will know right away if they worked. Your shoulders will be thanking you loudly. Come out slowly, and to release the shoulders, try pushing your hands far apart, as if you were attempting to push the walls of the room apart. This is a good time to mutter "om" and hopefully not "ow." Now you are ready for the other side.

You may add the option of folding forward while you hold the arm positions, but if you feel that folding forward reduces your stress in either the shoulders or the hips, don't bother. If folding forward intensifies the stress nicely, then go for it. Remember, you can do this in many different basic Yin Yoga postures, such as Square Pose or Straddle.

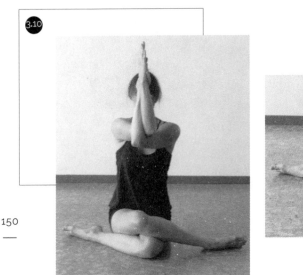

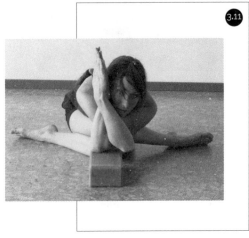

Eagle Arms

Another variation is called Eagle Arms: bring the right elbow out in front and under the left elbow. Try to wrap the arms as tightly as you can, and see whether you can bring your palms together. If you can't bring the palms together, just fake it. This is not yet Eagle Arms; eagles soar, so start to move your elbows up and away from you (figure 3.10). Notice where you are feeling this; we are now adducting the arms, but we are abducting the scapulae. This pose is a lovely antidote to the tight shoulders we develop from sitting at a computer all day. As we lift the arms we are adding flexion at the shoulders.

If you would like to go to a deeper edge, try leaning forward and resting your elbows on a block or a bolster (figure 3.11), or hooking the elbows over the front of the knees and trying to get them, over time, to the floor. Can you straighten the arms while they are crossed? Keep working to slide them away from you. Hold for a couple of minutes. When you are finished, sit up and open the arms really wide, creating a bit of a backbend, opening the heart. Now you are ready for the other side; make sure it is the other arm that is underneath this time.

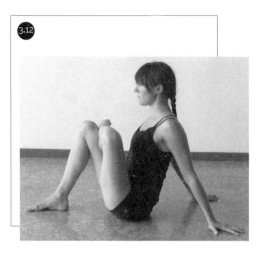

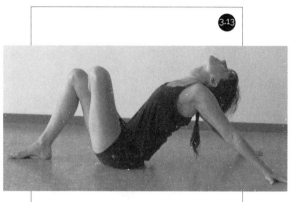

SHOULDERS AND ARMS

This next position adducts the scapulae, providing a lovely release to the front of the chest, and puts a deep stress into the arms, especially the elbow joints. We can do this movement while still in Shoelace, but it may be deeper to try it while in a posture we could call Sitting Swan (figure 3.12). Sitting Swan is an alternative way to work into the hips if the full Swan is too much, or anytime a hip-opening pose is not accessible. Let's use Sitting Swan as the basic template for this arm variation.

To come into the posture, take a sitting position where your legs are straight out in front of you, lean back slightly on your hands, place your left ankle over the right knee, bend the right leg and bring the heel in toward your hip. Keep the left foot flexed to stiffen the knee a little bit. As you hold the pose, you may find the intensity in your left hip diminishes; if so, slide the hips closer to the right foot.

Now, focus on the arms. Slowly move the hands backward away from you and lean into them (figure 3.13). Notice the stress points: you may feel this entirely in the shoulders, the elbows or the wrists. As long as you are feeling something, you are getting the benefits. Sensation is good, but don't make it sensational—when you have had enough, after 1 or 2 minutes, come out. Shake out the arms to relax them. In a moment, do this again but switch the legs.

A deeper option may not be available while in Sitting Swan, so try this with the legs straight out in front of you. See whether you can slide the hands further behind you and bring the hands closer together. If you desire, you can drop your head back, adding extension to the neck, but remember all the neck caveats discussed earlier. Eventually, your hands may touch or overlap; this is the juiciest version meant for students who don't feel anything in the shallower positions. Again, don't overstay your welcome.

151

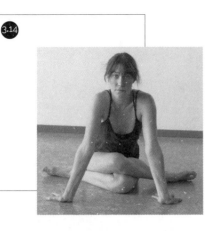

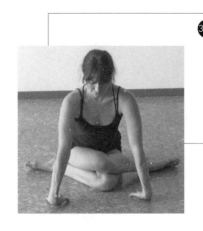

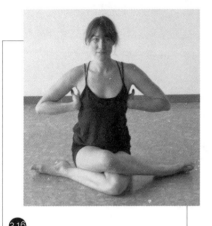

THE WRISTS

Body workers, typists, and musicians are just some of the people who suffer from repetitive stress syndrome (RSS), often in their wrists. A sleeve of fascia that envelops the arms becomes thicker around the wrists. This is called a retinaculum. There are also many layers of ligaments, such as the carpal ligament, that pass over the tendons of the flexors of the fingers. Repetitive, yang-like movements of the hand can damage these yin-like tissues, creating problems with names like "carpal tunnel syndrome."[33] Yin-like exercises may help thicken and strengthen these tissues, if done properly.

If you suffer from any form of RSS, see your health-care professional before doing these exercises. As always, don't go to where it is painful or where it hurts after you come out of the posture.

Once again, we can work the hands and wrists while luxuriating in other Yin Yoga poses. Let's come into a sitting pose again and investigate a few options for working with the wrists in a yin manner. Raise your hands out in front of you with the palms turned up; lower the tips of your fingers to the floor and then lean over your hands, trying to bring the heel of your palms to the ground (figure 3.14). Move to the place where you feel a sensation inside the forearm. If this is too much, move your hands closer toward you. If, in time, the sensations ebb away, you can move deeper by moving the hands further away from you and folding your chest toward your thighs. These sensations can be quite intense: don't stay where you feel any burning. One minute here may be enough for now. When you are done, sit back up and shake out the wrists.

Now you are ready for the other side. Again, bring your hands out in front of you, but this time have the palms facing down (figure 3.15). Lower your fingertips to the floor, and lean forward so you are bringing the back of your hands to the ground. You may start to feel like some sort of prehistoric, gorilla yogi with your knuckles dragging on the ground; that just means you are doing it properly. If this is too much, move your hands closer toward you; as your edge moves, try sliding the hands further away. One minute may be enough here too. When done, sit back up and shake out the wrists.

This version of the wrist stretch is a nice counterpose for yang yogis who love flow-ing vinyasas that involve lots of Up Dogs and Down Dogs. You can do these two ver-sions of wrist stretches while in Dragon, Swan, Straddle or any seated posture.

Another variation for the back of the hands is Seagull (figure 3.16). Sit up tall (or come to standing if you like), and open your arms wide to the side, with the palms facing the back of the room. Now bring the back of the hands to your armpits, keep-ing the fingers facing the back of the room. Snuggle your hands backward a bit more. Add more juice by lowering your wings (your elbows). You may find this yin position for the wrists a nice way to end a series of Sun Salutations: it is similar to standing on your hands in *Padahastasana*. Hold for a minute or so, then release your hands and shake out the wrists.

These Yin Yoga positions by no means exhaust all the ways we can stress our upper body tissues. Feel free to develop other positions. Remember, the principles are simple—stress the tissues, play your edges, become still, hold for time, and when finished, relax and rest the area you just worked. Also remember, we are deliberately stressing these tissues: you need to feel it. Don't be too deep or hold too long—remember Goldilocks—but do hold long enough that you are getting something.

COUNTERPOSES

In Chapter 6, the physiology of tissues is discussed, and you will be introduced to the concept of creep, which is the elongation of tissues when subjected to a constant stress. Yin Yoga generates creep, which is why we feel so fragile right afterwards. Ideally, before moving on to other endeavors, we would like to reduce the creep we created, restoring stability in the joints. If you have been targeting the spine, stiffen it with Balancing Cat, the Mini Curl Up and Plank on elbows (aka Crocodile).[34] Another nice option for the spine is called spinal flossing (aka neural mobilization). If you have been targeting the hips, stiffen them with standing poses such as Warrior 2, or do the Golden Seed.

Feel free to listen to your inner guidance, and if prompted, spontaneously erupt into whatever organic movement feels appropriate. The list of counterposes below is certainly not exhaustive, and our intention is not to describe in detail how to do yang asanas. If you wish to dive deeper into these postures or find more options, seek out a good yoga teacher.

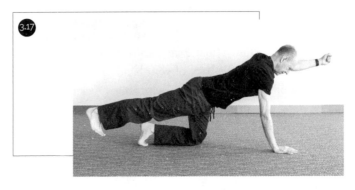

Balancing Cat: While on all fours (hands and knees), straighten one arm out in front of you while extending the opposite leg back behind you. Ensure that the lifted leg is not too high; we do not have to arch or extend the spine—keep it as close to neutral as possible. While the spine is neutral, the muscles are engaged all around your core, helping to stiffen the spine. Hold for 30 seconds, and then switch sides. You may want to repeat this again but holding for less time on each subsequent set of holds.

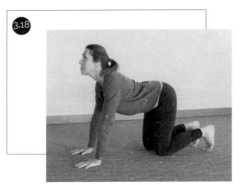

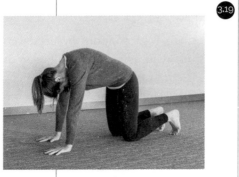

Cat's Breath: This is a nice counterpose to any spine work because it moves the spine in flexion and extension, getting rid of any kinks. As a counterpose, however, don't try for great range of motions now; be content to simply undulate the spine. To do so, come onto your hands and knees and surf your breath; as you inhale, lift your head and drop your spine. As you exhale, arch your back up while you drop your chin to your chest. Begin the movement from the tailbone, and allow the spine to ripple from tail to head.

Down Dog and all its variations: This may be the best counterpose after Swan or Dragon. Down Dog stretches the back of the body while toning the upper body. There are many ways to be a dog, but to keep it easy, come onto all fours, tuck the toes under, and lift your knees off the floor. Be a happy dog: lift your tail. Push the floor away with your paws, and draw your heels toward the earth. They may never reach the floor, but that is okay. Just move in that direction.

Golden Seed: Designed by Paul and Suzee Grilley, this lovely, flowing sequence is done standing, which can help to stiffen and stabilize the hips and legs. (Feel free to use this at any time, not just at the end of a Yin Yoga practice—perhaps as a replacement for Sun Salutations.) Ideally, each movement is done on either an inhalation or an exhalation. To begin, stand with your feet about 3 feet apart, toes pointed slightly outward, arms at your side (fig. 3.20).

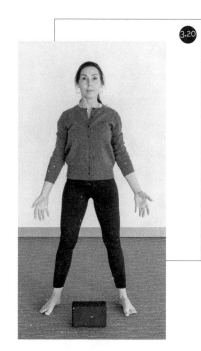

1. *Inhale* as you circle the arms up over your head.

2. *Exhale* as you push your palms to the sides of the room, turning your feet out. Squat lower while drawing the knees back so that they point over the toes. You are in the Goddess position (fig. 3.21).

3. *Inhale*, drawing your fingers to your shoulders, with your legs still in Goddess.

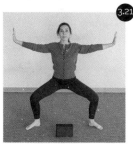

4. *Exhale* as you straighten your legs, square up your feet and fold, bringing hands to the floor or onto a block if the floor is too far away.

5. *Inhale* as you twist to the left, raising your left hand up to the sky, right hand pushing down (fig. 3.22).

6. *Exhale* as you switch sides: place your left palm on the floor or a block.

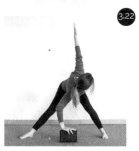

7. *Inhale* as you twist to the right, raising your right hand up to the sky, left hand grounded.

8. *Exhale* as you bring both hands to the earth. Turn the palms up, fingertips touching, and squat down so that your hips are the same height as your shoulders (fig. 3.23).

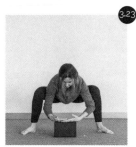

9. *Inhale* as you stand up, straighten the legs and draw your hands up to heart level, keeping the palms facing up and fingertips touching.

10. *Exhale* as you squat down (Goddess again). Keeping fingertips together, turn the palms to face the sky, and push your hands high above you.

11. *Inhale* while straightening your legs, standing tall with arms still over your head.

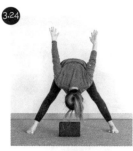

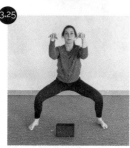

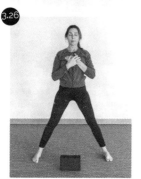

12. *Exhale* as you fold into the Dipping Bird: head down to the earth but arms up in the air behind your back, like wings (fig. 3.24).

13. *Inhale* to the Rocking Horse: squat down but bring your arms up in front of you, elbows bent, wrists relaxed, as if you were holding the reins of a horse (fig. 3.25).

14. *Exhale* as you fold again into the Dipping Bird.

15. *Inhale* as you stand up, knees soft (bent a little), arms rising up in front of you, also soft, wrists relaxed, until the legs are straight and your arms are over your head.

16. *Exhale* as you fold your wings: circle your hands to the heart center (fig. 3.26). Pause for one full breath, and begin again. Four cycles may be sufficient, but you can decide what is appropriate.

Mini Curl Up: This is another way to stiffen the core after spinal work. It is much better and far safer than sit-ups. The main emphasis for this is—less is more! Start with hands under the lumbar curve (*not* under the sacrum or pelvis); this will ensure that the spine stays neutral. One leg is straight along the floor, and the other leg is bent with the foot on the floor. The movement is subtle: lift the chest up 1 or 2 inches but no higher (fig. 3.27). Keep your gaze on the ceiling to prevent flexing the neck. The head will lift up with the chest, but there is no need to draw the chin to the chest. This makes for a nice counterpose anytime the neck has been stressed, such as in Snail Pose. For stronger students, the second track is to have the elbows come off the floor.

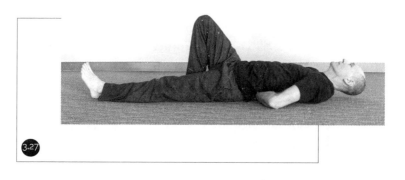

Pentacle (aka a mini Shavasana): Paul Grilley often recommends a brief rest between each posture. Lie down on your back, spread your arms and legs, and become still for a minute. Deliberately relax and enjoy the rebound or echo of the previous posture.

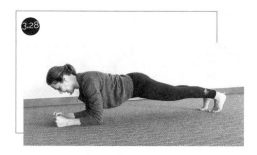
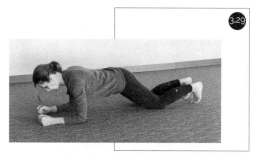

Plank on elbows (aka Crocodile): This is a nice way to release the knees and tone the core of the body: the butt and gut. It is great after Saddle Pose, which can really stress the knees. It is also ideal after a sequence of postures that stressed the spine. Basically, this is the push-up position but done on forearms. Start in Sphinx Pose on elbows, tuck your toes under and lift your buttocks to the same height as your shoulders (fig. 3.28). An easier option is to allow your knees to stay on the ground (fig. 3.29). In either case, don't let your hips sag to the floor: keep the hips at the same height as your shoulders. Thirty seconds to a minute here should be plenty. Students who need more challenge may work up to 90-second holds.

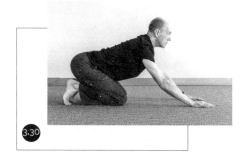
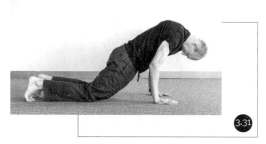

Spinal flossing (aka neural mobilization): Begin with Cat's Breath, but add movement of the hips. This may feel counterintuitive, but as you inhale and look up, move your hips back toward your heels (fig. 3.30). You may even touch your heels with your buttocks. As you exhale and look down, round your back up and move your hips forward; you can even bend your elbows a bit to allow yourself to come more forward, like a mini push-up (fig. 3.31). Repeat several times *slowly*. Spinal flossing can assist with mobilizing the spinal cord and the sciatic nerves, helping them to regain their natural amount of gliding through the surrounding tissues; this may reduce or eliminate adhesions or areas of stuckness, which can entrap the nerves, causing pain.

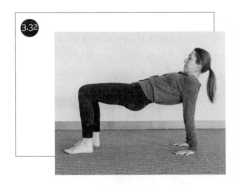 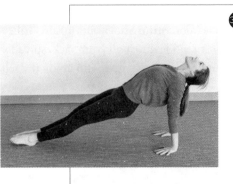

Tabletop (aka Hammock) or Slide: These 2 counterposes can be delicious any time you have been marinating in a forward fold posture, such as Butterfly or Caterpillar. With hands behind you on the floor, lift your hips up. Your feet can be on the floor with the legs bent (fig. 3.32) or straight (having the legs straight turns this into Slide—fig. 3.33). You can make this into a flow by raising and lowering the hips in time with the breath (up on inhale, down on exhale). After 3 or 4 cycles, hold the position for 3 or 4 breaths.

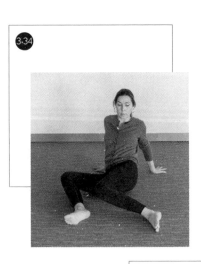 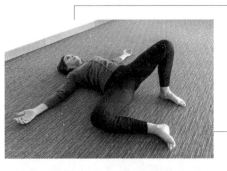 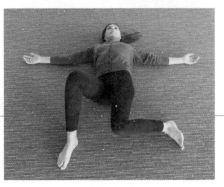

Windshield Wipers: This is actually a counterpose for both external rotations, such as Shoelace, and for internal rotations, such as Saddle, because we internally and externally rotate the hips. It can be done lying down or sitting. For the sitting version (fig. 3.34), sit leaning back a bit with your arms behind you and hands on the floor, your feet wide apart and on the floor, and slowly drop the knees from side to side toward the floor. Make sure the feet are apart! If the feet are together, there is very little internal rotation in the hips. If you want to emphasize only external rotation (as a counterpose for internal rotations), work one leg outward, knee toward the floor, but keep the other leg more vertical and then switch sides (fig. 3.35). If you want to emphasize internal rotation (as a counterpose for external rotations) work one leg inward, knee close to the floor with the other leg more vertical, and then switch sides (fig. 3.36).

While it is fine to spontaneously move into any movement that feels right or that the body craves, don't overdo it. Yang movements between yin postures should be brief. It is possible to create fusion classes, where we combine both yin and yang asanas in one class; however, we want to avoid constant switching from yang mode to yin mode and back again. If you are creating a fusion class, let each segment last for a while. Allow at least 10 to 15 minutes of constant yang practice and at least 10 to 15 minutes of yin practice to unfold at each time. Do not keep switching back and forth more quickly than that. During a Yin Yoga class, keep the yang counterposes brief: 1 to 2 minutes should be enough.

Endnotes

1 See Goldberg, *The Path of Modern Yoga*. The earliest texts on Hatha Yoga made outrageous claims about the health benefits of even simple postures. For example, the *Hatha Yoga Pradipika* claimed that Lotus Pose (Padmasana) could cure all disease! By the early 1900s, a veneer of scientific reasoning was added to the marketing of yoga to appeal to a broad cross-section of potential practitioners. Yoga was being sold as a health cure rather than a path to spiritual liberation. These medical claims continue to be proffered right up to the present day, but now a new sensibility is arising around such pronouncements. We cannot state categorically that yoga will have any particular benefit for everybody. At best, we can say that it might help someone with a particular condition, but equally it might not. There are many anecdotes of yoga helping people with a particular condition, and rigorous scientific studies with double-blind controls are being done, which have dispelled many earlier, fanciful claims but have also pointed to some verifiable benefits for many or even most people. However, it is never possible to say that yoga will help everybody. At best, we can say that it has a potential to help certain people with certain conditions.

2 The goal of Yoga Injury Prevention (https://yip.guru) is to help people with a variety of physical conditions maintain a full and safe yoga practice by describing a list of contraindications for various postures. These contraindications are determined through searching the scientific and medical literature. As with all such efforts, the findings will evolve over time, so the dedicated student/teacher should check in with the site from time to time to see what is new.

3 Loosely translated this means "thank you Shiva." More formally it is translated as "O salutations to the auspicious one."

4 See B.K.S. Iyengar, *Yoga: The Path to Holistic Health* (London, UK: Dorling Kindersley, 2001), 84 and 188.

5 See Iyengar, *Yoga: The Path to Holistic Health*, 219.

6 See Iyengar, *Yoga: The Path to Holistic Health*, 88, 89 and 190.

7 See Iyengar, *Yoga: The Path to Holistic Health*, 94, 95 and 201.

8 See Iyengar, *Yoga: The Path to Holistic Health*, 102, 103 and 197.

9 See Iyengar, *Yoga: The Path to Holistic Health*, 202.

10 See Iyengar, *Yoga: The Path to Holistic Health*, 72 and 180.

11 The back leg's kneecap in lunging postures like Swan or Dragon can experience uncomfortable pain from pressure against the floor. However, if the knee is bent and the foot allowed to come off the floor, the kneecap slides under the end of the femur and thus is no longer in contact with the floor, which should reduce discomfort. If it is tiring to keep the knee bent, the shin can rest against a wall or on a block or bolster for support.

12 See B.K.S. Iyengar, *Light on Yoga* (New York: Schocken Books, 1979), 354.

13 For a detailed biomechanical explanation of why the stresses along the spine and in the pelvis may be different when the hips are pinned versus when the shoulders are pinned, see Bernie Clark, *Your Spine, Your Yoga*, 92–94.

14 Sitting on the heels means that the hips are flexed 90°, and for many students this reduces the amount of internal rotation available in the hip sockets. However, when the hips are fully extended, they do have enough room to internally rotate the femurs in the hip sockets. In these cases, it is better to come into the posture from lying down (via Windshield Wipers), which keeps the hips extended.

15 See Iyengar, *Light on Yoga*, 125.

16 See Iyengar, *Yoga: The Path to Holistic Health*, 146 and 228.

17 For most people, when the hips are more flexed, there is more space for the femur to externally rotate in the hip socket, thus less stress is felt in the knee. See Bernie Clark, *Your Body, Your Yoga* (Vancouver, BC: Wild Strawberry Productions, 2016) for the biomechanics of this effect.

18 See Iyengar, *Yoga: The Path to Holistic Health*, 130 and 214.

19 Having your hands out to the sides makes you look more like a seal; if you feel the urge to bark, you have found the pose.

20 In physical therapy, this is known as McKenzie therapy. For people with flexion-caused problems in the low back (such as a slipped disc), backbends can ease the nucleus pulposus back into the middle of the disc.

21 See Iyengar, *Light on Yoga*, 108.

22 See Iyengar, *Yoga: The Path to Holistic Health*, 191.

23 See Iyengar, *Light on Yoga*, 266.

24 Benefits may include energetic stimulation, mindfulness practice and maintaining their current range of motion.

25 Groans coming out of Yin Yoga poses sound like "ommmm." Om is the first syllable of "OhmiGod!"

26 See Iyengar, *Yoga: The Path to Holistic Health*, 195.

27 The back leg's kneecap in lunging postures such as Swan or Dragon can experience uncomfortable pain from pressure against the floor. However, if the knee is bent and the foot allowed to come off the floor, the kneecap slides under the end of the femur and thus is no longer in contact with the floor, which should reduce discomfort. If it is tiring to keep the knee bent, the shin can rest against a wall or on a bolster for support.

28 See Iyengar, *Light on Yoga*, 392.

29 This is due to Lenz's law. Energy flow induces magnetic fields in metallic circles, which in turn weaken the energy flow.

30 Often teachers will ask students to end the class by lying on their right side to relax the heart. This is a great suggestion for ending a yang class. Lying on the right side helps to open the left nostril, due to a sinus reflex. However, the left nostril is the yin channel. After 90 minutes or so of yin practice, it is nice to balance the body by lying on the left side, allowing the right nostril, the yang channel, to open.

31 The 6 movements of the arm are flexion (which, if the arms are down at our side, means moving the arms forward and up), extension (moving the arms back and up), abduction (moving the arms away from the side of the body), adduction (bringing the arms closer toward each other), and internal and external rotation of the arm.

32 The 8 degrees of movement of the shoulder are adduction (the shoulder blades come together), abduction (the shoulder blades move apart), depression (where we drop the shoulder blades down the back), elevation (where we raise the shoulder blades up), upward and downward rotation, and tilting the top of the scapula backward or forward.

33 Carpal tunnel syndrome arises where there is pressure on the median nerve that runs under the fascia and ligaments of the wrist to the hand. There is debate whether repetitive movement actually causes carpal tunnel syndrome, and certainly there are many potential causes of this condition; the carpal tunnel may be smaller in some people, trauma or injury could have happened there, fluid retention, rheumatoid arthritis… The list goes on. However, it is well known that repetitive stress can create tendonitis, bursitis and inflammation of the wrist joint.

34 These 3 postures that serve to stiffen and stabilize the spine are sometimes referred to as the McGill Big 3, named after Stuart McGill, the spine biomechanic who determined that they are excellent and safe ways to strengthen the core.

4

YIN YOGA FLOWS

We have learned how to practice Yin Yoga safely and how to set an intention for our practice. We've discussed many postures and why we would want to do each one, and we have learned how to begin and end our practice. It's time now to put it all together and do it!

The classes, or flows, offered in this section are just a small sampling of what is possible, but they do provide a good representation of ways to work the main fields of the body. Feel free to experiment with them and change them around. There are 10 flows, and most of them have variations for beginners and for more advanced students. Choose your track deliberately. If you are a beginner or are naturally fairly stiff, follow Track 1. Give your body, heart and mind time to open up. Track 3 is for students who are naturally more flexible and need something different to create the desired stress in the targeted areas. Track 2 is for those in between. The basic difference between Track 2 and Track 3 is simply the amount of time in each pose. To go deeper in Yin Yoga does not mean we need more difficult postures but, rather, that we stay longer in the simpler poses. For this reason, no flows are listed for Track 3, because they are the same postures as in Track 2, held longer.

The 10 main flows and their themes are as follows:

1. An Easy Beginner's Flow
2. A Flow for the Spine (working with the spine's 6 degrees of freedom)
3. A Flow for the Hips (working with the hips' 6 degrees of freedom)
4. A Flow for the Legs (working the 4 quadrants of the legs)
5. A Flow for the Shoulders, Arms and Wrists (and for the Heart and Lung meridians)

6. A Flow for the Kidney and Urinary Bladder Meridians

7. A Flow for the Liver and Gall Bladder Meridians

8. A Flow for the Stomach and Spleen Meridians

9. A Flow for the Whole Body (working the seldom-targeted parts of the body)

10. Wall Yin (a more restorative flow using the wall as a prop)

While there is a main intention for each flow, this does not mean that you will not affect other areas of the body at the same time: you will. The theme just guides your emphasis. You may add to any of these flows your own goal of mindfulness, breath work, healing imagery, soul work or any other intention that you wish to invoke.

It is easy to lose track of the time as you marinate and end up doing one side longer than the other, so you may want to use a watch that can be set to beep, buzz, flash or vibrate when time is up. The total time shown for each flow is an approximation: you can decide how long you want your practice to be. The time may be a bit longer or shorter, depending upon how long you wait between postures. You can use a separate clock or timer to keep track of the total practice time. We have allocated about 10% of the practice time to Shavasana, but you may want to extend this. We have also allocated 3 to 5 minutes for the opening meditation, but again, you may wish to lengthen this or even add a closing meditation after Shavasana.

1) AN EASY BEGINNER'S FLOW

In this gentle one-hour flow, you'll begin by working the spine and then the hips. You will finish with twisting the spine before final relaxation. Hold each posture for 3 minutes, and relax the body in any way that feels comfortable for 30 to 60 seconds between asanas. You can make this into a 90-minute practice by extending the hold times to 5 minutes.

Opening Meditation

Butterfly
Counterpose: Windshield Wipers

Straddles
Half Butterfly fold over right leg

Half Butterfly fold over left leg

Straddle fold down the middle

Counterpose: Windshield Wipers

Child's Pose (1 minute)

Sphinx

Seal

Child's Pose (1 minute)

Half Shoelaces
With right leg straight

With left leg straight

Counterpose: Windshield Wipers

Happy Baby

Reclining Twists
Two-knee twist to the right side

Two-knee twist to the left side

Shavasana

Finishing Meditation

2) A FLOW FOR THE SPINE

This flow will move the spine through its 6 degrees of freedom: flexion, extension, lateral flexions left and right, and twists left and right. Butterfly (or Dangling) at the beginning is a mild flexion to get started. Straddle deepens the flexion over each leg and targets the sides of the spine. Caterpillar (or Snail) is the deepest flexion. We move the spine into extension via Supported Bridge, Sphinx and/or Seal; Bananasana provides lateral flexions; and then we finish with twists of the spine. Add movement to the neck by allowing the head to move in the same direction as the torso. For flexion, the head drops forward. For extension, the head lifts up and back. For lateral flexion, allow the ear to come toward the shoulder; and for the twists, turn the cheek to the floor. Be careful if you have neck issues. For Track 3, extend the Track 2 hold times of each pose after the Straddle by an additional 2 minutes.

TRACK 1 — 60 minutes	TRACK 2 — 90 minutes
Meditation for 3 minutes	**Meditation** for 5 minutes
Butterfly for 4 minutes	**Dangling** for 3 minutes
» Counterpose: Windshield Wipers	**Squat** for 2 minutes
	Dangling for 3 minutes
	Squat for 2 minutes
Half Butterfly: fold over right leg for 4 minutes	**Straddle** fold over right leg for 3 minutes
» Counterpose: Windshield Wipers for 1 minute	» Next, add the side-bend option for 2 minutes
Half Butterfly: fold over left leg for 4 minutes	**Straddle** fold over left leg for 3 minutes
» Counterpose: Windshield Wipers for 1 minute	» Next, add the side-bend option for 2 minutes
	Straddle fold straight down the middle for 5 minutes
	» Counterpose: Windshield Wipers for 1 minute
Caterpillar for 4 minutes	**Caterpillar** for 2 minutes
» Counterpose: Cat's Breath	**Snail** for 3 minutes
	» Counterpose: Windshield Wipers

Supported Bridge for 4 minutes

» Counterpose: hug knees to chest and circle them

Sphinx for 4 minutes

» Counterpose: relax on abdomen, turn head to one side, and draw that knee up beside you on the floor for 1 minute

Sphinx for 5 minutes

» Counterpose: relax on abdomen, turn head to one side, and draw that knee up beside you on the floor for 1 minute

Seal for 5 minutes

» Counterpose: relax on abdomen, turn head to other side, and draw that knee up beside you on the floor for 1 minute

---

Bananasana to the right for 4 minutes

» Counterpose: hug knees to chest and circle them

Bananasana to the left for 4 minutes

» Counterpose: hug knees to chest and circle the knees

Bananasana to the right for 5 minutes

Bananasana to the left for 5 minutes

» Counterpose: hug knees to chest and circle them

Two-knee Reclining Twist on right side for 4 minutes

» Counterpose: hug knees to chest and circle them

Two-knee Reclining Twist on left side for 4 minutes

» Counterpose: hug knees to chest and circle them

One-knee Reclining Twist on left side for 5 minutes

» Counterpose: hug knees to chest and circle them

One-knee Reclining Twist on right side for 5 minutes

» Counterpose: hug knees to chest and circle them

Shavasana for 7 minutes

Shavasana for 10 minutes

3) A FLOW FOR THE HIPS

This flow moves the femurs in the hip sockets through all 6 degrees of freedom. It includes gentle external rotation, abduction and flexion via Butterfly, abduction and flexion via Straddle, pure flexion through Caterpillar, and external rotation with Shoelace—which also combines mild adduction and flexion. With the Dragon cycle the flexion for the front hip is combined with extension for the back hip, and when you get to the Winged Dragon, external rotation and abduction happen at the front hip socket. The Saddle (or Half Saddle) adds some extension along with internal rotation. Reclining Twisted Roots combines adduction with more internal rotation. For Track 3, extend the Track 2 hold times of each pose after the Caterpillar by an additional 2 to 3 minutes.

TRACK 1 — 60 minutes	TRACK 2 — 90 minutes
Meditation for 3 minutes	**Meditation** for 5 minutes
Butterfly for 5 minutes	**Butterfly** for 5 minutes
» Counterpose: Windshield Wipers	Go straight into next pose
Straddle for 5 minutes	**Straddle** for 10 minutes
» Counterpose: Windshield Wipers	» Counterpose: Windshield Wipers
Caterpillar for 3 minutes	**Caterpillar** for 5 minutes
» Counterpose: Tabletop	» Counterpose: Tabletop
Shoelace with right knee on top for 3 minutes	**Shoelace** with right knee on top for 5 minutes
» Counterpose: Windshield Wipers	» Counterpose: Windshield Wipers
Dragon Cycle for 3 minutes	**Dragon Cycle** for 5 minutes
» Step right foot forward	» Step right foot forward
» Baby Dragon for 1 minute	» Baby Dragon for 1 minute
» Winged Dragon for 2 minutes	» Low-Flying Dragon for 2 minutes
» Counterpose: step back to Down Dog	» Winged Dragon for 2 minutes
	» Counterpose: step back to Down Dog

Shoelace with left knee on top for 3 minutes

» Counterpose: Windshield Wipers

Shoelace with left knee on top for 5 minutes

» Counterpose: Windshield Wipers

Dragon Cycle for 3 minutes

» Step left foot forward

» Baby Dragon for 1 minute

» Winged Dragon for 2 minutes

» Counterpose: step back to Down Dog

Dragon Cycle for 5 minutes

» Step left foot forward

» Baby Dragon for 1 minute

» Low-Flying Dragon for 2 minutes

» Winged Dragon for 2 minutes

» Counterpose: step back to Down Dog

Half Saddle

» With right leg forward and left leg bent backward for 2 minutes

» With left leg forward and right leg bent backward for 2 minutes

» Counterpose: Child's Pose for 1 minute

Saddle, sitting between feet, for 5 minutes

» Counterpose: Plank on elbows for 1 minute

Reclining Twist (Twisted Roots)

» Twist to the right side for 3 minutes

» Twist to the left side for 3 minutes

» Counterpose: hug knees in and circle them

Reclining Twist (Twisted Roots)

» Twist to the right side for 5 minutes

» Twist to the left side for 5 minutes

» Counterpose: hug knees in and circle them

Shavasana for 7 minutes

Shavasana for 10 minutes

4) A FLOW FOR THE LEGS

The upper thighs have 4 sides: the top (quadriceps), inner legs (adductors), backs of legs (hamstrings), and outer hips (IT band and abductors). This flow targets the fascial bags within each of the major muscle groups in all 4 quadrants. By targeting the fascia through long-held stresses, we can help stress the whole myofascial group and regain or maintain the range of motion and health of these tissues. The key to this flow is to relax: keep the muscles soft; perhaps work with your ocean breath for a few moments at the beginning. Again, for Track 3, if you wish, simply luxuriate in each position after Caterpillar for a couple more minutes.

TRACK 1 — 60 minutes	TRACK 2 — 90 minutes
Meditation for 3 minutes	**Meditation** for 5 minutes
Butterfly for 5 minutes	**Butterfly** for 5 minutes
» Counterpose: Windshield Wipers	» Go straight into next pose
Straddle for 5 minutes	**Straddle** for 10 minutes
» Counterpose: Windshield Wipers	» Counterpose: Windshield Wipers
Caterpillar for 3 minutes	**Caterpillar** for 5 minutes
» Counterpose: Tabletop	» Counterpose: Tabletop
Full Swan with right knee forward for 2 minutes	**Full Swan** with right knee forward for 2 minutes
Sleeping Swan for 2 minutes	**Sleeping Swan** for 3 minutes
Shoelace with left knee on top for 3 minutes	**Shoelace** with left knee on top for 5 minutes
» Counterpose: Windshield Wipers	» Counterpose: Windshield Wipers
Full Swan with left knee forward for 2 minutes	**Full Swan** with left knee forward for 2 minutes
Sleeping Swan for 2 minutes	**Sleeping Swan** for 3 minutes
Shoelace with right knee on top for 3 minutes	**Shoelace** with right knee on top for 5 minutes
» Counterpose: Windshield Wipers	» Counterpose: Windshield Wipers

Saddle, sitting between feet, for 3 minutes	**Saddle**, sitting between feet, for 5 minutes
» If Saddle is not available, do Baby Dragon on each side for 2 minutes	» If Saddle is not available, do Baby Dragon on each side for 3 minutes
» Counterpose: lie still with legs straight	» Counterpose: lie still with legs straight
Bananasana to the right for 3 minutes	**Bananasana** to the right for 5 minutes
» Counterpose: hug knees to chest and circle them	» Counterpose: hug knees to chest and circle them
Bananasana to the left for 3 minutes	**Bananasana** to the left for 5 minutes
» Counterpose: hug knees to chest and circle them	» Counterpose: hug knees to chest and circle them
Two-knee Reclining Twist on right side for 1 minute	**One-knee Reclining Twist** on right side with the top leg (left) extended out to the side for 3 minutes
» Counterpose: hug knees to chest and circle them	» Counterpose: hug knees to chest and circle them
Two-knee Reclining Twist on left side for 1 minute	**One-knee Reclining Twist** on left side with the top leg (right) extended out to the side for 3 minutes
» Counterpose: hug knees to chest and circle them	» Counterpose: hug knees to chest and circle them
Shavasana for 7 minutes	**Shavasana** for 10 minutes

5) A FLOW FOR THE SHOULDERS, ARMS AND WRISTS

This flow works the spine and hips at the same time that it works the shoulders via Eagle Arms and Cowface Arms, the elbows via Sitting Swan and the wrists while in Butterfly or Straddle. While we stress these upper body tissues, we may also stimulate the upper body meridian lines, especially the Heart and Lungs. Review the asanas we will be using for the shoulders, arms and wrists (see Chapter 3) to help you choose the options that work best. Remember, if you feel any tingling in the fingers, back off or come out of the pose. For Track 3, if you wish, simply luxuriate in each position after Anahatasana for a couple more minutes.

TRACK 1 — 60 minutes	TRACK 2 — 90 minutes
Meditation for 3 minutes	**Meditation** for 5 minutes
Child's Pose with arms overhead for 3 minutes	**Frog** » Start in Tadpole for 2 minutes » Move hips forward to Full Frog for 3 minutes » Counterpose: slide onto your abdomen for 1 minute
Anahatasana for 3 minutes	**Anahatasana** for 4 minutes
Sphinx for 3 minutes » Counterpose: relax on abdomen, turn head to one side, and draw that knee up beside you on the floor for 1 minute **Seal** for 2 minutes » Counterpose: relax on abdomen, turn head to other side, and draw that knee up beside you on the floor for 1 minute	**Sphinx** for 5 minutes » Counterpose: relax on abdomen, turn head to one side, and draw that knee up beside you on the floor for 1 minute **Sphinx** for 3 minutes **Seal** for 2 minutes » Counterpose: relax on abdomen, turn head to other side, and draw that knee up beside you on the floor for 1 minute

Half Shoelace with right leg on top, left leg extended

» Cowface Arms with right hand behind back for 2 minutes

　» Counterpose: release arms and push hands apart

» Eagle Arms with left arm under the right for 2 minutes

　» Counterpose: release arms and push hands apart

Stretch legs out straight and lean back on the hands for 1 minute

» Or do **Sitting Swan** variation

Half Shoelace with left leg on top, right leg extended

» Cowface Arms with left hand behind back for 2 minutes

　» Counterpose: release arms and push hands apart

» Eagle Arms with right arm under the left for 2 minutes

　» Counterpose: release arms and push hands apart

Stretch legs out straight and lean back on the hands for 1 minute

» Or do **Sitting Swan** variation

Shoelace with right leg on top

» Cowface Arms with right hand behind back for 3 minutes

　» Counterpose: release arms and push hands apart

» Eagle Arms with left arm under the right for 2 minutes

　» Counterpose: release arms and push hands apart

Sitting Swan with right ankle on left knee

» Leaning on hands, move the hands as far away as they can go

» Hold for 2 minutes

Shoelace with left leg on top

» Cowface Arms with left hand behind back for 3 minutes

　» Counterpose: release arms and push hands apart

» Eagle Arms with right arm under the left for 2 minutes

　» Counterpose: release arms and push hands apart

Sitting Swan with left ankle on right knee

» Leaning on hands, move the hands as far away as they can go (see if you can bring them together)

» Hold for 2 minutes

Butterfly

» Bring hands out in front, turn palms up, and lower fingers to the floor. Lean forward until the heel of the palm is near the floor or until you feel stress in the inner forearm. Hold for 1 minute

» Release and shake out the wrists

» Bring hands out in front, turn palms down, and lower fingers to the floor. Lean forward until the back of the wrist is near the floor or until you feel stress there. Hold for 1 minute

» Release and shake out the wrists

» Stay in Butterfly for another 3 minutes

Straddle

» Bring hands out in front, turn palms up, and lower fingers to the floor. Lean forward until the heel of the palm is near the floor or until you feel stress in the inner forearm. Hold for 2 minutes

» Release and shake out the wrists

» Bring hands out in front, turn palms down, and lower fingers to the floor. Lean forward until the back of the wrist is near the floor or until you feel stress there. Hold for 2 minutes

» Release and shake out the wrists

» Stay in Straddle for another 5 minutes

Two-knee Reclining Twist on right side for 2 minutes with left arm alongside the ear

» Counterpose: hug knees to chest and circle them

Two-knee Reclining Twist on left side for 2 minutes with right arm alongside the ear

» Counterpose: hug knees to chest and circle them

One-knee Reclining Twist on right side for 5 minutes with left arm alongside the ear

» Counterpose: hug knees to chest and circle them

One-knee Reclining Twist on left side for 5 minutes with right arm alongside the ear

» Counterpose: hug knees to chest and circle them

Shavasana for 7 minutes

Shavasana for 10 minutes

6) A FLOW FOR THE KIDNEY AND URINARY BLADDER MERIDIANS

This flow includes forward and backbends that may stimulate the Kidney and Urinary Bladder meridians. The Track 2 flow adds more stimulation to the inner groins. Any flow focusing on the spine may be very effective at stimulating and nourishing the Kidneys. Note that we start with extension of the spine; this allows a nice compression of the kidneys. For Track 3, if you wish, simply luxuriate in each position for a couple more minutes.

TRACK 1 — 60 minutes	TRACK 2 — 90 minutes
Meditation for 3 minutes	**Meditation** for 5 minutes
Sphinx for 5 minutes	**Sphinx** for 5 minutes
» Counterpose: relax on abdomen, turn head to the right, and draw that knee up beside you on the floor for 1 minute	» Counterpose: relax on abdomen, turn head to the right, and draw that knee up beside you on the floor for 1 minute
Saddle, sitting on feet or a block, for 3 minutes	**Saddle**, sitting on feet or a block, for 6 minutes
» If Saddle is not available, do Half Saddle on each side for 2 minutes	» If Saddle is not available, do Half Saddle on each side for 3 minutes
» If Saddle still doesn't work, do another round of Sphinx	» Counterpose: Plank on elbows for 1 minute
» Counterpose: Child's Pose	
Sphinx for 5 minutes	**Sphinx** for 3 minutes
	Seal for 2 minutes
» Counterpose: relax on abdomen, turn head to the left, and draw that knee up beside you on the floor for 1 minute	» Counterpose: relax on abdomen, turn head to the left, and draw that knee up beside you on the floor for 1 minute
Butterfly for 4 minutes	**Butterfly** for 5 minutes

Half Butterfly: fold over the right leg for 3 minutes

» Counterpose: Windshield Wipers for 1 minute

Half Butterfly: fold over the left leg for 3 minutes

» Counterpose: Windshield Wipers for 1 minute

Straddle fold straight down the middle for 3 minutes

» Counterpose: Windshield Wipers for 1 minute

Straddle fold over right leg for 5 minutes

Straddle fold over left leg for 5 minutes

Straddle fold straight down the middle for 5 minutes

» Counterpose: Windshield Wipers for 1 minute

Caterpillar for 5 minutes

» Counterpose: Tabletop

Caterpillar for 3 minutes

Snail for 2 minutes

» Counterpose: Tabletop

Anahatasana for 4 minutes

Dragon Cycle: start with right foot forward

» Baby Dragon for 1 minute; High-Flying Dragon for 2 minutes; Winged Dragon for 2 minutes; Counterpose: Down Dog for 1 minute

» Do the other side with left foot

Reclining Twist (Twisted Roots)

» Twist to the right side for 4 minutes

» Twist to the left side for 4 minutes

» Counterpose: hug knees in and circle them

Reclining Twist (Twisted Roots)

» Twist to the right side for 5 minutes

» Twist to the left side for 5 minutes

» Counterpose: hug knees in and circle them

Shavasana for 7 minutes

Shavasana for 10 minutes

7) A FLOW FOR THE LIVER AND GALL BLADDER MERIDIANS

Any flows that include hip openers and twists may stimulate the Liver and Gall Bladder meridians. We can enhance the flow of energy along these lines with our breath and our attention, as described in Chapter 7. To help activate the Liver and Gall Bladder, it is useful to activate the Kidneys first. The Kidneys' energy supports all the internal organs. You will notice that we stimulate the Kidneys early in this flow via the Bridge, Sphinx and Seal poses. For Track 3, if you wish, simply luxuriate in each position for a couple more minutes.

TRACK 1 — 60 minutes	TRACK 2 — 90 minutes
Meditation for 3 minutes	**Meditation** for 5 minutes
Supported Bridge for 3 minutes	**Supported Bridge** for 5 minutes
Sphinx for 3 minutes	**Sphinx** for 5 minutes
» Counterpose: relax on abdomen, turn head to a side, and draw that knee up beside you on the floor for 1 minute	» Counterpose: relax on abdomen, turn head to the right, and draw that knee up beside you on the floor for 1 minute
	Sphinx for 3 minutes
	Seal for 2 minutes
	» Counterpose: relax on abdomen, turn head to the left, and draw that knee up beside you on the floor for 1 minute
Swan	Swan
» Full Swan with right knee forward for 1 minute	» Full Swan with right knee forward for 2 minutes
» Sleeping Swan for 3 minutes	» Sleeping Swan for 3 minutes
» Child's Pose for 1 minute	» Lean to your right and come into Shoelace

Shoelace with left knee on top for 4 minutes

» For 2 minutes, twist to the left

» For 2 minutes, side bend to the left

» Counterpose: Windshield Wipers

Swan

» Full Swan with left knee forward for 1 minute

» Sleeping Swan for 3 minutes

» Child's Pose for 1 minute

Shoelace with right knee on top for 4 minutes

» For 2 minutes, twist to the right

» For 2 minutes, side bend to the right

» Counterpose: Windshield Wipers

Straddle fold over right leg for 3 minutes

» Counterpose: Windshield Wipers for 1 minute

Straddle fold over left leg for 3 minutes

» Counterpose: Windshield Wipers for 1 minute

Straddle fold straight down the middle for 3 minutes

» Counterpose: Windshield Wipers for 1 minute

Bananasana to the right for 3 minutes

» Counterpose: hug knees to chest and circle them

Bananasana to the left for 3 minutes

» Counterpose: hug knees to chest and circle them

Shoelace with left knee on top for 5 minutes

» For 2 minutes, twist to the left

» For 3 minutes, side bend to the left

» Counterpose: Windshield Wipers

Swan

» Full Swan with left knee forward for 2 minutes

» Sleeping Swan for 3 minutes

» Lean to your right and come into Shoelace

Shoelace with right knee on top for 5 minutes

» For 2 minutes, twist to the right

» For 3 minutes, side bend to the right

» Counterpose: Windshield Wipers

Straddle fold over right leg for 5 minutes

» Add a twisting/side bend halfway through the pose

Straddle fold over left leg for 5 minutes

» Add a twisting/side bend halfway through the pose

Straddle fold straight down the middle for 5 minutes

» Counterpose: Windshield Wipers for 1 minute

Bananasana to the right for 5 minutes

» Counterpose: hug knees to chest and circle them

Bananasana to the left for 5 minutes

» Counterpose: hug knees to chest and circle them

Two-knee Reclining Twist on right side for 2 minutes

» Counterpose: hug knees to chest and circle them

Two-knee Reclining Twist on left side for 2 minutes

» Counterpose: hug knees to chest and circle them

One-knee Reclining Twist on right side with the top leg (left) extended out to the side for 2 minutes

» Bend top leg and come into one-knee twist for 3 minutes

» Counterpose: hug knees to chest and circle them

One-knee Reclining Twist on left side with the top leg (right) extended out to the side for 3 minutes

» Bend top leg and come into one-knee twist for 3 minutes

» Counterpose: hug knees to chest and circle them

Shavasana for 7 minutes

Shavasana for 10 minutes

8) A FLOW FOR THE STOMACH AND SPLEEN MERIDIANS

Any flows that include spinal or hip extensions may nourish the Stomach and Spleen. Deep twisting of the spine can also help to massage the internal organs. We can enhance the flow of energy along these lines with our breath and our attention, as described in Chapter 7. To help stimulate the Spleen and Stomach meridians, it is useful to activate the Kidneys first. The Kidneys' energy supports all the internal organs. You will notice that we stimulate the Kidneys early in this flow via the Bridge, Saddle and Sphinx poses, but we start with Child's Pose to compress the abdominal organs. For Track 3, if you wish, simply luxuriate in each position for a couple more minutes.

TRACK 1 — 60 minutes	TRACK 2 — 90 minutes
Meditation for 3 minutes	**Meditation** for 5 minutes
Child's Pose for 3 minutes	**Child's Pose** for 5 minutes
Supported Bridge for 3 minutes	**Supported Bridge** for 5 minutes
Saddle, sitting on feet or a block, for 4 minutes	**Saddle**, sitting on feet or a block, for 6 minutes
» If Saddle is not available, do Half Saddle on each side for 2 minutes	» If Saddle is not available, do Half Saddle on each side for 3 minutes
» If Saddle still doesn't work, do Sphinx Pose	» Counterpose: Plank on elbows for 1 minute
» Counterpose: Child's Pose for 1 minute	
	Sphinx for 3 minutes
	Seal for 2 minutes
	» Counterpose: relax on abdomen, turn head to a side, and draw that knee up beside you on the floor for 1 minute
Shoelace with left knee on top	**Shoelace** with left knee on top
» For 2 minutes, twist to the left	» For 2 minutes, twist to the left
» For 2 minutes, fold forward	» For 3 minutes, fold forward
» Counterpose: Windshield Wipers	» Counterpose: Windshield Wipers
Shoelace with right knee on top	**Shoelace** with right knee on top
» For 2 minutes, twist to the right	» For 2 minutes, twist to the right
» For 2 minutes, fold forward	» For 3 minutes, fold forward
» Counterpose: Windshield Wipers	» Counterpose: Windshield Wipers
Caterpillar for 3 minutes	**Caterpillar** for 3 minutes
» Counterpose: Tabletop	» Snail for 2 minutes
	» Counterpose: Tabletop

Dragon Cycle for 4 minutes

» Step right foot forward

» Baby Dragon for 1 minute

» Low-Flying Dragon for 2 minutes

» Bowing Dragon for 1 minute

» Counterpose: step back to Down Dog

Dragon Cycle for 4 minutes

» Step left foot forward

» Baby Dragon for 1 minute

» Low-Flying Dragon for 2 minutes

» Bowing Dragon for 1 minute

» Counterpose: step back to Down Dog

Dragon Cycle for 6 minutes

» Step right foot forward

» Baby Dragon for 2 minutes

» Low-Flying Dragon for 2 minutes

» Dragon Splits for 2 minutes

» Counterpose: step back to Down Dog

Dragon Cycle for 6 minutes

» Step left foot forward

» Baby Dragon for 2 minutes

» Low-Flying Dragon for 2 minutes

» Dragon Splits for 2 minutes

» Counterpose: step back to Down Dog

Two-knee Reclining Twist on right side for 4 minutes

» Counterpose: hug knees to chest and circle them

Two-knee Reclining Twist on left side for 4 minutes

» Counterpose: hug knees to chest and circle them

One-knee Reclining Twist on right side for 4 minutes

One-knee Reclining Twist on left side for 4 minutes

» Counterpose: hug knees to chest and circle them

Shavasana for 7 minutes

Shavasana for 10 minutes

9) A FLOW FOR THE WHOLE BODY

This flow targets many areas of the body that get missed in our normal yoga practices, yin or yang. We will work from the tips of the toes to the top of the head and touch many places in between. Try it all. Don't skip the face yoga practice.[1] Heart tapping, which we do at the beginning, may stimulate the immune system. The thymus gland is located right above the heart and beneath the sternum: when we tap, we may stimulate the cells in the thymus, whose job it is to mature the white blood stem cells. You can also imagine that you are massaging your heart. Zipper requires you to bring the soles of your feet together and interlace your toes, thus stimulating all 6 lower body meridians, which begin or end in the toes.[2] If you are not familiar with poses such as Ankle Stretch, Toe Squat and Happy Baby, review them in Chapter 3. We end with a lovely yang movement called Tantrumasana. For Track 1, hold for the minimum times shown; for Track 2 and 3, increase your hold times appropriately. Consider the times given as suggestions, not demands.

A WHOLE-BODY YIN WORKOUT
60 to 75 minutes

Meditation for 3 minutes

Heart tapping for 2 minutes

Use the tips of the fingers of your right hand to tap up and down along your sternum. Go slowly at first.

Butterfly with Toes in Zipper

Track 1: 3 minutes; Track 2: 5 minutes

» Neck circles: Allow your head to drop to the right shoulder, then lower your chin to your chest and raise your left ear to the left shoulder. Repeat these half circles several times.

» Track 2: Do full circles by dropping your head back. Allow your chin to make a full circle. Switch directions after 2 or 3 orbits.

» Shoulder circles: Keeping your head centered, draw your shoulders forward, up, back and down. Let your arms move freely. Switch directions after 2 or 3 orbits.

Dangling for 2 minutes

Track 1: If Dangling is too intense, do Caterpillar instead.

Squat for 2 minutes

Track 1: If Squat is too intense, sit in a tight Butterfly with the feet drawn in close to the body.

If time allows, repeat the Dangling and Squat one more time.

Toe Squat

Track 1: 3 minutes. Track 2: 5 minutes

» During this pose, we have time to work the shoulders and our face. First, bring your arms into Cowface, with the left hand behind you and the right arm up in the air. If you can't clasp hands, use a strap or a belt. Hold for 2 minutes.

» Face Yoga 1: Allow the biggest, goofiest smile you can manage to envelop your face.

» Release the arms into Eagle Arms with the right arm underneath. Move the elbows up and away. Hold for 2 minutes.

» Face Yoga 2: While in Eagle Arms, add the Scream—open your eyes and mouth as wide as you can. Stretch your face!

» Release the arms straight up in the air, interlace the fingers, and push the palms away for 1 minute.

» Face Yoga 3: Stick your tongue out so that it touches your chin, look up, and roar like a lion.

» When done, give your scalp a nice massage for 1 minute.

Ankle Stretch for 2 minutes

Counterpose: Plank on elbows for 1 minute

Toe Squat, part 2

Track 1: 3 minutes. Track 2: 5 minutes

» Bring your arms into Cowface, with the right hand behind you and the left arm up in the air. If you can't clasp, use a strap or belt. Hold for 2 minutes.

» Face Yoga 4: Keep your head centered and slide your face to the right as far as you can. Look to the right, but don't turn your head. Move your jaw to the right. You will feel like Popeye.[3]

» Release the arms into Eagle Arms with the left arm underneath. Move the elbows up and away. Hold for 2 minutes.

» Face Yoga 5: While in Eagle Arms, keep your head centered and slide your face to the left as far as you can.

» Release the arms straight up in the air, interlace the fingers, and push the palms away for 1 minute.

» Face Yoga 6: Stick your tongue out so that it touches your chin, look up, and roar like a lion.

» When done, give your scalp a nice massage for 1 minute.

Ankle Stretch for 2 minutes

Counterpose: Plank on elbows for 1 minute

Sphinx for 5 minutes

Track 2: add Seal after 3 minutes

Counterpose: Child's Pose for 1 minute

Happy Baby

Track 1: 3 minutes. Track 2: 5 minutes

Bananasana to the right

Track 1: 3 minutes. Track 2: 5 minutes

Counterpose: hug knees to chest and circle them

Bananasana to the left

Track 1: 3 minutes. Track 2: 5 minutes

Counterpose: hug knees to chest and circle them

Reclining Twist (Twisted Roots)

Twist to the right side for 4 minutes

Twist to the left side for 4 minutes

Counterpose: hug knees in and circle them

Tantrumasana

» Lying on your back, bend your knees so that your feet are flat on the floor. Place hands beside your feet, palms flat on the floor.

» For 15 seconds, slap the floor with your hands and feet as fast as you can.

» Pause for a little bit and then repeat for 10 seconds.

» Pause again and do a final burst for 5 seconds.

» Go fast! Channel your inner brat.

Shavasana for 7 minutes

10) WALL YIN

Ever have one of those days where you didn't want to do anything but collapse? Your get-up-and-go has got up and gone? Your yoga buddy, whom you rely on for moral support, has bailed on you? Where can you go for that support now? Well, it may be as close as that wall over there! Put on some soothing music, clear a space by your longest wall, grab a watch (preferably with a timer) and a cushion or two, and settle into some wall yin.

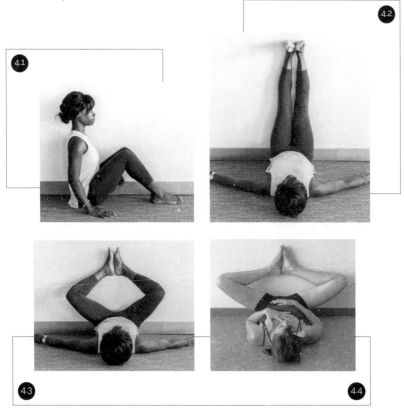

Wall Butterfly: Like all yoga journeys, you can start with a brief meditation, but this time with the wall supporting your feet. An easy way to get into postures against the wall is to sit sideways against the wall (fig. 4.1) and then swivel: swing your legs up the wall and lie down (fig. 4.2). Next, try to snuggle your buttocks to the corner of the wall and the floor. For Wall Butterfly, bring your feet together and let your heels come as low as they can, allowing the knees to go as wide as they can (fig. 4.3). Since this is your meditation position, place your hands where you feel most comfortable: over your heart or your belly (or one hand over each—fig. 4.4), or let your arms fall to the sides. Wait here for as long as your intuition suggests. Breathe: allow a few sighs to slip out, and be present.

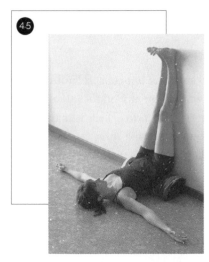

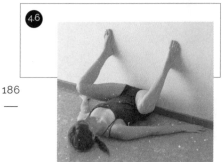

Wall Caterpillar (fig. 4.5): From Wall Butterfly, simply straighten your legs up the wall. If you find that you can't keep your legs straight, wiggle a little away from the wall. A nice option here may be to place a cushion under your sacrum. Hold this position between 3 and 10 minutes. It is very restorative and great for people who have been on their feet all day.

Wall Squat (aka Wall Happy Baby—fig. 4.6): Starting from the legs straight up the wall, bend both knees and slide your feet down. Have the feet comfortably far apart, which may be approximately hip width. If the feet and knees are more than hip-width apart, the pose gets juicier. Your buttocks may have lifted off the floor when you slid your feet down; for some people, this is quite alright and they like the hips up a bit. Others may not like this because it puts too much stress into the sacrum. Feel free to wiggle a bit away from the wall so that your sacrum can be flat on the floor. The intention here is to wake up the hip sockets; so as long as you are feeling something there, you are getting the pose. Three to 5 minutes here should be enough. For the last minute or so, try coming into the traditional Happy Baby by grabbing your feet or holding the backs of your thighs and pulling your knees to the floor. When you have had enough, straighten the legs up against the wall and release any tension from the previous posture. Wiggle, move and do whatever feels organic. Try a version of Tantrumasana that you may have perfected when you were a child. Let your arms and legs flail in the air!

Wall Straddle (fig. 4.7): You will need a bit of space for this one, especially if you are quite flexible. Start with your legs straight up the wall (or your variation of that) and then let gravity draw the legs apart, your feet sliding down the wall. Reach the Goldilocks Position where the sensations are just right. When you want a little more, try resting your hands on your inner thighs. No need to pull: let your muscles relax. Stay here for 3 to 5 minutes. If the sensations are too intense, here are 2 options: 1) place bolsters or blocks under the thighs for support (fig. 4.8); 2) loop together 2 straps around your feet and adjust the length of the strap and width between the legs (fig. 4.9). When you are ready to come out, use your hands to push your legs together, like closing a book. Wiggle and move. Remember, a bit of yang movement between the yin poses helps to free up stuck energy.

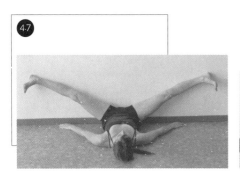

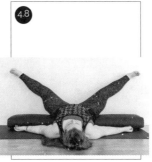

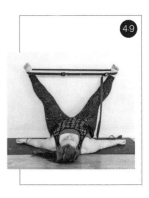

Wall Eye-of-the-Needle (aka Wall Swan): We will start on the right side; however, if your left hip is the more open one, feel free to start on the left side first. Begin with your legs straight up the wall and then place your right ankle on your left knee (fig. 4.10). Since you are upside down, the words above and below can be confusing, but ideally, we want the ankle just below the knee, which means closer to the floor or on your thigh, but not your shin. Flex the right foot, which helps to support the knee, and then slowly bend the straight leg, sliding the foot down the wall (fig. 4.11). See if you can get to a position in which your left foot is at the same height as the left knee. This may be the position of maximum stress in your hip.

187

If you need to, slide your buttocks away from the wall so that the sacrum can remain flat on the floor. Either way can be okay; you may want to stay there and let your hips be off the floor, or you may choose to move a bit away from the wall until your sacrum is again flat on the floor. One position is not better than the other. Notice the differences in where you feel each variation, and then choose which one you want to do.

Ease into this in stages: don't slide your left foot down the wall too quickly. You can also use your right hand to press into your knee and wing it out a few times to loosen up the joint before you hold in stillness as shown in fig. 4.11. Another option is to wedge a bolster between your chest and thigh (fig. 4.12). Hold here for 3 to 5 minutes, and come out of the pose by moving into a twist.[4]

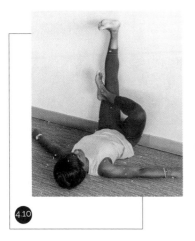

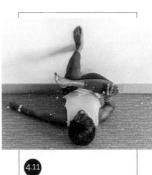

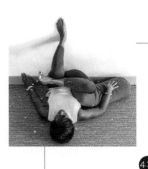

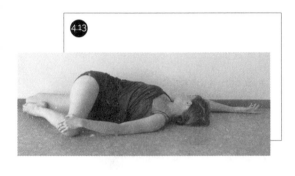

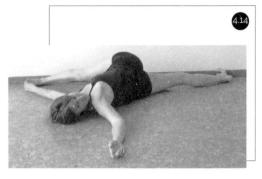

Reclining Twist: From Wall Eye-of-the-Needle we come into a reclining twist by simply lowering the legs and hips to the left, to the floor, while keeping the upper body where it is. You may want to spread your arms wide apart to help anchor your shoulders, then drop your right foot and left knee to the left and find a comfortable twist. Keeping your left foot (ideally the top of it) against the wall will keep your right knee closer to your chest (fig. 4.13), which can make this more an upper body twist. Even more challenging is to straighten both legs in opposite directions and have the feet still pressing against the wall (fig. 4.14). Hold here for 3 to 5 minutes. Come out of this pose by returning the legs up the wall and shaking them out for a bit.

Wall Eye-of-the-Needle (left side) and **Reclining Twist** (right side): Do the previous 2 postures again but on the other side. Start with your left ankle on your right knee for the Wall Eye-of-the-Needle and when done, go into the twist.

Wall Arch: Skip this posture if you don't want to invert today. The standard cautions and contraindications for inversions apply: students with neck issues, high blood pressure, glaucoma or diabetes, women who are menstruating, or anyone who just doesn't want to go upside down, leave this one out![5] You can go back to Wall Caterpillar if you prefer. If you have a stiff neck or concerns over flexing the neck too much, place a thick layer of blankets under the shoulders.

If you are ready to try the arch, straighten your legs up the wall and then slide both feet down the wall, as if you were coming into Wall Squat, but don't lower the

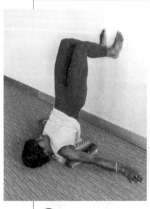

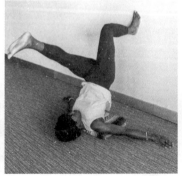

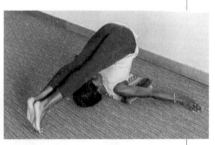

feet that far: 12–18 inches should be enough. Place your hands beside you, palms pressing into the floor. Press both feet into the wall and lift your hips high off the floor. Come into an arch (fig. 4.15). Keep your hands on the floor. Don't worry if your hips are not over your shoulders. By pressing into the wall with your legs instead of using your back muscles or arms, you should find it easy to stay upside down for quite a while. Stay here for a minute before trying the second variation.

The second variation is to allow your right foot to come off the wall and let that leg dangle over your head toward the floor (fig. 4.16). Keep the left foot on the wall. Stay here only if your neck is not complaining. After a minute or so, switch legs.

The final variation, again not for everyone, is to have both legs fall over your head and come into Snail Pose for the last minute or two (fig. 4.17). Come out of Snail by returning one leg at a time to the arch, and then lower down slowly. You may want to shake out your legs or do a mild spinal lift here to relax your spine.

Wall Sphinx: We finish in Sphinx but with our shins up against the wall. To come into this, roll over onto your belly. Bend your knees and scoot yourself back to the wall so that your knees are now at the corner between the wall and the floor. Your

shins will be against the wall (fig. 4.18). For a few minutes, allow the back to soak into this shape, and if you want a bit more compression or sensation in the lumbar spine, feel free to rest your elbows on a cushion (fig. 4.19). Stay for 3 to 5 minutes. The deepest version of this pose is to extend the arms into Wall Seal (fig. 4.20).

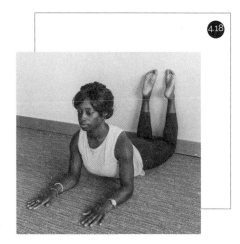

Shavasana and Closing Meditation: Now relax! Since this whole sequence has been rather relaxing already, you may choose to skip a reclining Shavasana and just sit quietly for several minutes.

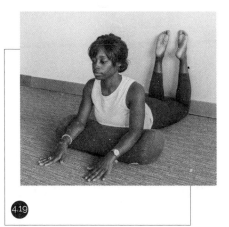

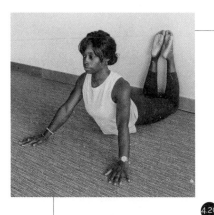

CREATING YOUR OWN FLOWS

The earlier flows make it easy to start your own Yin Yoga practice, but in time, you may need to add different flows with different emphases and intentions. It is not that difficult! In general, Yin Yoga targets the area from the navel to the knees because these are the yin areas of the body (the lower portions). As we grow older, the low back and hips tend to shrink-wrap and tighten much more than the upper body. As we have seen, we can apply the philosophy of Yin Yoga to all joints of the body, including the upper body; however, it is natural to choose the hips and spine as the primary targeted areas for our practice.

To plan your own flows, you can begin by considering the ways joints move and then select postures that take them through all their degrees of freedom. The following table shows these degrees of freedom for the major joints we affect in a yoga practice. (The shaded areas are the ones we normally target in a Yin Yoga class.)

Joint	Movement
Cervical spine	Flexion, extension, rotation, side flexion, protraction, retraction
Thoracic spine	Mainly rotation with limited but still important lateral flexion, forward flexion and extension
Lumbar spine	Mainly flexion and extension, with a bit of side flexion and minimal rotation
Hips	Flexion, extension, abduction, adduction, external rotation, internal rotation
Knees	Flexion and extension, but when the knee is bent, some rotation is possible
Shoulders – Scapula	Abduction (protraction), adduction (retraction), elevation and upward rotation,* depression and downward rotation,* tilting backward, tilting forward
Shoulders – Upper arm	Flexion, extension, abduction, adduction, external rotation, internal rotation
Elbow	Flexion and extension between the humerus and ulna; pronation and supination between the ulna and radius

* While these two movements often occur together, they can occur separately.

Yin Yoga for the Hips

Thus, the 6 main movements of the femur in the hip socket are:

1. Flexion (aka forward folding): where the front of the torso and legs come closer together. Simply sitting on the floor will flex the hips 90°, but deeper flexion may occur by folding further forward.

2. Extension (aka backbending): where the back of the pelvis and the back of the legs come closer together.

3. Abduction (aka spreading the legs): where the top of the femur, called the greater trochanter, comes closer to the top and side of the pelvis, called the ilium.

4. Adduction (aka bringing legs together): where the top of the femur moves further away from the ilium.

5. External rotation: where the inner thighs roll open outward and to the front.

6. Internal rotation: where the inner thighs roll inward and toward the back.

Our next step is to notice which of the postures described in Chapter 3 create which movement, as shown in the next table.

Movement at the Hips	Asanas that Cause Such Movement
Flexion to 90°	Reclining Twist, Shoelace, Square, Straddle (Dragonfly), Toe Squat
Flexion past 90°	Butterfly, Half Butterfly, Caterpillar, Child's Pose, Dangling, Dragon (front leg), Happy Baby, Reclining Twist with knees drawn to chest, Shoelace with forward folding, Square with forward folding, Squat, Straddle (Dragonfly) with forward folding, Swan (front leg)
Extension	Bridge, Cat Pulling Its Tail, Dragon (back leg), Saddle, Seal, Swan (back leg)
Abduction	Bananasana (inside leg), Butterfly, Half Butterfly, Deer, Dragon (Winged—front leg), Frog, Happy Baby, Straddle (Dragonfly), Swan (front leg)
Adduction	Bananasana (outside leg), Reclining Twist (top leg of one-knee twist and Twisted Roots), Shoelace
External rotation	Butterfly, Half Butterfly, Deer (front leg), Dragon (Winged—front leg), Frog, Happy Baby, Shoelace, Square, Squat, Straddle (when folded forward), Swan (front leg)
Internal rotation	Deer (back leg), Reclining Twist (Twisted Roots), Saddle (with feet apart)*

* There is also a version of Half Butterfly, sometimes referred to as Half Frog, where the back leg is in internal rotation.

With this table, we can now decide which area(s) we want to target and select the appropriate posture that creates stress in the chosen direction. Remember to start shallow and work deeper over time, and to group the key postures/movements together, leaving counterposes for later as a separate group.

Often, more than one movement occurs in the hip joints at the same time. For example, Butterfly will create flexion, abduction and external rotation in the hip joints. Similarly, Shoelace places the hips into external rotation, flexion and adduction. This is handy because it means we do not need 6 different postures to move the hips in all 6 possible directions. And this means that we can choose fewer postures and linger longer in them while still getting the kind of stress we desire in the targeted area.

Yin Yoga for the Spine

The movements of the lumbar and thoracic spine are flexion, extension, lateral flexion (also called side-bending) and rotation. The lumbar spine has 5 vertebrae (in most people), while the thoracic spine has 12 vertebrae connecting to 12 ribs (in most people). The upper vertebrae articulate over the lower ones via bony joints, which I will refer to as facet joints.[6] The orientation of the thoracic facets is back to front, making rotation the easiest motion. Flexion and extension is much less in each thoracic vertebral joint than in the lumbar spine, but because there are 12 thoracic vertebrae, the total amount of movement along the full thoracic spine is similar to that found in the full lumbar spine.[7] The lumbar spine's facets are oriented to the side, enhancing flexion and extension movements but greatly restricting rotation.

Postures that round the upper body forward will cause lumbar and thoracic flexion, while those that move the upper body backward will cause extension. Given the postures shown in Chapter 3, you can select the asanas that create each possible movement of the spine. These are shown in the following table.

Spinal Movement	Yin Yoga Postures that Cause Such Movement
Flexion	Butterfly, Half Butterfly, Caterpillar, Child's Pose, Dangling, Happy Baby,* Shoelace, Snail, Square, Squat,* Straddle**
Extension	Anahatasana, Bridge, Cat Pulling Its Tail, High-Flying Dragon, Frog,* Saddle,** Seal, Sphinx, Swan
Side flexion	Bananasana, Half Butterfly with side bend, Shoelace with side bend, Straddle with side bend
Rotation	Half Butterfly*, Cat Pulling Its Tail, Deer with twist, Dragon with twist, Reclining Twist, Shoelace with twist, Square with twist

* These will probably be mild movements for most people.
** For very flexible students, these will be very mild movements.

While we can achieve movements in multiple directions at the same time at the hips, we are much less likely to move the spine in multiple directions at the same time.[8] This fact means that if we want to move the spine through all 6 degrees of freedom, we will usually need 6 postures to do so. However, we can add movements at the hips while we target the spine. For example, in Saddle Pose, we are internally rotating our hips while extending the spine. In Butterfly, we are flexing the spine while working the hips in flexion, abduction and external rotation. So feel free to add some bonus stresses in the hips while you primarily target the spine.

Endnotes

1 There are more than 40 muscles in our face, depending on how you count them. We can do yoga for these muscles just as we can for any others. Who says our hamstrings are more important that our zygomaticus minor?

2 If you can't interlace your toes, that is not a good sign! You are probably wearing unsensible shoes. There is an old Daoist saying, "A man with open toes has an open mind." This applies to women too! If you can't interlace your toes, use your fingers.

3 Popeye, for those who do not know him, is a famous American Zen master but unfortunately a fictional one. He often would say, "I am what I am." Brilliant.

4 A note from Lorien in the YinYoga.com Forum on this pose: "The students with really open hips may need a little help to get any sensation in Eye-of-the-Needle pose. Let's say the right foot is resting on the left thigh; as I bend my left knee and slide my foot down the wall, my right knee falls into my chest and I feel no sensation around my hips unless I open my right knee toward the wall. I've found that if I brace my right elbow on the floor and prop open my right thigh with my hand, I can hold this position without a lot of muscular effort. Some students place a block on their ribcage to prop the thigh, but I don't like what that does to my breath. Did I mention yet how much I love using the wall?"

5 The Yoga Injury Prevention website (https://yip.guru) suggests the following conditions are contra-indicated for the inversion of Shoulder Stand: cervical disc, hypertension, imbalance, menstruation, nosebleed, osteoporosis, posterior total hip replacement, retinal tear, spinal fracture (vertebral body) and compression fracture.

6 The proper anatomical name for these flat, bony bits at the top and bottom of each vertebra is "zygapophyseal facets." That is an awkward name to spell, let alone pronounce, so let's just call them facet joints.

7 An average thoracic spine can flex between 30° and 40°, while it can extend 15° to 20°. By contrast, the average lumbar spine can flex 52° and extend 16°. These figures and their ranges, due to simple human variation, are explained in detail in Clark, *Your Spine, Your Yoga*.

8 This does not imply that we shouldn't move the spine in multiple directions at once, just that it rarely happens in most postures. Indeed, if we can add a flexion or extension to the spine while it is twisting, often the twist is deeper than when no flexion or extension occurs.

5

SPECIAL SITUATIONS

Yin Yoga is soft, yielding and nourishing—many of the qualities that draw people to restorative yoga. While restorative yoga incorporates many yin elements, the form of Yin Yoga described in this book is not restorative yoga: the intentions are quite different. Restorative yoga principally tries to heal specific problems and regain health, while Yin Yoga makes an assumption that you are already healthy and want to go beyond this to wellness and optimal health. We can, however, use the system of Yin Yoga described here to help us out when we are not currently experiencing optimal health or when we have special conditions to take into consideration.

Numerous special conditions may arise in any random group of yoga students. In the Forum at YinYoga.com, students often ask questions about how Yin Yoga may help with their own special injury or circumstance, and through community feedback, valuable suggestions are made. In this chapter, we will go over 3 of the most common issues: knees and hips; the low back; and pregnancy and fertility. What is presented is far from the final word, but it may give some guidance for those with challenges in these areas. Feel free to ask about your own situation in the Forum or offer wisdom to those who are working through their own challenges. Remember, talk to your health-care provider before trying any of these suggestions!

Before diving in, one other point is worth making: you are unique! While we can say what many people or even most people have done to remedy a particular problem they had, your experience may be unlike theirs. For example, pregnancy: no two women have the exact same experience. Indeed, even for a single woman, no two pregnancies are exactly alike. Human variation must be taken into consideration. What worked for one person may be harmful for another. Should a pregnant woman never lie on her back? Maybe. It depends! Many women have no problem doing yoga postures on their back throughout their pregnancy, but many other women cannot and should not. Beware of dogmatic prescriptions, and always check out how something feels and works for you. If it doesn't work, don't do it! If it does work, don't let other well-meaning advice scare you off what you know to be good.

HIP AND KNEE ISSUES

Yin Yoga predominantly targets the area from the knees to the navel. Often, knee issues are caused by hip problems; working to safely open the hips has been found to reduce knee pain in some cases. (A note on "hip openings"—what does that even mean? I will assume we are referring to improving the range of motion for external rotation, although increasing abduction could also be included.) The most common problems with the knees are tears to the ligaments and cartilage, and arthritis. Although we cannot cover all the pathologies related to the knees, one particular problem that crops up often in yoga classes is a torn meniscus.

The knee is a complex joint with many ligaments wrapping it to give it structural support. Between the two bones that form the knee joint (the femur and tibia) are two C-shaped cushions of cartilage called the menisci. These allow the bones to join together snugly and provide some cushioning so that the ends of the bones do not come into abrasive contact. The inner meniscus (called the medial meniscus) is anchored to the medial collateral ligament, as shown in the illustration. This means that unlike the lateral meniscus, which is not anchored, the medial meniscus cannot slide too far and often gets trapped and crushed when the knee is forced into Lotus Pose (Padmasana). This shows up as a burning pain in the inner knee. For some students, however, pain arises in the outer knee; this may be due to an overstretching of the lateral collateral ligament rather than damage to the lateral meniscus. Injury to the lateral meniscus is usually due to a sports trauma or accident.

If the hips are tight and won't easily rotate (common for most Westerners), the stress from the external rotation tends to transfer to the knee. Fortunately, our bodies are designed to warn us with pain when the stress in the knee joint becomes dangerous. Unfortunately, we don't always listen, we push into the pain, and the result is a torn meniscus.[1]

If the pain is severe and continuous, surgery may be the only choice, although recently studies have found that surgery's success may be due more to the placebo effect than to the trimming or removing of the meniscus.[2] If the pain is minor and

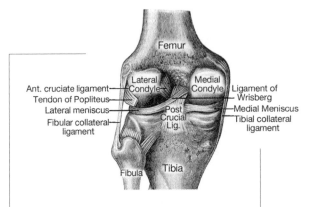

Femur
Lateral Condyle
Medial Condyle
Ant. cruciate ligament
Tendon of Popliteus
Lateral meniscus
Fibular collateral ligament
Ligament of Wrisberg
Medial Meniscus
Tibial collateral ligament
Post Crucial Lig.
Fibula
Tibia

manageable, you may be advised to simply live with the tear, but what else can you do to make sure you don't make it worse? Yin Yoga! By working to open the hips, slowly and over time, we can reduce stress on the menisci and minimize discomfort. By gently and persistently stressing the knee, we may also be able to stimulate regrowth of the supporting tissues.[3]

We can use Yin Yoga to open the hips and reduce knee stress in two ways: by doing lots of the hip-opening postures during our asana practice and by living on the floor. Poses that are great for opening the hips (increasing external rotation) include Shoelace, Square, Swan and the Dragons. Remember, we want zero tolerance of any pain in the knees with these poses. Spending as much time as possible on the floor is the other way to open the knees. A major cause of tight hips is the fact that we spend so much time sitting in chairs, which does not externally rotate the hips. Sitting on the floor does, so do it. Don't worry about how to do it: change your posture as frequently as you like—just get down there. Sit cross-legged sometimes, stretch one leg out for a while in Half Butterfly, have both legs out in Straddle, come into Shoelace, wiggle back into Swan. It doesn't matter.

The more external rotation available at the hips, the less the knees are stressed; however, sometimes stressing the knees is exactly what we do need. Stress can stimulate healing if done intelligently. The absence of stress will create fragility. Again, check with your doctor and listen to your body, but Straddle is one way to create a therapeutic stress to the inner knees: when the legs are spread wide apart, there is a lovely tugging on the medial collateral ligament. The medial meniscus is continuous with that ligament, so when you feel a nice stress there, you are helping to stimulate the cells that build ligaments, joint capsules, fascia and cartilage—the fibroblasts, fasciacytes and chondrocytes. Again, if there is pain when you do this, stop and bring the legs closer together.

A great pose to create appropriate stress in the knee is Saddle, but you do not have to do the full reclining version. In the yang yoga world, sitting on the heels is known as Thunderbolt or *Vajrasana*. If this is not possible, put a couple of blocks between your feet and sit up higher. If your ankles complain, try putting a folded towel under them. You will be able to sense the stress in the knees, which can be very therapeutic for the kneecaps. But you will also feel some stress in the ankle and arch of the foot. You can make it juicier, if that is appropriate, by rolling up a cloth or towel and tucking it tightly behind the knees; this will feel like you are creating more space in the knee joint, but in reality you are simply increasing stress on those tissues. Many people with meniscus problems or osteoarthritis have found this variation highly beneficial.

We have to be careful now: too much stress makes the condition worse, but no stress also makes the condition worse. Remember our antifragility curve from Chapter 2. As always, check in with your health-care provider and let her know what you are planning to do.

HIP REPLACEMENT

The most common problems with our hips are tears to the ligaments and the labrum, and osteoporosis.[4] Osteoporosis is investigated in the next chapter, so for now, let's look at how to help strengthen and lengthen the ligaments of the hips.

Often, students will complain about how tight their hips are, and no wonder—in the West, our hips *are* tight! The joint has been shrink-wrapped (restricted) to a very small range of motion, especially in rotation. The joint capsule and the ligaments holding the joint together have gotten smaller, shorter and tighter. This is normally caused by not using our full range of motion, thanks to sitting all day in chairs with our legs together. Again, living on the floor will help immensely with opening the hips. We did not lose our hips' normal range of motion overnight, and we will not regain it quickly either. But by applying the Yin Yoga principles to our hips, we may be able to recover what was lost.

When we regain the range of motion in our hips, we take a big load off our knees and ankles. The hip-opening poses described in the previous section work well: Shoelace, Square, Swan, Dragon, Straddle and Saddle. But what if we have some special conditions, such as having had a hip replaced? Is Yin Yoga advisable in this case?

Since every body is different, every hip operation is different. There are several ways that the surgeon can cut and enter the body to install the new hardware, so the surgeon is the best one to tell you what is possible for your new hip. Generally, external rotation and abduction should be no problem, but caution is needed if you are trying to adduct or internally rotate the hip. You should not be trying to recover range of motion but to thicken the ligaments and heal from the surgery. Many patients find they automatically have a greater range of motion after surgery.

When you are given the all-clear sign from your health-care team, then you can start to stress this area. The most common (because it is cheapest) approach surgeons take is to enter the hip with a long cut from the side, which weakens the capsular ligaments that resist adduction and internal rotation of the hip. If this was your surgeon's approach, you may be advised to avoid postures with those movements. No Saddle sitting between the legs, no Deer Pose, no Twisted Roots, no Shoelace either (because of the adduction). Instead, focus on easy external rotations such as Butterfly or Square Pose before you move into deeper external rotations such as Winged Dragon. If the surgeon used a different technique that involved smaller incisions, avoiding

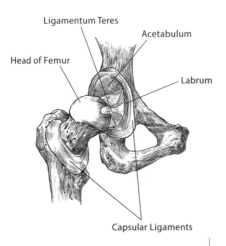

Ligamentum Teres

Acetabulum

Head of Femur

Labrum

Capsular Ligaments

the side of the hip, you may not have these restrictions. Again, listen to the surgeon and follow her advice.

At some point, hip replacement or not, what will stop your hip movement is not going to be tension of the ligaments or muscles, but impingement of the neck of the femur against the labrum of the hip socket, pinching of the front of the pelvis to the thighs, or squeezing of the muscles between the top of the femur (called the greater trochanter) and the side of the pelvis. These restrictions are due to *compression*, which is the ultimate dictator of how far we can go in any pose. Once you have reached the point of compression in your hips, you are not going to go any further in that direction for that pose. To know whether you have reached your ultimate edge, pay attention to the sensations you are experiencing. If tight muscles or ligaments are still stopping you—that's tension—continue to work there; but if you feel compression, you are not going to get more open, so don't try to go further.

The shape and orientation of your bones are the ultimate determiners of how open you will get. If your knees are still up by your ears when you sit cross-legged on the floor, and you feel sensations in the outside of the hips, that may be it for you. You may never get more open than that, thanks to your bone structure. Don't let this be an excuse for not trying to get as open as you can: this is only a stopping point once you have worked through all your tension resistance in the muscles and liga-ments. But many yoga students have severely hurt themselves by trying to push past their point of compression to get deeper into a pose than their body can ultimately tolerate. Knee damage occurs when the hips won't open any further and the student cranks on the lower legs to get the foot into Lotus position.[5] If the hips won't open, the knee twists and the pressure goes into the joint. Soon, we are asking our doctor about meniscus surgery.

Pay attention: any pain is a no-no. Listen to the little tweaks your body is sending you. Little tweaks lead to big tweaks, and big tweaks lead to expensive operations.

LOW BACK DISORDERS

The discomfort of anyone who suffers from low back pain certainly feels real, but the cause of that pain is often mysterious.[6] Medicine traditionally has looked for a bio-mechanical cause of back pain, but in the last few decades, our understanding of pain in general and back pain specifically has moved the spotlight away from purely bio-mechanical causes to a more multidimensional approach. Today, we have a broader model for understanding pain and disease, called the *biopsychosocial* model.

As shown in the graphic on the next page, there are 3 broad areas that can cause, contribute to, or exacerbate pain and suffering: the biological, the psychological and the sociological. For the past 300 years, medicine in the West looked mostly at the biological factors of health: our anatomy, infections, biological functions and

Biological Factors
Prenatal care
Genetics
Disease/infections
Immune responses
Medical therapies
Stress response

Psychological Factors
Education
Memory
Perceptions
Beliefs
Emotions
Thinking style and thoughts
Stress management strategies
Adaptability
Self-esteem

Social Factors
Social support
Family background
Interpersonal relations
Workplace conditions
Culture & traditions
Access to medical care
Socio-economic status
Poverty
Ethnicity

symptoms. Today, that has expanded to include genetic predispositions. But as the ancient Greek physician Hippocrates noted, "It is far more important to know what person the disease has than what disease the person has." This means that our psychology also plays an important role in our well-being—how we perceive and understand our world, our strategies for coping, our education level, our memories and our adaptability. Still, genes and psychology are not enough. George Engel, a 20th-century physician and the developer of the biopsychosocial model, discovered that the social lives we lead also play a formidable role in our health: our network of friends, family and co-workers, our ethnic background and cultural traditions, our income levels and access to health care, and our working conditions.

Mechanical and movement factors can certainly be a cause of low back pain, and when the mechanical deficiencies are caused by unskillful movements, retraining oneself in the movements and developing better technique can help prevent future pain. However, psychological or sociological factors may be a larger cause of pain than structural or mechanical factors. One way the psychological or sociological factors can affect us is through changes in our soft tissues (muscles, ligaments and fascia), but before we can understand those (in Chapter 6), we should look at the way pain can arise in the soft tissues.

Pain is experienced through a complex cascade of communication. Physical stress may stimulate the sensation of pain, while chemical messages can sensitize the nerve endings that create pain; the nerves that create the sensation of pain are called *nociceptors*. These nociceptors send signals to the brain, which can ignore, attend to, or amplify the signals, depending upon many psychosocial factors. You may not notice the pain signals if you are under acute physical stress—running away from a hungry tiger, or competing in a triathlon. However, you may notice the pain even more if the stress is emotional—for example, if you are feeling anxious.[7]

Acute low back pain almost always resolves itself without intervention.[8] However, for many people, acute episodes start to recur, leading to a chronic vulnerability. It is beyond our scope to investigate all the possible ways psychological and sociological factors can create chronic back pain and dysfunction, but it is probably not a surprise that meditation and a mindful practice of yoga can help ease the psychological causes of pain. This will be looked at in Chapter 8.

Pain in the back can be put into two broad categories: *back-dominant* pain and *leg-dominant* pain. Back-dominant pain occurs in the back or hips, and while it may radiate into the buttocks or legs, it is predominantly felt in the back. This pain often accompanies specific types of movements and can occur in spasms. Of the two types of pain, this is the better one to have, because there is no sign of nerve damage or injury to the spinal cord. A common example of leg-dominant pain is sciatica, where pain may be felt in the back but is most strongly felt in the buttock, the legs or even the feet. This is more of a constant pain than a spasmodic one and often eases when the person lies down. Another type of leg-dominant pain occurs only when we're standing, walking or running, easing when we're bending over or sitting down.

Sciatica can be caused by tightness in the buttock muscles (referred to as piriformis syndrome) or by disc bulges or herniation. A disc bulge, tear or herniation often points to movement patterns that caused the injury. For example, twisting often causes a tear in the annulus of a disc, while bulging or herniation of the disc is most often caused by flexion.[9] Due to extensive and repetitive pressure on the intervertebral discs, the nucleus may extrude into the rings of the annulus, creating the bulge or, more seriously, a hernia. But these bulges are not always a problem per se. About 30% of healthy, pain-free 20-year-olds have a bulging disc! The rate increases as we get older, but a bulging disc does not necessarily cause pain. Over 84% of individuals over 80 years of age with no pain or discomfort have disc bulges and yet lead fully functional lives.[10]

If you have been diagnosed with a bulging or herniated disc, you may have been told to avoid all flexion of the spine: this means no more forward folds. However, everyone is different. It may be possible to do flexions of the hips, as we find in Butterfly, Caterpillar, etc., without rounding the spine. Flexion of the hips can continue to work the backs of the legs, while keeping the spine neutral avoids exacerbating the disc issues (think of the Wall Yin postures where the spine remains neutral while you work the legs and hips). Twists may also be contraindicated at this time, depending upon how severe the disc issue is.

However! As we have seen with the antifragility curve in Chapter 2, no stress is not a good prescription either. If you never flex the spine, then there is no stress on the discs, and they will atrophy. With the injury to your back, you will have to take care that you do not overstress the spine, but you do want to have some stress. With care, intention and attention, you may be able to navigate the narrow band between too little and too much.

For students with a bulging disc, there is some good news: Sphinx Pose may be just what you need! Robin McKenzie, a New Zealand physical therapist, discovered in the 1960s that Sphinx can in some cases push the protruding jelly back into the middle of the disc. This doesn't work with all disc bulges (it depends upon the exact nature and direction of the bulge), but it does for many patients. Stuart McGill, a Canadian professor who specializes in low back disorders, agrees with the approach of using extensions to help with bulging discs but also asks his patients to do strengthening exercises to stabilize the core muscles. Postures such as Plank on elbows, Side Planks (Vasisthasana) or Balancing Cat, with one arm extended forward and the opposite leg stretched backward, strengthen the back, sides and front core muscles while—and this is the important part—keeping the lumbar spine in a neutral position.[11]

If you have a low back disorder, check with your doctor about what is safe to do. Let your yoga teacher know about the problem and your doctor's thoughts before the class starts so that you can work together to decide which poses to avoid and which ones to add. Experimentation may be required. Remember to practice with intention and attention, and also remember that the pain may not be physical at all. This doesn't mean it is not real—it is! It just may have nonphysical causes.

HAVING BABIES [12]

Infertility is defined as being unable to conceive after one year of trying. The cause may be the woman or the man.

Through our yoga practice, we can focus on structural, hormonal and even psychological issues that can affect a woman's ability to conceive. Structural problems for women may include fibroids (which interfere with processes within the uterus), endometriosis, ovarian cysts, polycystic ovary syndrome (an endocrine disorder that affects approximately 5% of all women), vulvodynia (chronic vulvar pain with no known cause) and vaginismus (vaginal tightness). Other structural problems that can interfere with conception include compression of nerves that innervate the reproductive organs. These nerves wind their way from the lumbar spine and through the inferior mesenteric ganglia. Bulging discs, derangement of the spine, and herniated discs can impinge these nerves. Alongside the nerves are the arteries that feed the pelvis and organs, which can also be compressed.

Men have similar structural issues regarding the nerves and arteries. These can include inflammation of the testes, low sperm count and poor sperm motility.

Hormonally, stress can reduce women's fertility. This is a well-known dilemma: stress interferes with conception, and not being able to conceive creates more stress! Yoga definitely helps to manage and reduce stress, as discussed in Chapter 8.

We can reduce some structural pressure on the nerves and arteries by lengthening the psoas; hip-extension poses such as Swan, Dragon and Saddle may be helpful.

We can also look to the energy body to help bring energy to the right places. Energy workers recommend that the focus here be placed on the heart chakra and the svadhisthana, which controls the sexual organs. Twists are great (for the Heart), and Kidney work may help the second chakra, the svadhisthana. Massage of the Liver 2 and 3 acupressure points may also help with conception.[13] Stressing the Kidney 5 acupressure point may assist with irregular menstruation.[14]

From a physical perspective, the following 90-minute Yin Yoga flow may be helpful. Hold each pose for 3 to 5 minutes. If you have less time, drop Happy Baby and Swan rather than shorten the amount of time in the poses. While in the postures, feel free to also reach out and apply some acupressure on the key points mentioned above.

- Opening meditation: focus on relaxing and becoming de-stressed. Ocean Breath for 2 minutes may help.
- Butterfly: massage the Kidney points.
- Half Butterfly: massage the Liver points.
- Anahatasana
- Sphinx and/or Seal
- Saddle with arms overhead
- Shoelace with twist
- Swan with psoas release (Screaming Swan option)
- Happy Baby
- Reclining Twists
- Shavasana

Remember, stress is a big factor in not being able to conceive. Relax, and vary the time in the poses to suit your level of practice. The intention now is to stimulate the meridian lines, not to be able to bring your foot behind your head.

Pregnancy

Every body is different, and what may work wonderfully for one woman's pregnancy will be ineffective for another's. Indeed, what worked in your last pregnancy may not work this time. Listen carefully to your body, and find out what works for you.

The suggestions in this section come from many women who shared their experiences in the YinYoga.com Forum. This is not an exhaustive investigation into prenatal yoga, and it is a very good idea to seek out a qualified prenatal yoga teacher who will teach you the basic do's and don'ts of yoga as you progress through the trimesters. As always, check with your health-care provider about what you are planning to do!

Intentions are important. While you are pregnant, the intention in your practice should not be to go further into poses than you have ever gone before. Range of motion is not the issue now; your baby's health and your own comfort are key. Due to the release of a hormone called relaxin, especially in the first trimester, your connective tissues will start to become softer. It may be easy to overstress the ligaments and cartilage in your body and possibly stretch and damage them. Whatever range of motion you had before becoming pregnant, stick with that—don't try to go further. Check the contraindications mentioned in the asanas in Chapter 3, and notice the options offered there.

First Trimester

The baby is just getting nicely settled in now; generally, women are told not to do inversions, so that the embryo can implant firmly into the wall of the uterus. We don't have to worry too much about this in Yin Yoga because aside from the Snail Pose and Wall Arch, there are no inversions. In the first trimester the belly is not so big that it gets in the way of forward folds or twists, but you should start to reduce compression here anyway. Pressure on the belly can be reduced through strategic uses of props.

It is in the first trimester, and again just before delivery, that relaxin is released in high concentrations. One area that really starts to soften is the pubic symphysis, the cartilage between the pubic rami. This area will need to open a little bit to allow the baby to pass through the birth canal, but in our yoga practice we can inadvertently overstress this area. Take care in any poses involving abduction of the legs (Butterfly and Straddle) to not go further than you could go before you became pregnant.

Second and Third Trimesters

As the baby grows, there is a lot of weight on the low back. Many women crave release in the spine and just love some nice backbends. However, lying on the belly is no longer an option, and Sphinx Pose, as nice as it would be, is not available… at least, not in the normal way. Now is the time to rely upon bolsters and props. Try an easy Seal or Sphinx Pose with a bolster across the top of the thighs, allowing space for the belly to drop down but not press into the floor. Some women report that a block or support under the pubic bone feels better. Experiment. Feel free to rest your hands or elbows on bolsters or blocks too. The full Swan may be a nice way to stress the spine and start to work the hips as well. Sleeping Swan can be managed by resting your upper body on a bolster.

Squat, Butterfly and Straddle provide lots of space for your growing belly and help to keep the hips open. Just remember, don't go too far. Stay where it is mildly juicy. Twists are okay and can also release the spine, but due to the growing belly, we don't want to twist too deeply. Keep it in the upper chest rather than in the abdominal area. Saddle is probably not a good idea right now but may be accessible if a bolster is used to recline upon, or if you lean back against a wall. Women are often advised not to lie on their backs because the weight of the baby compresses the vena cava, a vein that brings blood back to the heart. However, this caveat is often overdone. If all the blood returning back to the heart was being stopped, you would notice that! No woman would stay in a place where this was happening, so don't become overly protective. Pregnant women are not fragile glass figurines: they are a lot stronger than most people (I am thinking mainly of male teachers) give them credit for. If you find lying on your back nice, go for it. If it doesn't work for you, don't do it.

Another benefit of Yin Yoga during pregnancy is the effect on the energy body. We want to stimulate the meridian lines and send chi throughout the body and to the baby. The following flow may be one way to achieve this.

- **Opening meditation:** focus on relaxing and becoming de-stressed.
- **Butterfly:** may stimulate the Liver, Kidney and Urinary Bladder meridians.
- **Straddle** (fold over the left leg, right leg, and then down the middle): may stimulate the Liver, Kidney and Urinary Bladder meridians.
- **Square Pose:** may stimulate the Gall Bladder and Liver meridians.
- **Full Swan:** may stimulate all 6 lower body meridians.
- **Sphinx and/or Seal Pose:** may stimulate the Urinary Bladder, Kidney and Stomach meridians.
- **Wide-knee Child's Pose:** may stimulate the Liver, Gall Bladder and Kidney meridians.
- **Easy Frog or Tadpole:** may stimulate the Liver, Gall Bladder, Urinary Bladder and Kidney meridians.
- **Shavasana,** which now may feel better if done lying on the left side, perhaps with a bolster between the legs.

Here is one woman's feedback from this flow:[15]

> I'm 5 months pregnant, and last night I did the series of yin pregnancy poses Bernie suggested. Then I crawled into bed. I slept better than I have in a while. And the ache I had been feeling in my upper back was gone. I wish I had done a regular yoga routine during my first pregnancy. I'm sure I would have had a more enjoyable and comfortable experience!

As your pregnancy advances, don't hold the poses as long as you did before you were pregnant. The following are several suggestions from a Yin Yoga prenatal teacher who was 8 months pregnant with twins as she related this.[16] Note her recommendation to hold the poses for only 1 to 3 minutes! That is a good rule of thumb now: 3 minutes, maximum.

> I still love practicing Yin Yoga poses, but because of the loosening in the groin's connective tissue, holding the poses for only 1 to 3 minutes now is more beneficial. Some of the poses, such as Half Butterfly, I will hold for 5 minutes, occasionally, but to be on the safe side I put a blanket under the folded leg to prevent overstretching. In Swan, 1 to 2 minutes seems to be

quite enough. I do this pose in almost every prenatal lesson, as the release on the sacroiliac joint is heavenly for most women. Due to the relaxed tissues of the pelvis, some may find it very uncomfortable.

For me, at about 3 months the backbending poses such as Swan and Seal became too much. Saddle with a bolster I enjoyed for longer; still 1 to 3 minutes, maximum. However, from about 6 months onward, lying on my back for more than 5 minutes was very uncomfortable. A nice way to release the upper back and reduce heartburn is to stand facing a wall with your feet about 2 to 3 feet away and walk your hands up the wall. Lean into the wall to stretch your upper back and shoulders.

I found that vinyasa (a flowing yang style) practice was not suitable for me during this pregnancy; it exacerbated a lot of symptoms, including heartburn. Another thing worth mentioning is that during pregnancy my legs become stiff very easily: to avoid cramping, I try to keep the fluids moving and I rotate my ankles after coming out of yin poses, and shake them out. The yin stretches for the legs have really helped prevent stiffness. I have been focusing more on the lower body than the spine. I find yang movements, such as Cat/Cow variations, work well for keeping my spine mobile.

As for forward folding and compressing the belly, as Bernie says, it will get to a point where your belly is too big to allow such a thing. I have never "hurt" myself by compressing my belly; its size means that I just can't forward fold in the same way as before. I just meet with it earlier, so taking the legs wide has become the only option.

For constipation, the Cat/Cow flow, side bends and gentle twists work well. (A good one whilst pregnant is standing and letting your arms swing by your sides as you rotate left and right.) Twists are beneficial for the whole spine and sacroiliac joint, especially if you are having constipation; you need to be very slow and gentle. Use a bolster under the knees in the reclining twists, and turn your head to the same side as your knees rather than looking away from the legs.

Postnatal Yin Yoga

Now you have the lovely bundle of joy in your arms. Time to get your body back! Roberta Hughes, an excellent pre- and postnatal Yin Yoga teacher, provided these observations:

The 6 weeks following delivery is a time of healing for the mother. After delivery, most women will notice that their bodies are very stiff and tight. After I delivered, I could hardly do a forward fold. However, yin postures can be used to gently stretch the body, as well as massage the belly and stimulate abdominal muscles in a gentle way. Here is my recommendation to women who have had a healthy vaginal birth:

- **Week 1:** Lots of Kegel exercises[17] and belly massage! When taking a shower, do Kegel exercises continuously as you wash and rinse your hair. Spend 1 to 2 minutes massaging the belly in a clockwise motion with moderate to deep pressure.
- **Week 2:** Add in forward folds to stretch the hamstrings and compress the belly. Seated forward folds such as Caterpillar and Legs Up the Wall are perfect. Avoid hip openers and inner-thigh stretches for now.
- **Week 3:** Continue with forward folds. Add in reclining twists to help massage the belly, shrink the uterus and stimulate the abdominal muscles.
- **Week 4:** Continue with above. Add inner-thigh forward folds such as Half Butterfly and, later, Straddle.
- **Week 5:** Continue with above. Add deeper twists (seated) to work the abdominals gently.
- **Week 6:** After getting a check-up and clearance from your doctor, begin core-strengthening work (yang) and continue with the postures above (yin).

Just 1 to 2 yin postures a day from those listed above can be very nourishing for a new mom. Practicing consistently will make a difference. Remember to be flexible with expectations, and try to feel satisfied if you only have 5 minutes here and there throughout the day to do yoga, rather than 30 to 60 minutes for a complete practice.

Endnotes

1 Not all torn menisci are a problem. Many people have tears there and feel no pain at all. They live full and happy lives. Indeed, one study found that 19% of women in their 50s and 56% of men in their 80s have torn menisci but no pain or problems at all. See Martin Englund et al., "Incidental Meniscal Findings on Knee MRI in Middle-Aged and Elderly Persons," *New England Journal of Medicine* 359.1 (2008): 1108–15.

2 See J. Bruce Moseley, et al. "A Controlled Trial of Arthroscopic Surgery for Osteoarthritis of the Knee," *New England Journal of Medicine* 347 (2002): 81–8 and the more recent Raine Sihvonen et al., "Arthroscopic Partial Meniscectomy Versus Placebo Surgery for a Degenerative Meniscus Tear: A 2-year Follow-up of the Randomised Controlled Trial" in *Clinical Orthopaedics and Related Surgery* 476.7 (2018): 1393–5.

3 I have seen no studies that verify this statement, but I have experienced its benefits and heard other anecdotal evidence as well.

4 The labrum is a special kind of cartilage that forms a rim around the hip socket, making the socket a bit bigger and helping to hold the femur in place.

5 Interested readers seeking more insight into the hips and knees may find my book *Your Body, Your Yoga* useful.

6 The bulk of this section is an extract on low back pain from the appendices of my book *Your Spine, Your Body.*

7 See Robert M. Sapolsky, *Why Zebras Don't Get Ulcers*, 3rd ed. (New York: St Martin's Griffin, 2012), 186–201.

8 See A. Qaseem, T.J. Wilt, R.M. McLean, M.A. Forciea, and Clinical Guidelines Committee of the American College of Physicians, "Noninvasive Treatments for Acute, Subacute, and Chronic Low Back Pain: A Clinical Practice Guideline from the American College of Physicians," *Annals of Internal Medicine* 166.7 (2017): 514–30, doi:10.7326/M16-2367.

9 See the November 15, 2013, interview with Stuart McGill by Brent Contreras at https://bretcontreras.com/transcribed-interview-with-stu-mcgill, accessed on January 18, 2019.

10 See W. Brinjikji et al., "Systematic Literature Review of Imaging Features of Spinal Degeneration in Asymptomatic Populations," *American Journal of Neuroradiology* 36.4 (2015): 811–16.

11 Stuart McGill, author of *Low Back Disorders*, is professor emeritus at the University of Waterloo. He discovered that too often, core strengtheners end up flexing the low back: poses such as sit-ups or crunches are the worst ways to work the lower spine. See his book for a description of safer and more appropriate exercises.

12 I am indebted to Nataly Pluta for much of this information. In her workshops on fertility and yoga, Nataly cites work by Alice Domar.

13 The Liver 2 acupuncture point is between the big toe and second toe, on the webbing. One inch (or finger width) above Liver 2 is the Liver 3 point. To massage these points, simply press a finger or your thumb down on the spot and massage deeply.

14 Kidney 5 is on the inner ankle, behind the medial malleolus, and one finger width down.

15 With thanks to Sunny Mom in California.

16 With thanks to Hannah Marie.

17 For more on Kegel exercises, read pages 76 and 77 of my book *Your Spine, Your Yoga.*

6

THE PHYSICAL BENEFITS

We have looked at *what* Yin Yoga is and *how* to practice it. Now is the time to discuss *why* we would want to do this form of practice. We will look at the benefits of Yin Yoga in 3 major areas: physical (in this chapter), energetic (in the next chapter) and mental/emotional (in the final chapter). There are other reasons for doing any yoga practice, such as assisting in our spiritual growth, but how yoga can assist us spiritually depends greatly on which path we are following. Not everyone's spiritual practice is affected in the same way through yoga, but everyone can benefit physically, energetically and mentally/emotionally.

STRESSING OUR TISSUES

Stress is good! We need some stress in life, and in our tissues. Stress is what we apply to our tissues in our yoga practice, and its health benefits have long been known. In 1892, Julius Wolff wrote a paper called "The Law of Transformation of the Bone." Today, we call his findings Wolff's law. Wolff discovered that bones are transformed by the stresses placed upon them. When the stress placed upon bone increases, so too does its structural resistance: it becomes thicker and stronger. Especially effective is cyclical loading and unloading, which inhibits bone absorption and increases bone formation.

The process by which this happens includes both *mechanotransduction* and *piezo-electricity* at a cellular level. Mechanotransduction occurs when cells convert mechanical stress into biochemical and electrical signals. Piezoelectricity is the creation of a small electrical current when a material is deformed. When we stress our bones, these

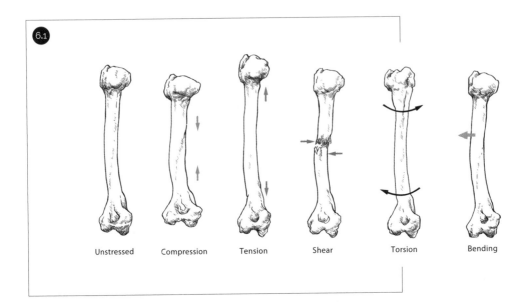

| Unstressed | Compression | Tension | Shear | Torsion | Bending |

currents flow through our tissues and signal specific cells to become active or inactive. (We will revisit this form of energy in the next chapter, as it may be the basis for what in the East is called prana or chi.) This effect also happens when we stress our cartilage, teeth, tendons, blood vessel walls, muscles and even our skin. Stress is essential to health, and that is what we do in our yoga practice—we create stress in our tissues.

Technically, according to biomechanics there are 5 kinds of stresses we can apply to the tissues of our body: compression, tension (stretch), shear, torsion (also called twisting) and bending. These are shown in figure 6.1. However, closer investigations show that the 3 latter forms of stress are combinations of tension and compression applied in different ways. So for our purposes, we can consider all the physical stresses we apply to our bodies during a yoga practice to be either tension (also called stretching[1]) or compression. That makes life simpler. In backbends, we compress the facets of the vertebrae into each other, which can be very healthy for the bones; in forward bends, we apply a stretching stress to the fascia, ligaments and muscles along the back of the spine; and in twists, we provide a shearing stress between the vertebrae and the ribs, which both compresses and stretches the tissues between the ribs.

The results of these stresses affect the body in many ways, through creating communication signals via piezoelectricity and mechanotransduction, or through the physical twisting, elongating and compressing of tissues. Through these forces our bodies become rejuvenated in the same way an old sponge can be resurrected—by soaking it in warm water and twisting, squeezing and stretching it; the old, grungy particles trapped in the tissues of the sponge are released and carried away by the warm water. Similarly, our tissues are massaged by asana practice, releasing toxins and wastewater. Even old scar tissue may be broken down and removed.

OUR TISSUES

Our physical bodies are made up of many types of tissues that respond in different ways to exercise. As we discussed in Chapter 1, yang yoga is excellent at working the yang tissues, which are our muscles.[2] Yin Yoga is especially effective at working the deeper connective tissues of the body, which we can call the yin tissues. To fully understand the physiological benefits of Yin Yoga, we need to understand the nature of these tissues.

Tissues are aggregations of cells in our body that have a similar purpose and arrangement. Generally, there are 4 main kinds of tissues:

- Epithelia (skin, linings of our organs, etc.)
- Nerve
- Muscle
- Connective

Yoga most obviously affects these last 2, although it actually affects the whole body and all of our tissues. Every time we move, we engage muscles to create the movement, and each movement stretches, twists, or compresses all the tissues in the area, as well as areas farther away. For our investigation of how Yin Yoga affects and benefits the physical body, we will look more closely at our connective tissues. But before we head into that closer examination, it is helpful to understand one more facet of our physical body: flexibility.

THE LIMITS OF FLEXIBILITY

Physically, we reach the limit of how far we can move (our "edge") when one of two things occurs: our tissues can elongate no further, or our body is hitting itself. We will use the term *tension* for the former and *compression* for the latter. Tension arises when the body's tissues experience a stretching force. This tension can arise in our muscles but also in our fascia, ligaments, tendons and joint capsules. A common example of tension occurs for many people in their hamstrings. If your hamstrings are short and tight, when you try to come into a seated or standing forward bend with straight legs, you feel the tension in the back of your legs. The tension in your hamstrings restricts your range of motion.

Compression occurs when one part of the body comes into contact with another part and further movement in that direction is therefore not possible. There are several kinds and causes of compression. The first we will call *soft* compression; this occurs when flesh comes into contact with other flesh, as can often happen to flexible students when they fold forward in Caterpillar: their chest hits their thighs. The second is *medium* compression; this arises when our bones compress our flesh. An example is when the pelvis (specifically the ASIS, or anterior superior iliac spine) compresses into the flesh of your thigh in a lunge posture. The third kind we will call *hard* compression; this is the unyielding compression of bone hitting bone, which many students feel when doing backbends: their spinous processes kiss each other.

	TENSILE RESISTANCE			COMPRESSION		
Surface Tensions	Myofascial Meridians	Muscles & Tendons	Ligaments & Joint Capsule	SOFT: Flesh on Flesh	MEDIUM: Bone on Flesh	HARD: Bone on Bone

6.2

The stress of tension and compression can be arranged in a spectrum that starts, on the left, with the weakest form of tensile resistance to movement and moves all the way to the finality of bone-on-bone compression on the right. This is the *What stops me? spectrum* shown in figure 6.2. We can view our yoga practice as moving us from the far left of the *WSM? spectrum* to the far right, at which point the progress stops—you can move no further. But for many people, the progress is not so linear. Our biography dictates how fast we move along this spectrum, but our biology may reorder the major stopping points. For example, due to your unique anatomical biology, you may not be able to stretch out your tensile resistance in one particular posture, because your hard edge is so close that you get stopped before you even get started.

For many students, it is not easy to determine what is limiting their movement. Part of our practice is to pay attention to what is happening in the body when we move. A useful mantra to repeat during asana practice is "What stops me?" The answer to that question may influence your practice considerably.

If the range of motion (ROM) we have in our joints is limited by tension, it can be increased through asana practice, breathing and even diet. When the limit to the ROM has been reached because compression stops further movement, no amount of yoga will increase it; you have reached the limit for that pose, in that direction. It may be possible to do a different pose to move further by going around the point of compression, but eventually, after you have worked through all the tensile resistance in your tissues, compression will stop you.[3] Diet, injury, surgery and other interventions may reduce the point of compression, thus increasing ROM. For example, a woman 9 months pregnant may not be able to touch her toes due to compression of her belly and legs. Yoga will not help her now! Once she delivers her baby, the point of compression changes, and her range of motion in that direction will increase.

Tension

Tension may arise in a variety of tissues, not only in our muscles. Tension can be found in our muscles, tendons, skin, ligaments and the fascia that envelops and invests all of our tissues. One study found 4 main contributors to tension in the mid-range of a joint's movement:[4]

- Skin: 2%
- Muscles: 41%
- Tendons: 10%
- Joint capsule: 47%

A progression from minimal tension to significant tension is reflected in the study's findings and in our *WSM? spectrum*. The *WSM? spectrum* shows that tension can arise minimally in the skin (referred to as surface tension), then more significantly within the superficial fascia and deeper fascia, and in the muscles and tendons. After these tensile restrictions have been worked through, tension in the ligaments and the joint capsule becomes the limiting cause of restriction to motion.

The study cited above showed that tightness in the muscles is not the major factor in limiting our range of motion: the joint capsule has a greater effect on our mobility than the muscles. As we reach the end range of our movement, the muscles have even less effect on further movement; now, the connective tissues are fully responsible for tensile resistance. Missing from this study, however, are many other factors that also contribute to limitations in our mobility, such as restrictions between fascial boundaries. Often, what keeps us stiff and tight are adhesions between the otherwise sliding surfaces of the body. Scar tissue is a common example of such adhesions. When an injury results in scar tissue forming between the normally sliding surfaces of our muscle fibers, we grow tighter and less able to move. This form of tension is not removed by lengthening our muscles because it is not shortness in the muscles or the joint capsule that is stopping us now, but a contraction or stuckness in one area of our fascial network. Another cause of fascial tension is contracture of the fascia itself. Fascia may shrink, causing tension, which again restricts our natural mobility.

How do you know whether tension is stopping you? Pay attention. Tension is felt in the side opposite from the movement. For example, in Caterpillar, the tensile resistance to going forward may be felt in the *back* of the body (in the hamstrings or along the spine). When tension restricts movement, it shows up in the opposite direction of the movement. This is important—training is required to help us recognize when tension is stopping us. Once we realize that tension will always arise in the opposite direction from which we are trying to move, we are able to pay attention and discern when tension has arisen. Remember that tension can be changed, over time, with diligent practice. If what is stopping us is not tension, then we have reached compression, and our journey will require different strategies: either going around that point of compression or humbly accepting that we have reached our ultimate limit.

Compression

Compression is defined to be when one part of the body comes into contact with another part of the body, making further movement impossible. A trivial but illustrative example is the elbow joint: extend your arm out to the side, then investigate why you can't move your forearm further away from your shoulder. What is happening at your elbow joint to restrict further movement? The answer will probably be compression: your ulna is hitting the humerus and can't go any further. We can define this form of compression, where the bones impinge upon each other, as *hard* compression. It has a firm, solid, final feel.

Bone hitting bone is one example of compression, but it can arise in other ways. Remember the flexible student doing Caterpillar? A flesh-on-flesh form of compression stops her. This is *soft* compression. It has a spongy or bouncy feeling to it. Yoga is not going to change this: she has reached a fundamental limit in how far she can fold in that pose, in that direction. In her case, it may be possible to go around the points of soft compression by abducting her legs. But there is no going around the elbow's points of compression. Wisdom suggests that she not try and instead accept this as a limitation of her body.

A third form of compression occurs when bone hits flesh. This is *medium* compression. It has a pinching, uncomfortable feeling to it. An example of this often occurs for many students when they flex their hips. Due to the shape of their pelvis and the size of their thighs, the pelvis hits the thigh. This point of compression often shows up in poses like Child's Pose (Balasana) and low lunges (Dragons), or any time the thighs are drawn toward the chest. Fortunately, in this case there is an easy option for going around the point of compression: students can simply abduct the leg a bit (or a lot). This abduction allows the pelvis to go inside the thigh, and the point of compression is bypassed, allowing greater movement.

Compression has a very different feel than tension, and it occurs in a very different area. As mentioned, tension is felt in the direction *away* from the movement; compression is felt in the direction *of* the movement.

FASCIA

As shown, the yin tissues contribute far more to tensile restrictions than muscles do. But 30% of our muscle tissues are made up of fascia, which is also a yin-like tissue. Indeed, by today's definitions, tendons, ligaments and joint capsules are all fascia. It is this yin tissue that restricts our range of motion when tension is stopping us, far more than our muscles. This fact makes fascia a very important tissue to understand.

The term *fascia* is from Latin and means "band" or "bandage." Fascia, and all of its components, creates an integrating mesh that envelops our bones, muscles and organs. It is like a 3-dimensional body stocking that invests and supports all our tissues. Our blood vessels and nerves are held in place due to the structure and support of our fascia. For a long time, Western researchers and doctors ignored fascia and considered it merely filling for the body, of little conse-

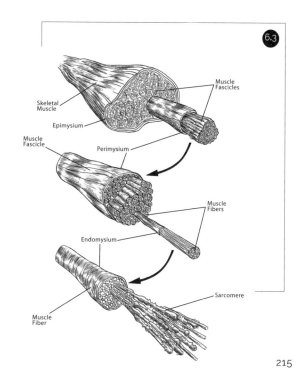

quence. Now, we are realizing that fascia is very important for our overall health, our ability to move and the proper functioning of our internal communication systems.

One map we could create for our body would show a series of tubes within tubes within tubes, where the tubes are made of fascia. A great metaphor for understanding fascia is a package of hot dog wieners. There is an outer plastic wrapper holding the hot dogs together: that is analogous to how our fascia wraps the muscle groups. Within this outer plastic wrapper, each individual hot dog has its own plastic bag.[5] This is the same within our body: each major muscle group is made up of smaller groups of muscles, each with their own fascial bag. And so it goes right down to the smallest muscle fiber—all wrapped in fascia, as shown in figure 6.3.

The understanding of fascia and its importance continues to evolve. In 2017, a committee took a stab at creating a consensus definition. Here is what they came up with:

> The fascial system consists of the three-dimensional continuum of soft, collagen containing, loose and dense fibrous connective tissues that permeate the body. It incorporates elements such as adipose tissue, adventitia and neurovascular sheaths, aponeuroses, deep and superficial fasciae, epineurium, joint capsules, ligaments, membranes, meninges, myofascial expansions, periosteum, retinacula, septa, tendons, visceral fasciae, and all the intramuscular and intermuscular connective tissues including endo-/peri-/epimysium. The fascial system interpenetrates and surrounds all organs, muscles, bones and nerve fibers, endowing the body with a functional structure, and providing an environment that enables all body systems to operate in an integrated manner.[6]

That is quite a mouthful! Here is a simplifying table showing the components of fascia.[7]

Cells	Extracellular Matrix	Nerves
Fibroblasts	Hyaluronic acid and water	Free nerve endings
Myofibroblasts	Fibers:	Pacini and Ruffini corpuscles
Fasciacytes	» Collagen	Muscle spindles
Telocytes	» Elastin and fibrillin	Golgi corpuscles

What each of these components does is summarized in this table.

Cells	Extracellular Matrix	Nerves
Regulation of fascial metabolism	Gliding and lubrication	Pain, pressure, vibration and heat perception
Adaptation of fascia to hormonal influences	Force transmission	Proprioception
	Networking: physical connections	Interoception

One of the component cells in fascia is a fibroblast. Fibroblasts build fibers, laying down the collagen and elastin strands that give fascia its form, rigidity and some mobility. Another type of cell is a myofibroblast. This cell can act like muscles, slowly contracting, increasing stress in the fascial network and shrinking the region, tightening us up. This can lead to problems. For example, the lumbar fascia has a high density of myofibroblasts, although the amount can vary between individuals. These contracting fibers can restrict the length of our fascia and lead to many pathologies, which in turn can lead to tissue remodeling (including shortening) and chronic instability in the lower back, headaches and fibromyalgia. Treatments targeting the deep fascia, such as Rolfing, acupuncture and Yin Yoga, may be able to reduce the symptoms of these pathologies and correct the underlying causes. Contracted myofibroblasts are another answer to the "What stops me?" question.

Fasciacytes are cells that produce the water-hugging molecules that keep our tissues moist, and that create lubricated, gliding surfaces between the tubes of the body. Too little water and we get stuck and can't move (another answer to the WSM? question!).

However, too much and the molecules start gumming up the work, which we will look at shortly. What exactly the telocytes are doing in our fascia is still being worked out. They seem to play a role in homeostasis (keeping things in balance) through tissue repair and regeneration.

THE MYOFASCIA-TENDON COMPLEX

The outermost fascial bag surrounding a muscle is called the epimysium (see figure 6.3), which wraps the entire muscle group and gives it shape and rigidity. Without this bag, all the other tubes inside would fall apart. Inside the epimysium we have a series of parallel tubes called fascicles wrapped in their own bags of fascia called the perimysium. And inside these we have muscle fibers (sometimes these are called muscle cells) wrapped in a bag of fascia called the endomysium.

At the lower levels, the active unit of the muscle, called a sarcomere, is also encased in a fascial bag, which attaches to the fascial bag that it lies within. When the sarcomere contracts, it pulls against the fascia, which in turn pulls against the larger enveloping bags. At the level of the epimysium, the fascia *becomes* the tendon. There is never a sharp dividing line between one tissue and the next; rather, the fascia becomes denser and eventually becomes the tendon. In the same manner, the tendon, which joins to a bone, eventually becomes the bone.[8] This point where fascia becomes tendon is called the myotendinous (MT) junction. As the contracting force is transmitted from the sarcomere through the fascial bags, it eventually reaches the tendon, and through the tendon the contracting force reaches the bone, resulting in a movement of the bone and an articulation of a joint.

Along this chain of becoming, where the fascia becomes the tendon, which becomes the bone, there are weaker and stronger areas. The muscle cells are very soft and fragile, but thanks to the connective-tissue covering of fascia, it is not the muscle that is damaged most frequently due to the forces of contraction or stretching. The weakest link in the chain is the MT junction. Most sports injuries occur there.[9]

If we were to take a sarcomere out of the body we would be able to stretch it about 3 times its resting length.[10] Inside the body, the muscle cell can normally only be stretched to about 1.5 to 1.7 times its resting length.[11] Clearly, what causes resistance to stretching our muscles is not the sarcomere itself; rather, it is the resistance of the fascia to elongation that provides the stiffness we experience in our tight muscles.

Collagen, as shown in figure 6.4, has fibers that are mostly straight, but they do have some sideways connecting links. The fibers are very yin-like: they resist elongation or stretching but can bend and slide along each other, which lengthens the whole unit. If there are a lot of cross-links between the fibers, there is less ability to slide. Imagine a ladder with only one rung between the two long poles; there would

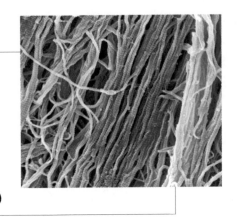

6.4

not be a lot of stability. But imagine dozens of rungs between the poles of many ladders all joined together; the whole group of ladders has much more stability. It is these collagen fibers that give our fascia its ability to resist stretching.

Elastin, as the name implies, is much more elastic. Elastin fibers can be stretched up to 150% of their normal length without breaking.[12] Fascia has varying amounts of collagen and elastin, which affect how flexible the fascia is. Our degree of flexibility relies upon both the number of elastin fibers we have and the organization of the collagen fibers. As we stress the fibers within the fascia, a rearrangement of the collagen, their cross-links and the elastin fibers occurs. The whole fascial bag can become permanently elongated. Within this new space, more sarcomeres will be created, normally near the MT junction.

When we add sarcomeres we create more strength in the myofascia–tendon complex. If we add the new sarcomere in series with the existing tissues, which means we add it to the end of the myofascia just before the MT junction, we also create more length. Through our yoga practice we create both strength and length. Body builders, who work on strength alone, tend to add new sarcomeres in parallel to the existing myofascia, thus making the muscle thicker and stronger but not longer. It is for this reason that body builders get big and cut, while yogis get long and lanky. Both become stronger, but yogis get longer.

It is beyond our scope to investigate the microscopic changes that occur as a result of stressing the myofascia–tendon complex, but it is important to note that fascia is a yin-like tissue and will respond best to yin-like stresses. A long-held static stress will help reorganize the fascia and allow it to become longer and thicker more than a short, yang type of stress will. Sitting in Straddle fold for long periods of time will lengthen your adductor muscles because of the effect of the stress on the fascial bags of the muscles. However, yang types of stresses are necessary for the muscle to become stronger. Again, balance is required—we need both yin and yang forms of exercise to be optimally healthy.

THE DEEP FASCIA

Fascia can vary in thickness and density depending on where it is and what it is being used for. Often it is found in sheets, tubes and bags, as already discussed. There is a type of fascia located just beneath the surface of the skin (called superficial fascia or hypodermis)[13] and another type directly beneath this, the deep fascia, which is usually tougher and tighter. Embedded inside this deep fascia are the tissues of the muscles, the blood vessels and all the other tubes that wind through the body. A third kind of fascia lines the body's cavities. For our purposes, we are mostly interested in the deep fascia and how it contributes to the restrictions of our range of motion.

There are many layers to the deep fascia, like multiple layers of a plastic wrap, but each of these layers can glide upon the others, at least in healthy, pain-free fascia. Between the layers are loose connective tissues containing an appropriate amount of hyaluronic acid (HA) produced by fasciacytes. Any increase in viscosity of the loose connective tissue between the gliding layers of deep fascia does not show up in MRIs or X-rays, but we now know that when fascia doesn't glide, nerves can become trapped, creating a burning pain.

Normal anatomy drawings rarely show the fascia and concentrate only on the muscles, leading to a misguided impression that the muscles (and the bones, circulatory system and nervous system) are distinct, separate systems within our body. Distinct they are; separate they are not. Everything is interconnected, and all the tissues work together. The deep fascia merges with all the other tissues embedded within it. Even the organs cannot be completely separated from the bed of deep fascia but are continuous with it. We can make only an arbitrary distinction between what is muscle tissue and what is deep fascia. They are one continuum. What we do to one, we do to all.

Some of the functions of the deep fascia include:

1. Binding muscle together, while ensuring proper alignment of the muscle fibers, blood vessels and nerves winding through the muscles, and other components of the muscle.

2. Transmitting forces applied to the muscle evenly to all parts of the muscle.

3. Lubricating the various surfaces that need to move or slide along each other.

Fascia is not only continuous with the muscles, organs and all tissues found within it; the fascia itself is connected throughout the body. Fascia holds us together. Fascia keeps the bones connected and upright. Without fascia, the bones would collapse to the floor like a medical-school skeleton without its wires.

This continuity means a small movement in one area of the body pulls on the whole web of fascia connected throughout the body. If you are paying attention, the slightest movement at one end of the body can be felt at the other end. This is what makes it possible to feel the movement of the breath everywhere in the body—but it requires attention and practice.

Fascia is another answer to the "What stops me?" question. Here is an illustrative example. Put on a shirt or sweater that covers your shoulder. Now, lift your right arm up to the sky. Notice how easy that is to do. Next, grab the bottom right side of your shirt and pull it down. Again, lift your arm up. Notice a difference? What are you feeling? What is stopping you from lifting your arm up as high as before? You may sense something tugging at the top of your shoulder, but in reality it is the restriction in your shirt far away from the shoulder that is resisting your movement. This would be analogous to someone who has scar tissue in their lower abdomen, perhaps from an appendectomy or a C-section. That scar becomes adhered fascia that tugs on all the other tissues in the area. It takes more attention to sense the line of resistance stopping you, but you can see it in your shirt.

Can we get rid of fibrosis or scar tissue? Yes, but it takes a long time! On average, it takes about 2 years to replace collagen. (Rates vary depending on which tissue you look at. Consider the superficial fascia where someone has a tattoo; if this was done as a young child, remodeling of this fascia eliminates the tattoo in time, but for adults, tattoos will remain for the rest of their lives.) Stress will dictate the direction of the new collagen fibers; thus, repairing scar tissue requires movement, stresses, pulling, etc. Otherwise the new fibers will just follow the chaotic orientation of the old fibers. However, even with the best therapy, the new tissues will never be as functional as the original tissues.

CONNECTIVE TISSUES

Prior to recent advancements in understanding fascia, anatomists would use the term connective tissues (CT) to describe tissues that bind, support and protect other tissues. CT is extracellular, which means the tissues are not cells in themselves but are the materials surrounding and between cells. Our definition of fascia, however, does include the extracellular fibers and water as well as the living cells in between our other tissues. It can be confusing to use both of these terms today, but there are still times when the term connective tissue can be useful, because it includes tissues not yet encompassed by the definition of fascia: bones and cartilage.

Figure 6.5 shows fascia, some connective tissue, nerve cells, fat cells (adipose), blood cells (macrophages, plasma cells, mast cells and lymphocytes) and blood vessels (capillaries). Weaving their way through all this are the fascial fibers we have already seen, collagen and elastin.

Cartilage and Bones

Bones are resistant to stress, especially compression, but also to shearing, bending and twisting; cartilage is softer than bone and is less resistant to these stresses but more so than fascia. Cartilage supports tissues and provides a degree of structure and firmness. Bones do exactly the same thing but to a different degree. Our bones are not at all like the bones you may have seen in labs, on a medical skeleton or even after a non-vegetarian meal. Usually, people see or notice only the "hard" parts of a

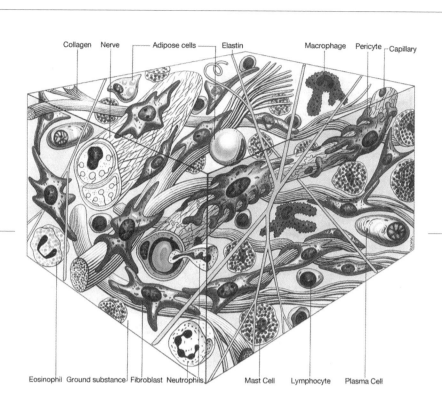

Collagen Nerve — Adipose cells — Elastin   Macrophage Pericyte — Capillary

Eosinophil Ground substance Fibroblast Neutrophils   Mast Cell   Lymphocyte   Plasma Cell

bone. This is the mineralized bone, which is generally made up of calcium salts that are deposited between the collagen fibers of the bone. What is missing is the mesh of collagen wrapping the outer part of the bone. It is much more leather-like. Living bone contains a significant portion of both collagen and calcium salts. The mineral salts help us tolerate compression of the bone, while the collagen helps us resist tension that would bend or break the bone.

If the bone was made only of mineral salt and was subjected to extreme pressure, it would snap the way a dead tree branch breaks: cleanly. However, healthy (especially young) bone, with a high degree of collagen meshing, breaks more like a living branch of a tree. If you have ever tried to snap off a living branch, you know that you have to do a lot of yang-like yoga to it until eventually it breaks, leaving the ends frayed.[14]

Examined closely, the inside of our bones appears porous. This sponge-like scaffolding allows the bones to be light and yet incredibly strong. The inner, spongy-looking part is called *trabecular* bone. It is more elastic than the harder outer skin of the bone, which is called *cortical* bone (this is the mesh mentioned earlier). The ratio of trabecular to cortical bone varies throughout the body depending upon the need. For example, close to a joint that experiences a lot of stress, the amount of trabecular bone is high. However, there is great variability in the levels of trabecular bone between people and over time within one person. It is difficult to identify sites where trabecular density is universally high or low.[15]

Cartilage is similar in makeup to bone but has a different ratio of collagen to mineral salts and other components. The cartilage in our nose, for example, has much more hydration than our bones. The cartilage in our ears is even more flexible thanks to the presence of more elastin fibers. In our intervertebral discs we have fibrocartilage with a higher proportion of collagen to chondroitin. This allows the cartilage in our spines to have greater weightbearing support than we would find in the cartilage in our ears.

Ligaments and Tendons

Ligaments traditionally are thought to bind bones together and act to restrain movement, and they certainly do this. For example, the cruciate ligaments in the knee prevent too much movement between the tibia and femur, but as we will see shortly, this is not the whole story. Ligaments are similar in construction to tendons, being formed of collagen, elastin and water. Unlike tendons, ligaments come in a variety of shapes: cords, sheets or bands. Ligaments can be pliant and flexible in the directions where they are not binding the body.[16] These qualities make ligaments ideal for protecting joints, which may move in a variety of ways. Ligaments are tough, strong and pliable, mostly inelastic but not totally so.

This is important: tendons and ligaments do stretch! The idea that we should not or must not stress our ligaments or tendons because we may stretch them is flawed. They do and in many cases must stretch. Some ligaments have a higher proportion of stretchy elastin to stiff collagen. For example, our Achilles tendons stretch 4–6% while we run. They need to do that. They act like springs that stretch and then release energy back to the body, helping us to spring forward. The same effect occurs in our hamstring tendons, which means they really should be called our ham-springs! The ligaments in the vertebral column of our lumbar spine and in our necks are especially elastic. One ligament, called the yellow ligament, or ligamentum flavum, is designed to stretch up to 50%![17] Even our tight iliotibial bands have been noticed to stretch, again acting like a spring to help us walk and run.[18] Like all tissues, our ligaments and tendons need stress to stay healthy, but they also need to stretch. Humans are the jumping and running primates because of the stretchiness of our fascia, tendons and ligaments.

Yes, we can do too much. Tendons or ligaments that are stretched suddenly and farther than their elastic limit will be damaged and tear or remain stretched. This is called a sprain. At these times, ligaments and tendons are said to be plastic rather than elastic. Elastic materials, like our muscles or an elastic band, can be stretched considerably, and once stretched they will still revert back to their original shape. Plastic materials, like Plasticine or our ligaments, if stretched too much will remain in the new shape. Once a ligament or tendon is overstretched, it will not recover its original shape or size quickly. However, the body may repair it over time. For these reasons, how we exercise plastic tissues must be different from how we exercise elastic tissues. This does not mean we should not exercise our ligaments; we just have to take care so that we don't exceed their limits.

Ligaments Revisited

Traditionally, ligaments are considered to link bone to bone, helping to prevent hypermobility in the joints. However, this is not always the case. A Dutch researcher, Jaap van der Wal, carefully dissected joints to determine the relationship between the joint capsule, tendons and ligaments. He discovered by doing this that the ligaments are not in parallel to the muscles but rather are in series with them, as shown in figure 6.6. This realization shows ligaments are not passive structures that only come into play at the extremes of our ranges of motion, and only then to prevent too much movement. Instead, ligaments are part of a dynamic system, contiguous with muscles, tendons and bones. Van der Wal has called these units *dynaments* (from dynamic ligaments). While the old model still applies when ligaments directly connect bone to bone and no muscles are found (again, think of the cruciate ligaments in the knees), in most cases, ligaments are actively involved in determining the range of motion around a joint.

Ligaments do not become tense only at the extreme range of the joint's movement; when the muscle tenses, the tendon and the ligaments both undergo stress. This stress may restrict our full range of movement long before the joint has reached its limits. We can no longer think of movement as being governed only by muscles. As we have already seen, the muscle is 30% fascia, which becomes the tendon. And now we see that there is no hard cutoff point between the muscle and our ligaments either. The newest model of an articulating limb is bone, fascia, muscle, fascia, bone—with the

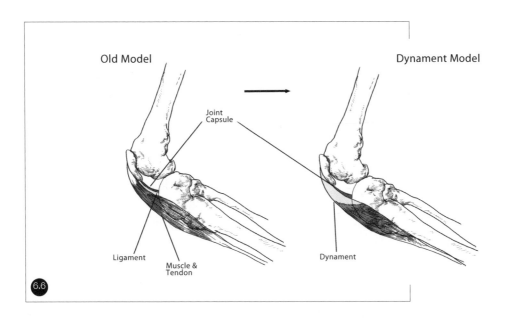

Old Model

Dynament Model

Joint Capsule

Ligament

Muscle & Tendon

Dynament

6.6

fascia consisting of the dynament of tendon and ligaments together. Tightness in the ligaments is simply one more form of tension that stops us.

Cold Muscles versus Warm Muscles

With this new appreciation of the nature of ligaments, we can now understand why so many yin yogis feel that they create more stress in their joints and connective tissues if they do their practice cold, before warming up their muscles. Invariably, the question is, "Why?" Why should the muscles be cool? Why don't we warm up before Yin Yoga? We warm up before yang exercises to allow the muscles to more easily stretch. When the muscles are cold, as everyone knows, we feel stiff and tight. Aggressive stretching of stiff, tight muscles could damage them. So it is a good idea, in a yang practice, to take time to warm up the body. But remember, yin is not yang. What works in one practice is not necessarily the best in the other practice.

Here is a simple way to demonstrate why doing your Yin Yoga while a bit cool is actually good for your body physically. Find 3 elastic bands of varying thicknesses and strengths, as shown in the figure below. Two of them should be of similar lengths but different thicknesses. As you can see in figure 6.7, the middle elastic is quite thin and is easily stretched. The bottom one is thicker and stronger. The top, shorter one is very thick and doesn't stretch easily at all.

Symbolically, the top elastic represents your ligaments: it is very stiff. The other two elastics represent your muscles at different temperatures: the bottom, thick elastic is your muscles when cold or cool, while the middle, thin elastic is your muscles once they are warmed up. As we know, warm muscles stretch further and more easily than muscles when cool, and the thinner elastic will also stretch further and more easily than the thicker elastic.

We now have all we need to simulate cold muscles versus warm muscles. Tension applied to our tissues will result in a stretch, to some degree, in the muscles and a stress on the ligaments and joint capsule.[19] How much the muscle stretches depends on how warmed up it is. However, the ligaments will stretch much less in response to the stress placed upon them because they are stiffer. The point of stressing the deep connective tissues in this way is not to stretch the tissues but to place tension on them so that the body responds by making the connective tissues stronger and thicker, and even longer, over time. To depict the stress on the ligaments, we will simulate that stress by showing a stretch in the thickest elastic band (the ligament).

We are almost ready. Once you have the elastics, loop them together as shown in figure 6.8. Then get a ruler so you can measure the effects of our little experiment. Now we are ready! Hold one end of the ligament (the thickest elastic) down at the zero point

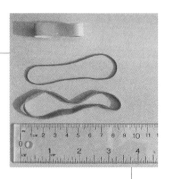

6.7

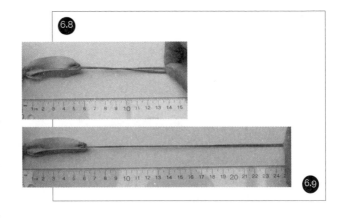

6.8

6.9

of your ruler. Loosely stretch the warm muscle (thinnest elastic) to the point where it is taut. Note how long they both are. In the example shown here, they both take up about 14 cm. Now, apply a stress and stretch them until they are about 25 cm long, as shown in figure 6.9. Next, carefully note how long the ligament has become. Do you see much change?

In figure 6.9 the ligament has only gone from about 5.5 cm to about 6.0 cm, which is about 9% strain; this means that not much stress has been applied to the ligament, even though we did apply a lot of stress to the combined structure of muscles and deep connective tissues. In other words, even though we stretched both elastics, the more flexible elastic "took up the stress."

Let's see how this would look if we did the same thing with "colder" muscles. Hold one end of the ligament (the thickest elastic) down at the zero point of your ruler, as shown in figure 6.10. Loosely stretch the cool muscle (the mid-thickest elastic) to where it is taut. Note how long they both are. Note in figure 6.10 that they both take up about 14 cm, which is about the same as in the first example. Now again, apply your stress to these tissues and stretch them until they are about 25 cm long, as shown in figure 6.11. Now, carefully note how long the ligament has become.

That is quite a change! In this picture, the ligament has stretched to 8.5 cm compared to only 5.5 cm when the muscles were warmed up, which is about 55% strain or 46% more than the warm example. If the muscles are warm, they take the stretch. When they are cold, the stress can go deeper. Graphically, then, this is why we want to do the yin practice while cooler if the objective of your practice is to obtain the maximum physical benefits of Yin Yoga. And you can feel this! You don't actually need to do a fancy experiment to rationalize your own experience, but it is interesting. All

this is not to say, however, that there are no benefits to doing a Yin Yoga practice while warmer. There are! Revisit the section in Chapter 2 on Hot Yin if you'd like a reminder.

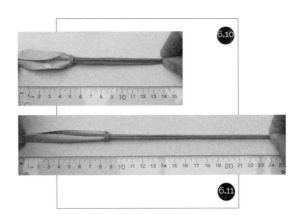

6.10

6.11

JOINTS

We have looked at fascia, bones, cartilage, ligaments and tendons. Now, let's look at our joints. A joint is simply the joining of two or more bones. Normally, joints allow movement of the body to occur and also provide support to the body. Muscles sometimes attach to the bones via tendons, which provide the force or leverage to move one bone relative to another, but sometimes, muscles are attached directly to bones (like the tibialis anterior).[20] Wrapping around the joints are ligaments and joint capsules that support and protect the joint. Inside the joints may be found synovial fluids or cartilage, or both, depending upon the type of joint and its function.

Not all joints are meant to provide large ranges of motion. Some do not allow any movement at all. There are 3 basic kinds of joints:

- Fibrous joints, where the bones are held together by connective tissues. An example of this kind of joint is the joining of the plates of our skull. No movement is desired here, so the joints are fibrous, held tightly together.

- Cartilaginous joints, where the bones are held together by cartilage and allow slight movement. One example is the pubic symphysis (where the two ends of the pubic bones are connected by cartilage). Slight movement is allowed, but large ranges of movement are not desirable.

- Synovial joints, where there is a space (the synovial cavity) between the bones. This type of joint provides the greatest degree of movement in a variety of ways.

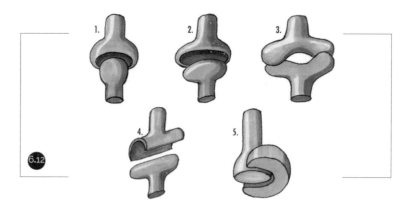

As shown in figure 6.12, there are several kinds of synovial joints:

1. Ball-and-socket joints, such as the hip joint. These allow the widest range of movement with a lot of stability.

2. Condyloid (or ellipsoid) joints, such as the knee. In a condyloid joint, 2 bones fit together but 1 bone's surface is concave while the other's is convex. (Some classifications make a distinction between condyloid and ellipsoid joints.) This

joint allows a rocking to-and-fro movement, like flexion and extension, but also allows some movements in other directions.

3. Saddle joints, such as at the thumb (between the metacarpal and carpal bones). Saddle joints, which resemble a saddle, permit a wide range of motion but with less inherent stability.

4. Hinge joints, such as the elbow (between the humerus and the ulna). These joints act like a door hinge, allowing only flexion and extension in just one plane.

5. Pivot joints, such as the elbow (between the radius and the ulna). This is where one bone rotates around another.

6. Gliding joints, such as in the carpals of the wrist. These joints allow a wide variety of movement but not much distance (not shown here).

Yoga does not try to increase the range of movement in all kinds of joints; however, for a cartilaginous joint that has grown too tight, Yin Yoga can help to restore the normal range of motion. Yin Yoga helps rebuild the synovial joints and even extend the current range of motion.

The Joint Capsule

In a synovial joint, the ends of the bones are coated in cartilage of varying and sometimes uneven thickness. Cartilage is softer and more pliable than the bone itself due to a higher proportion of proteoglycans to collagen. In some joints, even with the cartilage lining of the ends of the bones, the bones do not fit together snugly. In these cases, multiple folds of fibro-cartilage are employed, such as in the meniscus of the knee, to allow the bones to slide smoothly.

Around all the synovial joints is the synovium, a membrane that covers the entire joint. The synovium forms the capsule of the joint and secretes synovial fluid into it, to keep the articulating surfaces lubricated. As we age, the synovial fluid begins to dry up. Like a leaf in autumn, we dry up and curl up, becoming more and more yin-like until we crumble into dust. (This fluid is made up of water-attracting molecules such as hyaluronic acid and chondroitin sulfates. We will look at this watery substance shortly.) The important thing to remember about our joint capsules is that they too are fascia! Like ligaments and tendons, they are made up of collagen, elastin and water-loving molecules.

A Demonstration

As we pointed out in Chapter 1, the job of our muscles is to protect the joints. The muscles do this by tightly closing the joint (contracting). Remember how we demonstrated this? Again, take your right forefinger in your left hand. Relax the right hand and finger, and this time, apply a gentle pull with your left hand. Observe the base of the right finger; you may notice a slight dimpling or extension across the knuckle. Even if you can't see any movement, you will definitely feel an opening there. Now, contract the muscles of the right finger tightly and try to pull the finger. Notice the difference? There is no movement at all. The muscles have actively bound the joint so that no movement is possible.

The reason so much time and care are given to aligning the body and engaging our muscles properly in our active, yang styles of yoga is to make sure the joints are not damaged by our yang movements. This is wise. As the above demonstration showed, the muscles act to protect the joint and do not allow the joint to open.

As we will soon see, however, a chronically closed area of the body, whether it is in our muscles, our fascia, or our joints, can become permanently closed, a process known as contracture. If we only tighten our joints and never allow them to resume their full range of movement, we will lose the original range of motion. Yang yoga is not designed to open the joints. Yin Yoga is.

Hypermobility

There is a valid concern in yoga about whether it is a good idea for hypermobile people to stretch. They already have a large range of motion. Do they need more? Is any form of yoga, but especially Yin Yoga, a good idea for these people? The answer is—it depends! Specifically, it depends upon the cause of their hypermobility. In general, there are 3 reasons for hypermobility:

1. An injury to a joint, making the joint unstable and easily dislocated.
2. A specific condition, such as Ehlers-Danlos syndrome or Marfan syndrome. These people's collagen is different; it is not as stiff and thus allows a far greater range of motion in the joints.
3. Bone structures that allow greater ranges of motion than are normally available, but with no injury or alteration to the restraining tissues.

People in the first 2 categories should indeed be careful of doing Yin Yoga or any yoga practice. They could easily go too far and damage their joints. The key intention of their practice should be to build stability in the joints. Yoga can help them do this, but they must practice with clear intentions and great attention. This does not mean they shouldn't do Yin Yoga; it means they must do it with care. The postures in Yin Yoga are not deep in terms of large ranges of motion. We do not have "foot behind head" postures, Wheel Pose or deep backbends. Butterfly and Sphinx are gentle movements of the hips and spine and should be okay for even hypermobile students because they are not going into deep ranges of motion.

Student in the third category, while considered hypermobile compared to normal human beings, are able to do a full yoga practice, yin or yang style. Their hypermobility is due to the shape of their bones, not to a condition, disease or injury. Even though they are very mobile, they may also be very strong and stable in their joints. Think of the circus contortionist who can do a one-arm handstand while performing a deep backbend, bringing her foot to the back of her head. She is definitely hypermobile, but she is also very strong. A Yin Yoga practice is not risky for her at all. However, she doesn't need a yoga practice to increase her range of motion. She already has that. Her intention in doing yoga—again, yin or yang—is to stress her body in a safe, nurturing manner. Or perhaps she comes to the mat to chill, to meditate, to find her breath, to unwind before bed. There are many reasons to do yoga beyond gaining flexibility, and even hypermobile people can receive these benefits without having to go to or beyond their physical edges.[21]

COLLAGEN, CREEP AND COUNTERPOSES

Collagen has been referred to a lot already. The word comes from the Greek language and means "glue producer." That gives us a sense of what it does for us: it helps hold us together. It is ubiquitous, found throughout our fascia, ligaments, tendons and joint capsules. What makes this protein so useful are its strength and resistance to stretching. Unlike most proteins, which form clumps when gathered together, collagen is fibrous and can form mats, sheets or cord-like structures.

Collagen makes our bones and teeth strong, yet it gives our skin its strength too. When it degrades, it creates wrinkles. Collagen is found in scar tissue that is present after healing. It may take years for collagen to be reabsorbed by the body, but also, as we age, we are not as productive in replacing collagen. Dietary supplementation seems to help produce new, stronger collagen, but a better way may be to stimulate our own increased production.

Collagen is produced by fibroblasts.[22] If the rate of production is faster than the rate of absorption, then more cross-links are created, making the fibers stronger and more resistant to stretching. If the opposite occurs, and the rate of absorption is faster than the rate of production, then fewer cross-links are produced and the fiber is less resistant to stress. Researchers have speculated that exercise or mobilization may restrict the number of cross-links, thus increasing flexibility while reducing rigidity.[23] This is one model of why the practice of yoga can make us more flexible: it helps to remodel the stiffness of our collagen.

On the other hand, we do want some of the stability that collagen provides. As we age, or due to injury, our fascia, tendons and ligaments, all of which are predominantly made of collagen, can get weaker. Stimulation of the fibroblasts through yoga-induced stresses can activate the fibroblasts so that they lay down more collagen, allowing our connective tissues to become stronger.

Fibroblasts are not the only cells that create fibers. In our bones, osteoblasts are also laying down fibers of collagen, which are later mineralized to create mature bone. Other cells, called "osteoclasts," do the opposite; osteoclasts reabsorb collagen, cleaning up old bones by degrading the collagen and releasing its calcium and other material into the bloodstream. Health is the balance between creation and destruction: we need both to create new, stronger tissues and to clean up old, damaged ones.

Directional Stress on Connective Tissues

The direction of the collagen fibers is key. When the osteoblasts or fibroblasts create collagen fibers, they are randomly laid down in all directions. When a stress is applied along a predominant direction, electrical fields are generated by the fibers that experience the stress. These electrical fields prevent the body from reabsorbing those fibers, but fibers that are not being stressed, and thus have not created an electrical field, are reabsorbed. Over time, the body absorbs all fibers that are not supporting stress, leaving behind the fibers that are meant to do the work.

Astronauts in orbit live in a microgravity environment and have no stress upon the collagen fibers in their bones or muscles. Their osteoclasts and other cells continue to reabsorb tissues, but no new fibers are created. Studies of cosmonauts and astronauts who spent months on the Russian space station Mir revealed that space travelers lose, on average, 1–2% of bone mass each month.[24] In some astronauts, the lack of stress has resulted in a much greater loss of bone density—up to 20% over a 6-month stay in space! This loss of bone density generally occurred in the lower body and the lower back.

Connective tissues respond to demands. Stressing the body is essential to keep it healthy. Bones need stress to remain strong; so do ligaments and fascia. Simply walking is a great way to stress the bones of the legs, pelvis and spine. Yin Yoga is another way to provide this stress in an intelligent and safe way to targeted areas of the body. Specifically, Yin Yoga can target those areas where the astronauts suffered the most bone loss—the legs and lower back.

Aging or Damage of Connective Tissues

When the collagen fibers within the connective tissues are healthy, they generally line up quite straight and along the direction of the predominant stress. When elastin fibers age, they become mineralized, cross-linked with other fibers and stiffer. The relatively straight fibers become tangled or bent and, as a result, are shorter. These draw the muscle and bone closer together and decrease the range of motion. For example, when our lower back ligaments age, they become much stiffer, restraining our range.

Within the tangled area of the aging collagen fibers, particles can become trapped. When the fibers are long and straight, there is less likelihood of particles being trapped. What is trapped can be toxic to the body—waste products from the metabolism of nearby cells, free radicals or particles of pollution from outside the body, such as smoke or pesticides.

Once these particles are trapped, they can remain in the body for a long time, even forever (consider the ink of a tattoo: it is never reabsorbed once we are adults). Massage and yoga, which move the tissues of the body, can loosen up the bonds that trap these particles. Once freed, the particles can be swept into the lymphatic system and carried away, eventually eliminated from the body. Yoga stretches and compresses the collagen network of the body, which lengthens fibers and frees toxic particles.

Creep

Creep is the slow elongation that many materials undergo when subjected to stress. If you have ever left a blob of Silly Putty out on a table overnight, you may have awoken to find it flatter in the morning. Its plastic-like nature allowed it to undergo creep; it flattened under the stress of its own weight. Ice creeps—a glacier may slowly deform and flow under its own weight. The continents creep and flow very slowly beneath our feet. Concrete creeps, which is a good thing—the alternative is to crack under stress. Metal in buildings, bridges and airplanes creeps as well, which is not so good in the long term; as the materials creep, they become thinner and weaker, so the structure may eventually break. Within our own bodies, our tissues also exhibit creep when subjected to stress, especially with heat and over time, but unlike concrete or metal, our creepy bodies can return to normal.

Under a high-powered microscope, collagen fibers show up like pleats in an accordion: tiny strings of w's linked together—wwwwwwww. When a stress is sufficient and applied for a sufficiently long time, the w's start to spread apart, becoming longer, like a string of shallow v's—vvvvvvvv. This lengthening is called creep. How much and how fast our tissues creep may dictate how much stress we should subject our tissues to, how quickly, what is a safe amount of time to linger in a pose and what movements we should do next.

As we apply an external stress to tissues in one area, a balancing stress builds up within the tissues that exactly equals the external stress. Without this balance, the tissue would continue to lengthen until it ruptured. It is this inner stress that stops further strain (lengthening) from developing. However, due to changes in our tissues over time, the inner stress decreases, which allows the tissue to become a bit longer.[25] The decrease in the inner stress is technically called *stress relaxation*, but this is not Shavasana; it is a property exhibited by the tissues.

Ready for a few more definitions? Viscosity is a term used to describe how easily a fluid can flow. For example: honey flows more slowly out of a jar than water; honey is thus more viscous than water. A stretched elastic band returns to its original length once the stress is removed; as its name indicates, it is *elastic*. Our tissues are not quite elastic, but neither are they purely viscous: they are *viscoelastic*—both viscous and elastic. Under stress, our tissues flow, lengthen, stretch. Once stretched, and right after the stress is removed, our tissues remain a little bit longer than they were originally. In time—and it may take only a few minutes or up to several hours—this extra length may disappear, but how long that takes and how much creep occurs depends upon a number of factors:

- The rate of the stress being applied (faster stress creates less strain in a viscoelastic material).[26]

- The temperature of the tissue (warmer tissues exhibit more creep than colder ones).[27]

- The amount of time the stress is applied (the longer the stress is held, the more completely the material is deformed).[28]

- The nature of the tissues undergoing stress (for example, fascia undergoes creep much more than bone does).

It is interesting to notice how the factors manifest in different yoga styles. In an active power yoga or vinyasa/flow class, the stresses are quite dynamic and brief. There is little opportunity for the muscles and fascia to exhibit creep when the stresses are sharp, short and intense. However, the movements we make in these practices warm up the body considerably. The temperature of our muscles in our arms and legs is usually around 91°F (~ 33°C) when we have not yet warmed up, but after several Sun Salutations, the temperature can climb to around 102°F (~ 39°C). This increase in temperature increases viscoelasticity in our fascia, which means that our muscles are less limited by fascial resistance, so the limbs' range of motion increases.[29] Our muscles are more elastic when warm than cold, which is why warming up before any sporting activity is always a good idea. The degree of creep in our fascia is higher when we are warmed up, which is another reason our range of motion is greater.

In a "hot yoga" class, the temperature of the body is elevated due to the ambient temperature. When the room is hot, we don't need much in the way of muscular warm-up to increase viscoelasticity. This heat in turn increases the amount of creep that can occur, and the tissues do get noticeable longer—we are more flexible in a hot room than a cold one.

In an average Yin Yoga class, the room is not hot, the body is not pre-heated by any exercise or movements, and the postures are entered slowly. But the poses are held for many minutes at a time, allowing creep to flow to its maximum. One study found that "a time range of 240 seconds is sufficient to have an almost complete development of viscous phenomena. The stress-relaxation curves show that 90% of stress relaxation takes place in the first minute after the application of the strain."[30] In other words, time can do the job just as well as heat. This study implies that holding a posture for 1 minute takes the tissues to their maximum stress relaxation, but most of the creep happens in the first 4 minutes.

You have probably felt all this without knowing what was happening. As you held a posture in stillness, after about 1 minute you noticed a release, a letting go, an inner relaxation that allowed you to go a little deeper into the pose, to find your next edge. That may have been due to one of many things: maybe it was your nervous system reducing the tension in your muscles (your muscle tone), or maybe it was your collagen creeping. By about 4 minutes, you may have found your final edge, and no further depth occurs; you have reached the maximum creep your tissues will safely provide.

This is all good! We stress our tissues and then let them come slowly back to normal. During the stress, a lot of chemical, electrical and biological signals are created that help the body to heal or grow stronger. Our water may also change its nature, flushing out toxins and free radicals that impair cellular functioning. But after the pose is over, how do we regain normalcy? We need to consider the philosophy of counterposes.

Counterposes

Creep can occur through repetitive (cyclical) movements, through warming up, through practicing in a hot yoga room, and through long-held static stress.[31] In every case, the tissues that experienced creep will take time to recover their original stiffness and length. Static stress increases creep more quickly than cyclical stress.[32] Thus, Yin Yoga is more effective at generating creep than more active yoga practices. This can be very good and very therapeutic, but it does mean that yin yogis have to be more aware of the reality of creep and take care in deciding what to do after coming out of their postures. Sarah Powers defined the fourth principle of Yin Yoga to be "coming out slowly." There is a reason we feel so fragile after a yin pose: we have weakened and lengthened our fascia and joints. We need to take care how we move now.

One study found that the amount of flexion creep the spine experienced after 20 minutes of static stress was 6.8–9.6%. After 20 minutes of recovery, the amount of elongation had reduced to only 3–4%,[33] so less than half of the creep was gone after 20 minutes of relaxation. It took longer for the tissues to recover their normal stiffness than the time used to apply stress. In some cases, it took 7 hours or longer for the tissues to fully return to normal stiffness.[34] However, it must be pointed out that these studies were done in vitro (with a cadaver), not with living, moist tissues. Plus, in this study, the spine was first subjected to 10 cycles of dynamic stress before it received 20 minutes of static stress. (That was like doing 10 Sun Salutations before doing Yin Yoga postures.) The cyclical stress may have had a bearing on the recovery time needed. But the point to note is that time is needed after a long, static stress to allow the creep that occurred to dissipate. This fact has a bearing on choosing our counterposes and other activities after holding a posture for a long time.

Stressing an area by forcing it to bear significant weight right after it has experienced a lot of creep is not a good idea. The tissues are weaker and their tolerance to dynamic stress is reduced. After significant creep has set in, even bearing the body's own weight can cause damage. This means—don't do weight training or handstands or any other muscularly demanding exercises right after a long yin practice! Allow time for the tissues to regain their stiffness. One way to reduce this time is to move the body in the opposite direction. That is the basis of most counterposes in yoga. After a long period of spinal flexion, engage in mild spinal extensions. If you have been sitting for a long time, get up and walk around for a few minutes. Simply standing can help tissues recover more quickly.

These are good ideas for counterposes after we have been stretching out an area, as it needs time to shrink again. We can also do it by mild strengthening exercises! Strength building, or yang exercise, generally tightens us up. Runners and hikers notice this: after their long runs or walks, they feel noticeably stiff. Body builders also know this. Thus, after some yin exercise, we can do some light strength building. For example: if you did a Yin Yoga flow targeting the spine, strengthen the spine with some core work. If you worked the hips and legs, do a little bit of standing yoga. Don't go for big ranges of motion now; work on stability.

It is especially not a good idea to go right from your Yin Yoga practice to your sport! You will be way too loose and fragile. Give yourself time to get rid of all your creep and regain the springiness in your fascia and muscles. (However, doing Yin Yoga right *after* your sports may be a good idea.) If we have been doing a yang practice where we were strengthening an area, the counterposes will be different. Since strength building generally tightens up our tissues, we need to lengthen a little. Yin after yang can be just as good as yang after yin. This can be summarized as a little mantra for counterposes:

After stretching an area, strengthen it a bit.
After strengthening an area, stretch it a bit.

Yin Yoga Before Yang Yoga or Yang Before Yin?

There is no one right prescription that works for every body. However, although not every body will experience the same amount of creep and fragility in the fascia, the general principles still make sense. Stress and creep are healthy for most people, but we can do too much. Give yourself time to recover before subjecting your body to dynamic, large stresses after you have been doing long-held static stresses. Do counter-movements to help speed up the recovery time. Do not rely only on a long Shavasana; even a 20-minute Shavasana may not be sufficient to remove all the creep that crept in during your practice.

If you want to do an active (yang) practice and a yin practice together, it may be wiser to interlace the two styles, with 10–15 minutes of yin postures, followed by 5–10 minutes of yang movements, followed by another session of yin, then yang again, alternating but not going beyond 5 minutes in any one particular yin posture. This is not to say that 45 minutes of yin followed by 45 minutes of yang is wrong, but care should be taken to make sure that you don't stress the areas worked in the yin session when you do the yang practice. Work different parts. For example, if you worked the spine in your yin practice, do yang postures that do not require lots of flexions or twists of the spine. Standing postures may work best now, with a focus on ensuring the spine stays braced, neutral and strengthened. Keep the spine stiff and do not try for a large range of movement.

You can decide to do your yang practice first! That will build heat in the fascia and muscles, which will make creep happen more quickly. However, warm muscles may reduce the amount of stress that soaks into the ligaments and joint capsules (as mentioned above in the discussion on warm and cold muscles). Again, there is no right or wrong, there are just trade-offs and compromises. Try the alternatives for yourself and see which one works best for you.

There is the option to break up the long holds in your Yin Yoga practice into 2 or 3 shorter sessions. You don't need to do 20 minutes of flexion in one posture, but over several poses you can get to the same cumulative time. Here's an example. Start with Butterfly for 2 minutes, then Half Butterfly over one leg for 3 minutes, then Butterfly again for 2 minutes, Half Butterfly over the other leg for 3 minutes, again back to Butterfly for 2 minutes, then Straddle for 3 minutes, back to Butterfly for 2 minutes, then Caterpillar for the last 3 minutes. Spend 1 minute between each position for a short relaxation. You will have spent 20 minute with the spine in flexion, but the recovery time will be much faster than if you had held Butterfly, Straddle and Caterpillar non-stop for 20 minutes in a row.

Creep doesn't have to be creepy. We need to stress our tissues. While they are stressed, they undergo elongation and weakening. For most people, this is healthy and normal. When the stress ends, the tissues slowly revert to their original length and stiffness, and with a rest period, they should become healthier and stronger than before. However, right after the stress has ended, before the tissues have returned to normal, there is a danger period in which the tissues can be overtaxed, even by normal, everyday activities. During this period, it is advisable not to demand a lot of these tissues. However, it is possible to shorten the time in which the tissues are potentially at risk: move gently in the opposite direction of the original stress and reduce the temperature of the tissues (coolness reduces creep). Yin Yoga is especially good at generating creep, and we can sense the increased fragility of our tissues as we come out of these postures. Our own natural common sense will warn us not to move too strenuously or quickly. But this feeling of fragility may quickly go away, even though the tissues are not yet back to normal. Take care; be aware, and go gently into your next activities.

GROUND SUBSTANCES AND HYDRATION

One final topic will round out our investigation into how muscles, fascia and other connective tissues create stability, strength and elasticity in our body. This next topic involves ground substances, the fluids that fill the spaces between the fibers and cells in our tissues.

Imagine the inner tube of your bicycle wheel is deflated. Hold it in your hand and notice how limp and flexible it feels. You can bend it and twist it in any direction you like. Now imagine it is filled with water. Feel the rigidity that has suddenly appeared. Water, which normally seems to be quite yielding, is very difficult to compress. When constrained, water provides tremendous resistance to being squeezed. Ground substances, which are sometimes called cement substances, act very much like the water in the inner-tube analogy; they provide strength and support to the tissues. But they do so much more than that.

Ground substances are the non-fibrous portion of our extracellular matrix (the stuff outside the cells of our bodies). They are made up of various proteins, water and glycosaminoglycans (GAGs), which are water-loving molecules. Water can make up 60–70% of the ground substances. One of the most important GAGs is hyaluronic acid (HA), also called hyaluronan. Various researchers have estimated that HA can attract and bind 1,000 times its volume of water.[35] Another important kind of GAG is chondroitin sulfate.

When GAGs combine with proteins, they are called proteoglycans, and it is in this form that they attach to water molecules and hydrate our tissues. The proteoglycans are very malleable and move about freely. However, being made of water, they also resist compression tremendously.

With water as a principal component of our ground substances, we can see why they are excellent lubricants between fibrils and fascial sheets, allowing them to move or glide freely. Water also gives our tissues a spring-like ability, allowing them to return to their original shapes once pressure has ceased. This is crucial to our tissues' ability to withstand stresses; however, cyclic loading and unloading is important for maintaining tissue health. One study found that alteration between loading and unloading pressure, as long as it is not excessive, maintains cartilage health.[36] The synovial fluid in our joints is also a lubricant, and it too is made up substantially of GAGs. HA and two kinds of chondroitin sulfates are essential for keeping our joints working properly.

When the extracellular matrix is well hydrated, cells, nutrients and other components of the matrix can move freely. Toxins and waste products can migrate out of the matrix into the lymphatic system to be removed from the body. The ground substances, which are created in part by the fibroblasts (remember, fibroblasts also produce collagen), are also helpful in resisting the spread of infection and are a part of our immune system barrier.

Hyaluronic acid is a tricky substance. It is sometimes called a Goldilocks molecule because we can have too little, which is not good, but we can also have too much, which is also unhealthy. It turns out that exercise can increase HA levels, but this may not be good. If after exercise the HA is left alone, it aggregates, creating large, sticky blocks (this may be a primary cause of delayed-onset muscles soreness, known as DOMS). This macromolecular crowding leaves little room for water in the loose connective tissue, which may be a source of pain. For example, people suffering low back pain have 25% thicker deep fascia in their lower back and 52% less gliding available there.[37] Whether this is a cause of pain or a result of pain is not yet fully known.

So what can we do to disaggregate the HA blocks? Decreasing acidity levels (which means increasing pH levels) will do it. If we can lower the acidity in the tissues, the blocks are dissolved. However, this is difficult to do. Another technique is to increase temperature. HA is gel-like at around 100°F (~ 38°C), called the "gel state"—think of Jell-O – but becomes liquid at around 106°F (~ 41°C), called the solution state, or "sol state". In this liquid state, the adhesions can dissolve and toxic particles can be flushed out of the fascia into the lymphatic system. There are many ways to heat up our tissues: massage, movement, exercise, vigorous vinyasa yogas, steam baths, hot tubs, etc.

Another approach to reducing stuckness in the fascia is stress: fascial manipulation, including friction with pressure, over time increases stress and temperature in the deep fascia. This changes the gel state of the HA to the sol state and can permanently break apart the adhesions between the gliding layers. The residual particles of the broken up HA macromolecules can create short-term inflammation in the tissues, which in turn triggers the immune system to help clean up the area and heal any damage.[38] This approach to dealing with pain or a lack of movement due to fascial adhesions is what we can do in our yoga practice. Compression of the tissues, via yoga and other means, can temporarily transform the ground substance from gel to sol. During the fluid, sol state, toxins and wastes can be transported out of the matrix.[39] Even if this doesn't diminish adhesions or scar tissue, at the very least it can help to prevent these situations from arising.

Unfortunately, as we age, the ability of the body to create HA and other GAGs diminishes. We have fewer fibroblasts available to us, and those we do have produce less HA. Consequently, the extracellular matrix contains more and more fibers, and as these fibers come closer together, they generate cross-links that bind them to each other, so our tissues become stiffer, less elastic and less open to the flow of the other components in our matrix. Toxins and waste products (known as *ama* in yogic terms) become trapped in the matrix and cannot get out, harmful bacteria can multiply freely, and free radicals remain active. Immobility can also cause a steep drop in hydration: studies have shown a loss of up to 40% of HA, reducing our tissues' ability to slide across each other. Fortunately, exercise such as yoga and massage, which stress the extracellular matrix, can help us maintain the number of fibroblasts and keep them functioning properly. This helps to keep the matrix hydrated, open and strong.

INFLAMMATION

Research into the effects of long-held, static stretches on fascia has found a surprising immune system response: it reduces acute inflammation. Cyclical stresses, the kinds that generate repetitive stress syndromes, increase inflammation.[40] This is not good. However, eccentric exercises[41] create greater stimulation of fibroblasts, increasing their production of collagen, thus stimulating healing. Stretching causes a healthy increase in the alignment of fibroblasts in tendons.[42] Inflammation is reduced through moving our joints through their available ranges of motion.[43] One fascia researcher looking into the effects of very long stresses on fascia (similar to Yin Yoga stresses) discovered that a whole-body stretch held for 10 minutes twice a day reduces inflammation.[44]

Our knowledge and understanding of fascia and what it does is still growing. It is a complicated system that touches every part of the body, connecting, coordinating and communicating throughout the matrix. The more we learn about it, the more we know that we don't know enough. But we do know that movement and stress are healthy and necessary to keep the fascia functioning optimally. Whether that movement comes from exercise, yoga (yin and yang), massage or other physical therapies doesn't seem to be nearly as important as the simple requirement to keep moving and stressing the body.

OTHER PHYSIOLOGICAL BENEFITS OF YIN YOGA

If we consider our joints and bones for a moment, we can describe at least 3 big additional benefits of adding Yin Yoga to our practice:

- Fighting contracture of the joint capsules.
- Avoiding degeneration within the bones.
- Reducing fixation in the joints.

Contracture

Contracture is a loss of mobility in a joint. There are many possible causes of contracture: illness, nerve damage, muscle atrophy or problems with the joint's cartilage or ligaments.

Everyday life can create microscopic tears in our ligaments. These small wounds are healed by the insertion of ligament tissue in between the torn edges. However, if the body naturally lengthens ligaments due to their constant tearing and rebuilding, why then aren't our ligaments extremely long? As Paul Grilley likes to ask, "Why don't our knuckles drag on the ground when we walk?"

University of North Carolina Professor Laurence Dahners investigated this question and discovered a mechanism whereby the body shrink-wraps our joints by removing materials from our ligaments. He noted, "A common clinical finding is that unloaded ligaments not only atrophy, but also undergo contracture."[45] This is due in part to a lack of stress-generated electric signals.

There are similar findings about many other areas of our body; one part of the body creates materials (such as the osteoblasts in our bones, which create bone tissue), and another part consumes or removes materials (such as the osteoclasts, which dissolve bone). Health is the balance of these two functions.

An example of shrink-wrapping contracture is the classic frozen shoulder syndrome. Grandpa falls and breaks his arm, the bone is reset, and the arm rests in a sling for several weeks. When the time comes, the sling is removed, the bone has healed, but the shoulder is frozen. What happened? While there are multiple causes of frozen shoulder syndrome, such as inflammation, this cause was the lack of use of the shoulder joint. The body took away materials no longer needed, and when the time came to use the shoulder again, it couldn't respond.

The treatment for contracture is not surprising for any student of yoga: mobilization. You can do this yourself through Yin Yoga techniques and stretches, or through mechanical means. In the latter case, devices such as the Continuous Passive Motion machine move the limb through the patient's tolerable ranges of motion. This is exactly what we do in Yin Yoga: we gently but persistently move the body through its tolerable ranges of motions and hold it there. Eventually, we regain or even expand the original range of motion of the joint and combat contracture.

A study of contracture repair contrasted short, intense stresses like we find in our yang yoga practices with long-held, mild stresses like we find in our Yin Yoga practice. The researchers concluded that "the longest period of low force stretch produces the greatest amount of permanent elongation, with the least amount of trauma and structural weakening of the connective tissues. Consequently, permanent elongation of connective tissue results in range of motion increases for the patient."[46] The shorter, more intense stresses were observed to have resulted in "a higher proportion of elastic response, less remodeling, and greater trauma and weakening of the tissue."[47] If our objective is to remodel our connective tissue to fight contracture, Yin Yoga is one great way to go.

Degeneration

The body continually creates and absorbs bone. If this gets out of balance, we either gain bone mass, causing strengthening of the bone, or we lose bone density and the bone degenerates. Up until our mid-20s to mid-30s, we generally gain bone mass. If we exercise conscientiously, we can continue to maintain or even add bone mass past these earlier years. Eventually and unfortunately, we begin to lose bone density.

This condition is known as osteopenia or, in more severe cases, osteoporosis. This condition is more common in women than men, especially as women approach menopause.

One estimate suggests that 10 million Americans suffer from osteoporosis and another 34 million suffer from osteopenia, which leads to osteoporosis. Weakening in the bones results in almost 1.5 million fractures each year, with the majority occurring in the lower back. Other common sites for breakage are the wrists and hips.

Starting just before menopause, and over a 4- to 8-year period thereafter, women begin to lose bone density. Osteoporosis currently affects one in 4 women and one in 8 men. As we age, this ratio increases: by the end of menopause, 30% of women are osteoporotic. By the age of 80, the ratio is 70%.[48]

For a variety of reasons, osteoblast (bone-creating) activity may diminish or osteoclast (bone-absorption) activity may increase, causing osteoporosis. A lack of vitamin D or calcium can cause bone degeneration. Deficiencies of testosterone, estrogen or parathyroid hormones can also contribute to bone loss. So too can lack of use.

Fortunately, physical activity can cause bones to grow. It is well known that active people are less likely to develop osteoporosis. Autopsies have shown that attachment sites, where muscles join to the bone, grow bigger through continued use. One example is the lesser trochanter.[49] In runners, this site is highly developed. Too much stress, however, can be dangerous; marathon runners have been known to develop osteoporosis later in life.[50] As in everything, balance is needed.

The bones need to be stressed to remain healthy, and the stress needs to be appropriate. Yin Yoga provides compressive stress on the bones, especially the lumbar spine. Other forms of yoga also stress the bones; most standing postures will do this. In Yin Yoga, the stresses are held longer, allowing the bones more time to be stressed. This generates a larger recovery response—bones stressed longer will grow stronger. Very few active yoga postures will stress the lumbar bones like Yin Yoga does.

Fixation

Ever wonder what causes all those pops and cracks you hear as you move your body? There are lots of urban myths about the cause of these, but generally, there are 3: a release of gas, friction, or fixation.

Sometimes, gas bubbles will form in the synovial fluid of our joints. When these bubbles are reabsorbed, a pop may happen. Other cracking sounds from the joints are caused by friction when one part of the joint strikes another, such as when we crack our knuckles. Friction-created cracking is often heard in our knees when we lower down into a squat; this can be caused by cartilage or ligaments rubbing against each other and sometimes is an indication of misalignment in the joint or of the ligaments.

Fixation is a temporary sticking together of two surfaces. The cracking sound is generated when the surfaces are released. That nice pop you might get in your ribs or lower back when you go into a twist is probably caused by releasing fixation. Usually, it feels good because pressure has been released.

Fixation occurs under 3 conditions: first, the 2 surfaces that are getting stuck together must be smooth; second, there must be some liquid lubricant between the surfaces; third, the surfaces must be under some pressure that pushes them together.

Here's a good example of fixation. A frosty glass of ice water creates condensation (the liquid lubricant) all over the glass, including the bottom. The bottom of the glass is smooth, just like the surface of the coaster the glass is resting on. The water provides enough weight to press the glass onto the coaster. When we pick up the glass, the coaster comes along with it.

This is fixation. When you pop the coaster off the bottom of the glass, a sound may be audible. When you break the fixation between 2 bones in the body, a sound may be even more noticeable. You will definitely feel the release even without the sound.

Why do we care about breaking fixation? Well, it feels good, for one thing. But the main reason to break fixation is to prevent fusion of a joint. This is a permanent joining of the 2 bones, meaning that the joint has ceased to be mobile.

Fusion can happen to anyone. The joint between our hip (the ilium) and our tailbone (sacrum), called the sacroiliac joint, can become fused. A 2006 study in Israel showed that 34.2% of men had a bridge formed between their sacrum and ilium.[51] The rate for women was only 4.6%. This incidence of fusion was age related: older subjects had a higher incidence of bridging. For some older people, the joints of the lumbar spine also start to fuse.[52] Loss of flexibility here is very noticeable and a big problem.

Fusion begins with fixation, fixation is cured by mobility, and mobility of the joints is one of the big benefits of Yin Yoga.

SUMMARY

In this chapter we have seen a variety of reasons for adding Yin Yoga to our practice. This summary lists some of the main physical benefits:

- Improve our range of motion and flexibility.
- Passively lengthen our muscles through stressing the fascial bags that wrap the muscle fibers. This can be especially useful for the larger, more stubborn muscle groups such as the hamstrings and adductors.
- Reduce adhesions and scar tissue that restrict movement between the sliding surfaces of our muscles.

- Stimulate growth of fibroblasts, which are the cells responsible for creating collagen, elastin and the water-loving molecules that hydrate our tissues and joints.
- Make our ligaments thicker and stronger through greater collagen production.
- Improve lubrication through greater hydration of our tissues, which allows joints to move and fascia to slide more easily.
- Keep our skin younger looking through hydration, which provides room for cells to migrate through the extracellular matrix.
- Compress the extracellular matrix to liquefy the ground substance, which is often in a gel-like state, allowing toxins to flow out of the tissues.
- Reduce acute inflammation.
- Stimulate the chondrocytes and osteoblasts, which create cartilage and bone, helping to reduce degeneration of these tissues.
- Prevent or reduce contracture, where the ligaments and the joint capsule shrink and reduce the joint's mobility.
- Reduce osteopenia and osteoporosis, which are dangerous reductions in bone density.
- Reduce fixation, a condition that limits the movement of our joints and thus prevents fusion, a permanent loss of mobility in the joint.

Endnotes

1 The word tension comes from the Latin word tendere, which means to stretch. However, a tensile stretch doesn't always result in a stretch. That may depend upon the strength of the tension and the resilience of the tissues being stressed. But, even though an elongation may not happen, we loosely refer to this kind of stress as stretching.

2 We are limiting our discussion here to the effects of Yin Yoga on our physical body, so we will be only lightly investigating the nature of our muscle tissues or the impact of yang forms of yoga on the muscles.

3 "Always is always wrong, and never is never right," says Paul Grilley, and this is true here. Almost always we will be stopped ultimately by compression, but there are a few cases where this doesn't happen and tension remains the ultimate limitation. For example, for most people, extension in the hip sockets is only ever restricted by tension in the capsular ligaments. Compression here is not the ultimate cause of restriction.

4 R.J. Johns and V. Wright, "Relative Importance of Various Tissues in Joint Stiffness," *Journal of Applied Physiology* 17.5 (1962): 824–8.

5 At least to those who have a long memory. Modern hot dogs are no longer packaged like this.

6 From S. Adstrum, G. Hedley, R. Schleip, C. Stecco, and C.A. Yucesoy, "Defining the Fascial System," *Journal of Bodywork and Movement Therapies* 21.1 (2017): 173–7. It must be noted that not everyone loves this definition! It completely ignores bone, for example, which some researchers feel is directly continuous with fascia and should be considered part of fascia. It may be that we will never have one acceptable-to-all definition of fascia, but rather many working definitions appropriate to the avenue of enquiry undertaken.

7 These two tables were presented by Carla Stecco at the 5th International Fascia Congress in Berlin, Germany in November 2018.

8 Imagine a rainbow. There is a color that is easily identifiable as red and another as yellow, but it is not possible to find the exact point where red stops and yellow begins. Red becomes yellow gradually. So it is with fascia, tendon and bone. In our scientific methodologies, we love models that cut things apart and give them discrete names, but the body is not discrete; it is an integrated whole. To describe the body, it is very useful to give names to certain parts, but never forget that the body is not merely a collection of parts.

9 Mark Lindsay, *Fascia: Clinical Applications for Health and Human Performance* (Clifton Park, NY: Delmar Cengage Learning, 2008), 96.

10 Laurence E. Holt et al., *Flexibility: A Concise Guide* (New York, NY: Humana Press, 2008), 118.

11 Michael Alter, *The Science of Flexibility* (Champaign, IL: Human Kinetics, 2004), 31.

12 Lindsay, *Fascia*, 7.

13 If you rub the skin on the back of your forearm, you will notice some movement there; what allows the skin to move back and forth is the superficial fascia. Its lubricating nature allows movement between the surfaces of different tissue groups.

14 If this is hard to imagine, go find a green branch and try to break it cleanly. It can't be done. Only old, dried-out branches snap in half. The same difference is found in young and old bones.

15 See I.H. Parkinson and N.L. Fazzalari, "Characterisation of Trabecular Bone Structure," in M.J. Silva (ed.), *Skeletal Aging and Osteoporosis. Studies in Mechanobiology, Tissue Engineering and Biomaterials*, vol. 5 (Berlin: Springer, 2013), 31–51.

16 Imagine a credit card: it is pliant and flexible, you can bend it, and yet it will resist being stretched longer or wider.

17 See Neumann, *Kinesiology of the Musculoskeletal System*, 3rd ed. (Amsterdam: Elsevier, 2016), 326. Gray's Anatomy states that the ligamentum flavum can stretch 80% without damage [Henry Gray, Susan Standring, and B.K.B. Berkovitz, eds., *Gray's Anatomy*, 39th ed. (London, UK: Elsevier, 2005), 769].

18 Not by very much, however. A 2017 study found that the iliotibial band fibers could stretch 1–4%, depending upon where the fibers were; see Mark Wilhelm et al., "Deformation Response of the Iliotibial Band-Tensor Fascia Lata Complex to Clinical-Grade Longitudinal Tension Loading In-Vitro," *International Journal of Sports Physical Therapy* 12.1 (2017): 16–24.

19 I am again using the terms "stress" and "stretch" in a very technical way. Stress is the tension that we place upon our tissues. Stretch is the elongation that results from the stress. We could be even more technical and drop the word "stretch" in favor of the more precise word "strain," which is the ratio between the tissue's length after and before a stress is applied. We often say we are stretching our muscles, but to be more precise, what we are doing is applying a stress to our muscles that results in a stretch. A stretch, however, does not always accompany a stress, so they are not the same thing. We can stress ligaments, but because the ligaments are more plastic and less elastic than the muscles, that stress may not result in a stretch. The key is the stress, not the stretch.

20 Gil Hedley refers to this joining as "bone paint" because it seems like the muscles are painted directly onto the bone without any intervening tendons.

21 A more detailed and rigorous look at hypermobility and Yin Yoga can be found in the Web appendix of *Your Spine, Your Yoga.*

22 Fibroblasts also produce a wide variety of other substances found in the extracellular matrix, such as elastin.

23 W.M. Bryant, "Wound Healing," *Clinical Symposia* 29.3 (1977), 1–36; and R.J. Shephard, *Physiology and Biochemistry of Exercise* (New York, NY: Praeger, 1982).

24 See S.M. Smith, M.A. Heer, L.C. Shackelford, J.D. Sibonga, L. Ploutz-Snyder, and S.R. Zwart, "Benefits for Bone from Resistance Exercise and Nutrition in Long-duration Space-flight: Evidence from Biochemistry and Densitometry," *Journal of Bone and Mineral Research* 27.9 (2012): 1896–1906.

25 Two possible scenarios can play out when we hold a stress for a time: (1) the strain increases under a constant stress (meaning the tissues lengthen, which is what we are calling creep); or (2) if the strain is held constant (we don't lengthen any further), the internal stress decreases (which is called stress relaxation).

26 A viscoelastic material undergoes very little strain (elongation) when a quick, sudden stress is applied. Our joints are quite stiff, not elastic at all, when subjected to a sudden force. This is a good thing and provides us with stability in the joints when we shock them with quick, intense stresses, such as jumping and running. When the stresses are smaller and slower, the connective tissues around the joint become more pliable and allow some stretching to occur. Fast, jumping, ballistic movements will not cause creep, but long-held, static stress will. The rate of creep during static spinal flexion (yin poses), for example, is faster than during repetitive flexion (yang exercise). See Jesse S. Little and Partap S. Khalsa, "Human Lumbar Spine Creep during Cyclic and Static Flexion: Creep Rate, Biomechanics, and Facet Joint Capsule Strain," *Annals of Biomedical Engineering* 33.3 (2005): 391–401.

27 "Temperature increase in fascia of up to 105°F (~ 40°C) leads to reduced stiffness and more rapid elongation of the tissue, which in part can be attributed to higher extensibility of collagen"; see Werner Klinger, "Temperature Effects on Fascia," in R. Schleip, T. Findley, and P. Huijing (eds.), *Fascia: The Tensional Network of the Human Body* (London, UK: Churchill Livingstone, 2012), 421.

28 See Carla Stecco, *Functional Atlas of the Human Fascial System* (Philadelphia: Churchill Livingstone, 2015), 85.

29 See Klinger, "Temperatures Effects on Fascia," 421.

30 See Stecco, *Functional Atlas of the Human Fascial System*, 85.

31 Cyclical loading of the tissues does not create as much creep, nor do the tissues take as long to recover as they do with static stress, most likely because between each cycle of loading, the tissues have some time to recover. This can suggest another approach for a Yin Yoga practice: to have several shorter holds of the postures—for example, to come into a posture such as Butterfly for 2 minutes, come out and do another pose, then come back to Butterfly for another 2 minutes. By breaking up the postures into cyclical (but not dynamic) stress, we can reduce the overall recovery time.

32 See Little and Khalsa, "Human Lumbar Spine Creep."

33 Ibid.

34 See S.M. McGill and S. Brown, "Creep Response of the Lumbar Spine to Prolonged Full Flexion," *Clinical Biomechanics* 7 (1992;7): 43–46.

35 See E.F. Bernstein, J. Lee, D.B. Brown, R. Yu, and E. Van Scott, "Glycolic Acid Treatment Increases Type I Collagen mRNA and Hyaluronic Acid Content of Human Skin," *Dermatologic Surgery* 27.5 (2001): 429–33.

36 See R.F. Service, "Coming Soon to a Knee Near You: Cartilage Like Your Very Own," *Science* 322.5907 (2008): 1460–1.

37 H.M. Langevin et al., "Ultrasound Evidence of Altered Lumbar Connective Tissue Structure in Human Subjects with Chronic Low Back Pain," *BMC Musculoskeletal Disorders*, 10.151 (2009), doi:10.1186/1471-2474-10-151.

38 See Jaime M. Cyphert, Carol S. Trempus, and Stavros Garantziotis, "Size Matters: Molecular Weight Specificity of Hyaluronan Effects in Cell Biology," *International Journal of Cell Biology* 2015 (2015): 563818, doi:10.1155/2015/563818.

39 See Robert Schleip and Divo Gitta Muller, "Training Principles for Fascial Connective Tissues: Scientific Foundation and Suggested Practical Applications," *Journal of Bodywork and Movement Therapies* 17.1 (2013): 103–15.

40 Stecco, *Functional Atlas of the Human Fascial System.*

41 Eccentric exercises engage the muscles while the muscles undergo lengthening. This is different than concentric exercises, where the muscles shorten when engaged, or isometric exercises, where the muscles remain the same length while engaged.

42 See Stecco, *Functional Atlas of the Human Fascial System,* 7.

43 See Robert Schleip, *Fascial Fitness: How to Be Vital, Elastic and Dynamic in Everyday Life and Sport* (Jalandhar, India: Lotus Publishing, 2017), 81.

44 The subjects in these experiments were actually rats, but the principles uncovered are equally applicable to humans! See Helen Langevin's May 1, 2013 article "The Science of Stretch," The Scientist, at https://www.the-scientist.com/features/the-science-of-stretch-39407.

45 See Laurence Dahners, "On Changes in Length of Dense Collagenous Tissues: Growth and Contracture," available at http://laury.dahners.com/orthoprofessional.html.

46 Hepburn, "Case Studies: Contracture."

47 The elastic response occurs when the tissues return to the original lengths.

48 L.J. Melton III, "How Many Women Have Osteoporosis Now?" *Journal of Bone Mineral Research* 10 (1995): 175–7.

49 This "bump" on the upper, medial and slightly posterior side of the femur is an attachment site of the hip flexor muscles.

50 See arthritis.org for more on the risks of running.

51 Gali Dar and Israel Hershkovitz, "Sacroiliac Joint Bridging: Simple and Reliable Criteria for Sexing the Skeleton," *Journal of Forensic Science* 51 (2006): 480–3.

52 Sometimes with degenerative joints, a procedure called arthrodesis is used to deliberately fix joints by forcing them to fuse together.

7

THE ENERGETIC BENEFITS

We have been looking at the physical benefits of Yin Yoga from a Western point of view, but there are many potential models we can use to explain what happens as we practice yoga. In the West, we love to use scientific maps that explain, predict and test our hypotheses and findings. In the East, experience is primary and the explanations are more poetic. Unfortunately, to the Western mind, the Eastern maps do not ring true because they rarely follow the scientific method. This does not mean that the West is "right" and the East is not. The experiences of the Eastern yogis are real, even if their models explaining them do not meet the standards of proof Western science demands. If Western science consider the Eastern maps wrong, but the experiences are real, then it is up to Western science to modify their maps or develop new ones to explain the experiences, rather than simply ignore them. In this chapter, we will contrast 3 separate models of energy: the Indian yogis', the Chinese Daoists' and Western science's. We will discover that Western science can, indeed, explain at least some of the Eastern experiences of energy.

A YOGIC VIEW

In India, the practice called yoga evolved over thousands of years. The intentions of the practice were varied; there never was one yoga. There is no yoga tree showing the evolution of all the various forms of yoga we know today. Rather, there is a forest called yoga, within which many wondrous and frightening forms of practice have existed.

There are dozens of definitions of the word *yoga*. Long ago, *"yoga"* meant to hook up your chariot, upon your death on the battlefield, then rise up and pierce the disc of the sun, thereby becoming immortal. Many yogis were feared as magicians who could take over the bodies of the dead and bring them back to life. Other yogas allowed the yogi to fly through the air, split into many bodies at once, enter someone else's body and take control. Parents would frighten their children into obedience by warning them that the yogi would come and eat them if they misbehaved; this was not quite an idle threat, because some yogis did kill and eat people. Some yogis were mercenaries, feared warriors with weapons unknown in the West, such as deadly flying discs. A yogi could come into a man's home, take any food he pleased, take pleasure with the man's wife, leave with money or jewels, and suffer no rebuke or interference from the owner of the house.[1]

These yoga practices are obviously quite different from what we think of as contemporary yoga. Today, yoga is thought to be sweet, pure and practiced with intentions of health and spiritual progress. And these forms of yoga did and do exist in the yoga forest, but they were not the only trees in that mysterious land.

Around 200 C.E., a classical form of yoga was blossoming, summarized succinctly by a text known as the *Yoga Sutra*.[2] In this school of yoga, a yogi practiced to master his mind and still the whirling thought-forms fluctuating within. Once the mind was tamed, the yogi was able to enter a state of deep meditative absorption known as samadhi. The intention of this particular practice was to obtain liberation from the bonds of matter and, after leaving the body, become liberated. Only after death could liberation be achieved.[3] The body and mind were the enemies, formed of *prakriti*— created matter and energy, which entrap us and delude us into thinking we are our bodies or our minds.[4] Our true substance, called *purusha*, is pure consciousness: the witness. Nature entraps consciousness, so nature was our enemy. This fierce yoga of strict asceticism and meditation was not for everybody, and not all agreed that the mind and body were the enemies.

A new form of yoga grew in the forest as a reaction or counterpoint to classical yoga's life-denying practices: Tantra. Tantra Yoga embraced life. One could only become liberated if one had a body. To become liberated while alive, to become a *jivan-mukta*, required that we transform our body and channel our inner energies. Tantra created a sophisticated model of these inner energies, also called subtle energies because it is not easy to discern them, let alone master them. A later offshoot of Tantra Yoga, called Hatha Yoga, kept the subtle body model created by the tantrikas but dropped much of the more esoteric and socially unacceptable Tantra practices. With Tantra and Hatha, yogis now were practicing to enhance health and make the body stronger, rather than to starve the body, die and leave this squalid existence. A key to the managing of our subtle energies was the practice of pranayama, the management of our life force, known as prana.

Prana

The psycho-spiritual science[5] of *pranayama* developed around the concepts of energy (*prana*), the little rivers of energy flowing within our bodies (*nadis*), and the major energy plexuses (*chakras*). Energy allows us to be, live and act in the world. Just as Western science uses the term "*energy*" to denote all the various kinds of energies that exist (chemical, electrical, etc.), in the yogic models the term "prana" is used to encapsulate all of the various kinds of energies.

Prana is life and is also often considered to be our breath. It literally means "breathing forth." This understanding is not unique to India. Many ancient cultures equated life and breath. In Latin, the word *spiritus* also means breath. In the *Rig Veda*, the oldest Hindu text, prana is claimed to be the breath of the cosmic purusha.[6] *Prana* is an overarching term with many subcategories.

An understanding of prana is important for the yogi. The control of our energies, our prana, allows us to maintain or improve our health, to provide the energy needed to delve deeper into the mysteries of our existence, and to calm the inner winds that blow our minds from one thought to another.

Learning how prana works and how to free this energy is part of the psycho-spiritual practice known as pranayama. This is really two Sanskrit words: *prana* and *yama*. However, there are other yoga teachers who believe that the two words are *prana* and *ayama*.[7] As often happens in the yoga forest, there are a lot of contradictions and disagreements! *Yama* means to restrain or control, whereas *ayama* means to not do that. Thus, in one view, pranayama practice tries to free up the energy of prana (ayama), but in another view, the practice is to restrain it (yama). This can be confusing, so perhaps it is better to think of pranayama as regulating the breath in such a way that the prana is actually freed or extended in a controlled manner.

Why would we want to regulate the breath? If you have ever attempted to meditate and still the turnings of your mind, you know how difficult this is. Zen is one discipline that attempts to still the mind through sheer willpower. This is a very difficult practice, and it is not surprising that Zen was the way of the samurai. Yogis sought an easier route to the same goal, through regulating the breath. If the breath is quiet, the mind is still.

Inside the body there are 5 major and 5 minor kinds of prana.[8] We will look only at the major forms:

1. *Prana vayu*: the upward-lifting energy. This can be confusing; the prana vayu is a subset of the overall term for all energies, also called prana.[9] The prana vayu is responsible for the energy of the heart and the breath. When we see a tree's branches reaching upward to the sun, that is prana energy being expressed. When we feel our inhalations lift our spirit, along with our shoulders, that is prana. Try this. Stand in Mountain Pose. Tune into your prana as you inhale

and raise your arms overhead. Feel the lifting energy as your arms ascend. Repeat until you can really sense the prana lifting you.

2. *Apana vayu*: the downward, rooting energy. The apana vayu is responsible for elimination, through the lungs (carbon dioxide) and the digestive tract. The roots of a tree searching downward for stability are expressing apana. The rooting downward of our exhalations tap into the same energy. We can tune into apana while in Mountain Pose and after we have raised our arms overhead. Now start to bring the hands down to the chest; feel the rooting energy as your arms descend. Repeat until you can sense the apana rooting you.

3. *Samana vayu*: the balancing energy. The samana vayu is responsible for digestion and the metabolism of our cells. Its direction is inward. We can tune into samana when we draw our arms inward. Stand in Warrior 2 with your arms apart. As you exhale, draw your hands to your heart and feel the energy of hugging our muscles into our core. Repeat and sense.

4. *Vyana vayu*: the outward-moving energy. The vyana vayu is responsible for the movement of our muscles and for balancing the energy flow throughout our body. We can tune into vyana when we extend our arms out as we do in Warrior 2. Feel the outward-moving energy as you extend your limbs. Again, repeat the movement until you can really feel this energy moving you.

5. *Udana vayu*: the "up breath" or upward-moving energy. The udana vayu is responsible for producing sounds and is the energy of the 5 senses. Some texts place this only in the throat, but other texts say that it circulates in all the limbs and joints.

None of these energies exists in isolation. Sensing the flow of energy is a meditation practice all on its own. Just sitting for a few minutes watching prana and apana requires attention. As we hold our Yin Yoga poses for 5 minutes or longer, we are given the opportunity to practice this meditation on energy. As a result of this inner awareness, our thoughts will slow down, just as the sutras promise.

Energy does not simply exist; it flows. Just as a garden hose channels water, as our nerves channel electrical energy, and as our blood vessels channel chemical energy, so too is prana channeled in our bodies.

The Nadis

Water requires banks before it can become a river; prana also requires a path along which to travel. These pathways are the *nadis*, which means "little rivers." Some ancient texts, such as the *Shiva Samhita*, claim there are 350,000 nadis. Many texts claim there are 72,000. The *Tri-Shikhi-Braha-mana Upanishad* tells us that the number is countless.

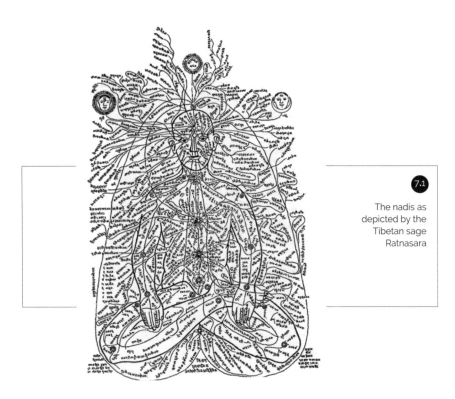

7.1

The nadis as depicted by the Tibetan sage Ratnasara

Despite the large number of nadis detected by the yogic sages (see figure 7.1), usually only 12 to 14 are named, and of these only 3 are really discussed. However, even here the texts vary considerably in the descriptions of each nadi.[10]

The 3 nadis of most importance are:

- The *sushumna* nadi
- The *ida* nadi
- The *pingala* nadi

The Sushumna Nadi

This is the most important nadi. Most texts agree that this channel begins in the muladhara chakra, which is located at the base of the spine. The channel corresponds to the Governor Vessel[11] meridian in the Daoist map. The sushumna flows inside the core of the spine, but it is not the spine; it is subtler than that. The perceived function of the sushumna depends upon the school of yoga one is studying.

In Tantra and Kundalini yoga, and in many Hatha Yoga schools, the sushumna is the key channel within which *kundalini* energy flows. Kundalini is said to be a special form of energy or the highest form of prana. The term refers to the power of the snake, which is envisioned as lying coiled up at the base of the spine, dormant and awaiting awakening. In some schools, the kundalini energy is known as shakti.

Georg Feuerstein suggested that prana may be considered like the energy in an atomic bomb, while kundalini energy is like that of a hydrogen bomb.[12] Shakti energy is directed upward from its home just below the *muladhara* chakra toward the *ajna* chakra (according to Dr. Hiroshi Motoyama, a Japanese Shinto priest, yogi and TCM scholar) or the *sahasrara* (according to Georg Feuerstein, a Western yoga scholar). The intention is to bring kundalini up the sushumna to the top of the head, where Shiva awaits reunion with Shakti.

Once the kundalini has been awakened and raised up the sushumna to the top of the head, many psychic phenomena may occur. Inner sounds, special sight and insights can be perceived. *Vibhutis* such as clairvoyance, telekinesis, telepresence and telepathy may be manifested.[13] Jivan-mukti (liberation while still residing in the body) is achieved in this manner.

The Ida and Pingala Nadis

Running alongside the sushumna nadi, on either side of the spine, are the *ida* and *pingala* nadis. Ida refers to the *chandra* (yin) energies of the moon, while pingala refers to the *surya* (yang) energies of the sun.[14]

The flow of these two channels is disputed. Modern teachers generally teach that the ida begins in the muladhara at the base of the spine and rises up the left side of the spine until it reaches a chakra. It switches sides at each chakra until it reaches the back of the head. Climbing over the head, it comes down the forehead until it ends in the left nostril. The pingala runs similarly but begins on the right side and ends in the right nostril. Together they form a caduceus, two snakes spiraling their way around the sushumna nadi.

Again, not everyone agrees! Dr. Motoyama's research reveals that none of the yogic texts actually describe in detail the paths of the ida and pingala. There is certainly no discussion of the nadis crossing at the chakras. Implied is that the nadis flow up alongside the spine much like the Urinary Bladder lines in Chinese medicine.

An interesting thing happens to the flow of energy in our ida and pingala channels: about once every 90 minutes or so, our breath switches sides. See if you can tell which nostril is more open right now. When we are healthy, the breath switches nostrils every 90 minutes or so. When we are ill, this happens maybe every few hours. It has been said that when death is near, the breath does not switch nostrils at all.

When the breath is flowing out of the surya (right) nostril, we are in a yang, energized state. When the breath is flowing out of the chandra (left) nostril, we are in a yin, passive state. There are several forms of pranayama that help to balance the surya and chandra energies, such as nadi shodhana (described below). These practices are normally done after asana practice, but they can be added to seated Yin Yoga poses.

According to many teachers, certain activities must be abstained from if the wrong nostril is open. For example, Pattabhi Jois, in the book *Yoga Mala,* warns that one must not make love when the sun is shining or when the right nostril is open. When the right nostril is open, it is the same as the sun shining.[15]

The Benefits and Practice of Pranayama

To achieve liberation, the tantric or Hatha Yoga traditions required cleansing and opening the major pathways, the nadis, and stimulating the flow of prana through them. The breath was the main tool used to stimulate the energy flow, while the physical practice of Hatha Yoga became the main tool used to dislodge any blockages to the flow of prana.

There are 2 key reasons for doing yoga, from an energetic perspective: the first is to stimulate or turn on the energy flow, and the second is to remove blockages.[16] This is analogous to a garden hose that has been left abandoned in a back yard for many years. Over time, mud and insect debris clog the hose. When we go to use the hose again and first turn on the water (which is analogous to stimulating the flow of prana), nothing happens. We have to do some yoga to the hose: we bend it and twist it to loosen up the blockages, turn on the water, and now the water is free to flow. This is what we do in our yoga practice: we move the body via our asana practice and turn on the energy via our breath.

Many forms of pranayamas are taught by the masters, but a number of these can be dangerous to play around with.[17] Like any tool, pranayama can be mishandled; the guidance of an experienced master is essential if we wish to explore the more esoteric pranayamas, especially the very yang-like versions. However, the more yin-like breath work describe below can provide a large measure of the benefit the yogis sought: a calm mind.

Nadi Shodhana

Shodhana means "purification." Thus, *nadi shodhana* is a cleansing of the energy passages. Other names for this practice are alternate nostril breathing or *anuloma viloma*.[18] The practice not only cleanses the nadis, it balances the energies on both sides of the body—yin and yang.

The hand position for nadi shodhana is shown on the next page in figure 7.2. The right hand is used, and the middle two fingers are either folded down to the palm or extended so they can rest on the spot between the eyebrows. As shown in figure 7.3, the right thumb is used to press in on the right side of the nose, closing that nostril. The little finger and ring fingers are kept together and are used to close the left nostril. Since the right arm will be lifted up during the practice, it may get heavy. You can use the left hand to support the right arm.

Basic Pattern

Exhale and begin with the left side by using the right thumb to press against the right nostril, closing it. Now inhale for a count of 4 through the left nostril; then release the right side while closing the left side, and exhale for a count of 4. Complete

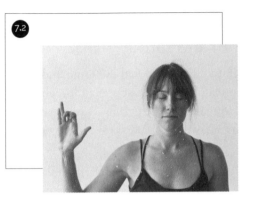
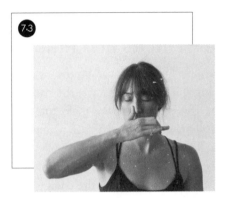

the cycle by inhaling on the right side; close it and open the left side, then exhale. Continue with a 4-count for 8 to 12 cycles. When you are finished, sit quietly.

Adding Kumbhaka and Lengthening the Exhalation

A more advanced version of nadi shodhana keeps the same inhalation timing but extends the exhalation for 8 counts. When this is mastered, you may wish to add retentions. Between the inhalation and the exhalation, pinch both sides of the nose closed and retain the breath for 4 counts. This is antar kumbhaka: retention with lungs full. As you gain experience, you may add bahir kumbhaka at the end of the exhalation, also for 4 counts. You can try a more advanced, extended nadi shodhana practice after a few months with these simple variations, if you experience no difficulties or side effects (visit www.YinYoga.com for a deeper discussion of these practices).

The Hamsa Mantra

Another form of pranayama practice easily adopted into our Yin Yoga practice is the recital of the *Hamsa* mantra. On average, we chant it 21,600 times a day. *"Ha"* is the sound of the breath on our exhalations, and *"sa"* is the sound of the inhalations. Some traditions reverse this, and the mantra is called *"so'ham"*—we hear *"hmmm"* on the inhalation and a sighing *"sa"* on the exhalation. Iyengar says they are actually combined; every creature creates so'ham on the inhalation (which means "he am I") and hamsa on the exhalation (which means "I am he"). This is called the *"ajapa mantra."*[9]

While we chant this barely audible mantra with each breath, we can feel energy moving within us. Close your eyes and notice the way your energy state is altered while you inhale and exhale. Experiment with hearing "ham" on the inhalation and "sa" on the exhalation. Does this feel energizing or calming for you? Next, reverse it. Hear "sa" on the inhalation and "ham" on the exhalation. Does this change the energetic feelings?

Like the ocean breath, hamsa breathing can be used outside of your yoga practice. We all have times in life when we are too stoked up and need to relax. The hamsa breath can be useful then. At other times, we need a quick boost of energy, and the opposite breath may be ideal.

Sometimes, even though we can feel the energy flowing through us, it feels unbalanced. After a long yin practice we can feel a bit "out of it." We need to perk ourselves up. Sometimes after a very yang practice, we may feel energized but overly buzzed. We need to calm down. If Shavasana has not brought you back to a calm but alert state, you may need some stronger medicine to come back to balance, such as nadi shodhana, described above.

Chakras

Within the human body are almost 100 plexuses. A plexus is a joining together (as opposed to a branching apart) of nerves forming a nerve net. The best known is the solar plexus, which is an autonomous cluster of nerve cells behind the stomach and below the diaphragm. Some scientists call the solar plexus our second brain. Blood vessels can form plexuses, such as the choroid plexus in the brain. And yogic sages tell us that nadis also form a network creating plexuses, which they call "chakras." Chakras are wheels or circles and are models of the way the subtle energy in our bodies can be networked into gathering points, in the same way nervous energy may be networked in our solar plexus.

Buddhist yogis developed one of the earliest models of the chakras 1,500 years ago. They helped develop the Tantra school of yoga. Their map showed 5 chakras, one for each of the meditation Buddhas. In the Tantra school of yoga, as practiced in India by Hindu yogis, 7 major plexuses were detected, one for each heavenly plane of existence (or *lokahs*), ranging from the earth to the highest heaven.[20]

The theories of chakras are varied and diverse. There is no consensus on the number of chakras we have (some texts describe 12 or more), their locations, descriptions, or even their purpose or function. Often chakras are depicted in diagrams as having a certain number of lotus petals, a particular color, sound and symbol. But here too there is wide diversity. Commonly agreed is that the chakras are energy centers of the subtle body.

Today we have many more maps than in centuries past. Long ago a *chakra* was not considered a term for nerve plexuses or endocrine glands of the physical body, even though today we notice that they reside in the same general locations. Similarly, chakras are not physical organs of the body. Much has been made of the close proximity and similar functions of the chakras and the endocrine organs, but the ancient yogic texts did not make such claims, and only in the last few decades have some teachers made this association.

There are many books available today that describe chakras in detail.[21] It is difficult to find a definitive explanation of what chakras are supposed to do, but it is safe to say that a chakra is a center of subtle energy (prana or kundalini) that needs to be manipulated to achieve complete physical and spiritual health, and eventual enlightenment. In ordinary individuals, the chakras are undeveloped or even dormant. The practice of yoga helps to awaken the chakras, allowing prana to flow through them. Eventually, when all 6 of the lowest chakras have been opened, energy is free (*ayama*) to reach the highest chakra, and liberation is possible.

Dr. Motoyama's View

One of the purposes of Tantra and Hatha Yogas is the gradual cleansing and opening of each chakra. Once these energies' vortexes are open, the flow of kundalini, or shakti energy, can rise up the central channel, and consciousness merges with God. The impression is easily gained that these chakras must be opened sequentially, beginning with the lowest and moving upward. This is not actually stated in any of the ancient texts on yoga. Many people may have one or two chakras already open but have lower ones blocked.

Paul Grilley's teacher, Dr. Hiroshi Motoyama, believed that the chakras should be opened in a specific sequence but not starting from the bottom one, the muladhara.[22] He strongly advises the student begin with the ajna, which is between the eyes. He says that "if the ajna is awakened first, the overpowering and potentially dangerous karmic forces hidden in the lower chakras may be safely controlled." After awakening the ajna, the yogi opens the muladhara and then the second chakra, the svadhisthana, and on up the line.

Dr. Motoyama reports that in his experience, chakras are less like wheels and more like cones, with the root of the cone in the spine and the top, open end of the cone on the front surface of the body. He calls the front of the chakra the receptor.

There is another major difference between Dr. Motoyama's view of the function of the chakras and the views of most authors on yoga: Dr. Motoyama determined that the chakras are bridges between 3 bodies we each possess:

1. The physical body and its mind: the consciousness associated with the physical.

2. The astral or subtle body and its mind: the consciousness associated with emotion. This is the home of prana or chi. It is interesting to note that chi obeys physical laws because it bridges both the physical and the astral bodies. Like the beam of a flashlight, chi weakens over space and time.

3. The causal body and its mind: the consciousness associated with wisdom and intellect. This is the home of a higher psychic energy Dr. Motoyama calls "*psi.*" It is also interesting to note that physical laws do not bind psi because psi does not touch the physical body. It does not weaken over space and time, but like a laser stays powerfully focused wherever it is directed.

Dr. Motoyama tells us that the physical body is yang compared to the yin nature of the astral and causal bodies. The chakras link these bodies together and allow information and energy to flow between them. It is due to this linkage that yogis throughout the ages have been reportedly able to perform impossible feats. For example, a master buried alive for weeks with no air, food or water survives because of his ability to transform astral energies into physical energy.

A DAOIST VIEW

In the first chapter, we began to look at a Daoist map that described the experience of the yogis of ancient China. We saw how, of the 5 major Daoist practices, inner alchemy became the practice of choice for the yogis seeking physical immortality.[23] A major component of the Daoist practice was controlling energy, just as it was in India. While the intentions were similar, the processes were different, and the maps created by the Daoists displayed different concepts and practices. In time, the maps blazed by the early Daoists became useful to doctors trying to treat their patients, and a branch of medicine evolved, which today we call Traditional Chinese Medicine (TCM).[24] Key to understanding Chinese medicine and the inner alchemical practices of the Daoist (and to understanding the benefits for us modern yinsters) is to be familiar with the important concepts found in the Daoist maps.

Chi

In Chinese medicine, a model of the body is used that is based upon energy and the passages along which energy flows to nourish the organs. These passages, similar to the yogic nadis, are called meridians.[25] And where the yogic models include psycho-energetic centers, the chakras, in the Chinese models the organs are the important centers for energy storage and distribution. In the Chinese model, the organs are functions residing not just within the physical location of the organs as we know them in the West—but within every cell of the body.

Chi (also spelled *Qi*) is derived from the word for *breath*, like *prana* or *spirit*, and denotes this essential life force. Unlike prana, chi is a much broader concept. It is not just life force: chi is the mystical, subtle force that moves the universe. One meaning for the word is "weather." Another is "heaven's breath." Chi is the pulsation of the universe itself. It is found everywhere, in all things animate and inanimate. It is not quite energy or matter; rather, it can be considered energy on the verge of becoming matter, or matter on the verge of becoming energy. Chi is becoming and being. Chi doesn't cause things to happen, as chi is always present before, during and after any change or event.[26] Another useful definition of chi is "organizational energy."[27] Whether chi is real or merely a metaphor is not important; thousands of years of successful medical use show how useful this map is.

When we looked at the Indian view of energy, we noticed that there were 5 main kinds of prana within the body. In a similar manner, the Daoist yogis and doctors discerned 5 kinds of chi, known as the fundamental textures:

- Chi
- Blood
- Jing
- Shen
- Fluids

Blood

Blood is what we would normally think of as blood in the West but with a bit more to it. Blood moves constantly throughout the body, flowing in both the blood vessels we are familiar with in the West and also through the meridians. Blood nurtures, nourishes and moistens. Blood is a yin complement to the yang chi. Where chi excites, Blood calms. Where chi advances, Blood remains.

Jing

There are many interpretations of what exactly jing is and does. Sometimes referred to as *essence*, jing can be considered the material basis of our body that nourishes and fuels our cells. Jing also cools the body and thus is yin in nature. Jing controls the long-term cycles of life rather than the quick daily rhythms. With an ample supply of jing, we grow wiser as we mature in old age; without enough jing, our aging is less graceful and we rage against the changes in our body.

One definition of jing notes that it is a form of chi found in sexual fluids. Another possible consideration is that jing is the carrier of our original physical nature. It is in the DNA that our cells build upon. Jing is stored in the Kidneys and is carried in the semen and menstrual fluids. From the Kidneys, jing is distributed to all other organs to help them in their normal, healthy functioning.

There are two kinds of jing: "before-heaven," the jing given to us before our birth, and "after-heaven," the jing we gain from living, eating and exercising. Unfortunately, our store of the prenatal jing is fixed and cannot be replenished. Once it is used up, life is over. Jing is consumed constantly just by being alive; however, some activities consume jing too quickly: stress, illness, too much sex or inappropriate sex, or abuse of substances. Some activities restore jing, but only the postnatal kind.

Think of jing as two bank accounts. One is a savings account into which you can never put more money. This account is filled at birth. The second is a checking account that allows deposits and withdrawals. When your checking account is overdrawn, funds are automatically transferred from your savings account. Once your savings account balance reaches zero, tilt! Game over.

The secret to longevity is to use up as little before-heaven jing as possible while building up a store of after-heaven jing through Daoist practices such as ch'i-kung, t'ai chi ch'uan, or Yin Yoga. Beyond these practices, just living mindfully will lengthen your life and develop wisdom: eat healthy foods, get plenty of sleep, hang out with inspiring people, and avoid unhealthy activities, individuals and practices. [28]

Shen

Shen is a broad term. A poor English translation would be *"soul."* Sometimes, Chinese Christians use *shen* as the word for *God*. Shen is the most refined and subtle form of chi. Shen is the inner strength underlying chi and jing, and it is closely associated with consciousness. Shen is awareness and is also associated with creativity. If shen is weakened, a person will suffer in many ways: forgetfulness and foggy thinking, insomnia or erratic behaviors may arise.[29]

Fluids

Fluids are all the other liquids we have not yet discussed. These include saliva, urine, perspiration and all the digestive liquids. Some fluids are dark and heavy, while others are light and clear. Fluids lubricate and nourish, feeding the skin, hair, muscles, joints, brain, organs, bones and marrow. While related to Blood, these other fluids are not as deep or as important as Blood.

Other Forms of Chi

The above categorization of chi is not the only model used. Some Chinese practitioners have different mappings for chi. Just as the yogis in India discovered 10 kinds of prana, some Daoist yogis have detected 32 different types of chi. Chi has been categorized as:

- Yuan chi: original chi given before birth, which governs our Organs.
- Gu chi: chi from food, also called grain chi.
- Kong chi: chi from air.
- Zong chi: gathering chi, created by combining gu chi and kong chi. Zong chi circulates the Blood.
- Zheng chi: true chi, created from zong chi when it is acted on by yuan chi. This is the chi most often referred to in texts.
- Ying chi: nourishing chi, which nourishes the Organs and produces Blood.
- Wei chi: defensive chi, which protects and warms the body.

- Organ chi: each Organ has its own form of chi.
- Earth chi: this form is often the main concern of feng-shui, the art of arranging your home in accordance with the flow of chi in nature.
- Sun or Sky chi: the energy we receive from above.

This is not a complete list. Many of the above forms of chi combine to create different types of chi. Like jing, a certain amount of chi is given to us before our birth, but we can also gain more chi through our diet, breath, exercise and meditation.

Function of Chi

One very important purpose of chi is to support the function of the organs. Chi helps to digest food and transform it into Blood and energy. Chi defends the body against infection and pathogens. Chi also maintains the body's temperature and circulation; it keeps the organs in place, keeps the Blood in its vessels, and governs the elimination of excess materials. Chi makes all movement and growth possible. When chi is out of balance, it can become deficient or stagnant; these are opportunities for disease and illness to arise.

There are 4 key pathological conditions of chi:

- Deficient chi: manifests as shortness of breath, dizziness, fatigue, paleness
- Sinking chi: manifests as prolapse of the organs
- Stagnant chi: manifests as various forms of pain
- Rebellious chi: manifests as coughing, belching, vomiting or hiccupping

It is clear how important chi is to our health. From a purely pragmatic perspective, learning to acquire and utilize chi properly, to keep it strong and mobile, will assist in extending a person's lifespan. The quality of that life depends upon other aspects of chi as well: the strength of the shen (spirit) energy and the health of the Organs.

To lay out the full extent of the maps that the Daoists created for energy would take several volumes. We will suspend our investigation into the Daoist concept of energy and move now to look at the next important concept, the Organs. Unlike the concept of chakras developed by Indian yogis, which are found in the subtle body, Organs are physical.

The Organs

As we have already noted, Chinese medical models often refer to the Organs with a capital letter to differentiate their model from the Western view of organs, which are denoted by a lowercase letter. When you see the word Heart, you will know you are dealing with the function of the Heart Organ rather than the physical heart organ, as we know it in the West.

In the Daoist concept of Organs, they are not merely physical entities—they are functions. These functions reside throughout the body, not in one place. Just as the body overall needs these functions to maintain health, each cell also requires the same functions. We cannot say that just the body needs oxygen and needs to eliminate wastes. The functions of respiration (via the Lungs) and elimination (via the Kidneys) are pervasive: every cell in our body needs to be nourished and have its waste removed.

The functions of the body are based upon the 5 solid Organs, referred to as the *zang* organs. These are the Heart, Spleen, Lungs, Kidneys and Liver. Everything in life requires yin and yang for balance; thus, these solid, yin-like zang Organs have their yang counterparts in the hollow *fu* Organs of the Urinary Bladder, Gall Bladder, Small Intestines, Stomach and Large Intestines. Each pair of Organs is connected via meridian channels. Each of the zang Organs is also associated with one of the 5 elements of Daoist cosmology and, through these elements, our emotions.

Zang Organs (Yin)

These are the viscera of the body, the solid organs that store our energies and fluids. These Organs can be considered yin relative to their partner fu Organs because they are solid. There are 6 zang Organs.

The Heart (and Pericardium)

The Heart is the ruler of all the zang Organs. The Heart controls our mental activities and the circulation of Blood. Problems with the Heart are often seen in the face, complexion and tongue. In this model, it is not the brain that controls our thoughts. The brain is simply the place where thoughts are received and stored. Our mental health, our ability to think, and the vigor of our Blood are directly related to the strength of the chi in our Heart. Weak chi here can result in insomnia and poor sleep, disturbing dreams, dullness and heart palpitations. If the Heart is weak, we may be easily startled or frightened, or experience inappropriate euphoria—the kind of joy exhibited by loud, drunk people singing in the streets late at night. If the Heart is strong, we can easily feel love. Feeling love and feeling loved can strengthen the Heart.

The Pericardium is considered an Organ in the Daoist philosophy, unlike in the West, where it is considered simply a fascial bag surrounding the heart. It is the gatekeeper to the heart, according to the Daoists. It prevents disease from entering the Heart, while allowing your loved ones in.

The Spleen

In Chinese medicine, the Spleen is essential for the digestion and distribution of nourishment. If the Spleen's chi is strong, the food's essence is spread throughout the body. If the chi is weak, the body becomes undernourished and weak. This same distribution occurs for water too; the Spleen ensures proper hydration of our cells and the elimination of water through the Kidneys. Because our Blood is mostly water, the Spleen directly affects the quality of our Blood. The Spleen also controls the proper functioning of our limbs and maintenance of our skeletal muscles. The Spleen affects our mental function, especially our intention, willpower and awareness of possibilities for change.

Weakness in the Spleen can often be seen in the lips and mouth. If things taste good, the Spleen is working well. If the Spleen chi is weak, worry may be a constant companion. Worry can weaken the Spleen (and create stomach problems).[30] If the Spleen is strong, we find great stores of creativity.

The Lungs

The Lungs control chi (breath), and since this is the first contact with the external winds, the Lungs have to be vigilant. They are associated with defensive chi to ensure nothing harmful enters the body. The Lungs help to control water and fluids. Edema (water retention) may be caused by a weakness in the Lungs.

The quality of Lung chi is often seen in the skin and hair. Sadness that won't go away may be a sign of weakness in the Lungs. A lot of grief and sadness can weaken the Lungs: just note what happens when we are sad and cry—the Lungs involuntarily spasm. Our ability to see and appreciate beauty indicates health of the Lungs. Noticing and enjoying beauty can strengthen our Lungs.

The Kidneys

The Kidneys store jing. Here this essence of our body can be converted into Kidney chi, which is used to help the Kidneys control water. The Kidneys send clear, healthy water upward to circulate in the body, and used, turbid waters downward for elimination. The Kidneys also govern water utilization. Because Blood and bones are so intimately connected to water, the Kidneys are also responsible for their proper functioning. Determination is said to be stored in the Kidneys, which are also directly connected to reproductive health and function.

Problems with the Kidneys can be seen in the ears and genitals. Problems may result in anxiety or emotions of fear arising at inappropriate times.[31] Too much fear can weaken our Kidneys, but they can also be the source of deep wisdom; when the Kidneys work well, we mature gracefully.

The Liver

The Liver is the home of hun, the ethereal soul (shen) that survives after death. When our shen is calm, the Liver is functioning well, and we can watch the world unfold dispassionately. The Liver has many physiological functions, and a prime one is to regulate the amount of Blood in circulation. While the Heart may govern the flow of Blood, the Liver stores and releases it. Because of this, Liver chi is important for the vitality of all parts of the body.

Weakness in the Liver can be seen in the eyes and tendons. Aching knees are one indicator of weakness; jaundiced eyes are another. When the Liver chi is weak, we may suffer from too much anger or irritation or be unable to express anger at all.[32] Anger management problems can lead to Liver problems. But when the Liver is healthy, we find kindness easy to offer; by offering kindness, we can help to heal our Liver.

The Fu Organs (Yang)

Each of the above zang Organs is yin-like and has a corresponding partner fu or yang Organ. The fu Organs are the receptor Organs. These hollow, yang-like Organs receive the fluids and energies from their zang counterparts. They excrete wastes and receive, digest, absorb and transmit nutrients. We can generalize and say that the fu Organs transform and transmit. There are 6 fu Organs.

The Small Intestines

Paired with the Heart, the Small Intestines receive and store water and food. Just as we understand in the West, the Small Intestines are believed to digest food, convert it into nutrition, and send the unusable bits downward for excretion. A Chinese doctor would call the bits for excretion "turbid" and the nutritious bits "clear." If we are suffering from too much heat or too much dampness, problems may arise in our urinary system, and turbidity will increase.

The Stomach

Paired with the Spleen, the Stomach receives and digests food. It also stores food and water. If Stomach chi is weak, food stagnates and all manner of digestive problems arise, such as flatulence and indigestion.

The Large Intestine

Paired with the Lungs, the Large Intestines compact our solid wastes. Just as the Lungs' chi controls water, the Large Intestines also affect water through the ability to absorb it. Too little absorption and we suffer loose bowels; too much and we become constipated.

The Urinary Bladder

Paired with the Kidneys, the Urinary Bladder stores and excretes urine. If there are problems with Kidney chi, they may show up in issues such as frequent urination or the need to get up at night many times to urinate.

The Gall Bladder

Paired with the Liver, the Gall Bladder stores and excretes bile. (In Chinese medicine, bile is considered Liver chi, not the byproduct of the liver's digestion of fats, as we believe in the West.) Together with the Liver, the Gall Bladder builds and controls the Blood and our overall chi levels. When weak, the Gall Bladder may cause us to be indecisive or hesitant. When strong, the Gall Bladder allows us to be decisive and bold.

The San Jiao

This Organ has no Western counterpart. Sometimes referred to as the Triple Burner, this Organ's function relates to digestion and overall elimination. There are many views of what the San Jiao is and does, but it is often considered to have 3 separable functions and locations:[33]

o The Upper Jiao, located above the diaphragm, distributes water in a mist form throughout the body, assisting the Heart and Lungs.

o The Middle Jiao, located between the diaphragm and the navel, assists the Stomach and Spleen with digestion and the transportation of nutrients.

o The Lower Jiao, located below the navel, assists the Kidneys and Urinary Bladder in their roles of elimination.

Beyond the zang and fu Organs listed here, there are 6 other miscellaneous Organs in the Chinese models. These organs of consciousness are associated with jing energy and include the Brain, Bone Marrow, Blood Vessels, Uterus, Gall Bladder (again!) and the Meridians.

The Five Elements and the Organs

The Greeks developed a model of the universe that posited 4 elements underlying all physical existence: earth, fire, water and air. The yogis of India within the Samkhya philosophy included space as a fifth element. The yogis, however, extended the model to all experience, not just physical forms. In China, the pragmatic Daoists also saw 5 base elements; however, they noted a couple of key differences. The 5 elements in their model are earth, fire, water, metal and wood. They developed this model from the patterns of the universe easily observable to anyone who watches.

Each element begets another. This birthing cycle is very natural. Rain (water) causes plants (wood) to grow. These plants and trees are scorched in summer and feed the flames when fire comes. From the fire, the plants turn to ash, which becomes earth. Within the earth are formed metal ores. Metals, when cold, cause water to condense, forming the rain that begins the creative cycle all over again. Each element not only nourishes; it also controls an element and in turn is controlled—thus, we also have a controlling cycle.

Here we find a universal method of checks and balances. Water promotes the existence of wood, which promotes fire, which burns things to the earth. In the earth we find metals, which through condensation promote the formation of water. In figure 7.4, you can follow the birthing cycle around the outside of the circle: each element nourishes its neighbor. However, we can have too much as well. Control is also need.

Follow the inner lines in the illustration and notice that water douses or controls fire, which melts or controls metal, which cuts or controls wood, which ploughs or controls earth, which soaks up or controls water. Harmony requires checks and balances. If any one element becomes too strong or too weak, imbalance occurs, illness sets in, and harmony is lost.

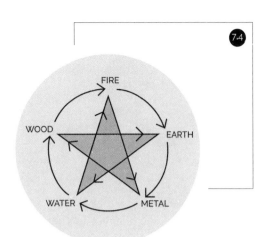

There is a time and a season for each element, as shown in the table below. Winter is a time of metal, while in summer wood predominates. While these observations were made of the external world, the Daoists noticed that the elements are inside us as well. Each of the major Organ pairs is the home of an element. Harmony in our internal world also requires checks and balances. If an Organ is suffering, that may be due to a deficit from its nourishing Organ, or from too much control by the controlling Organ. Physically we suffer if there is too much fire in our body or too little water. A Heart problem, according to a TCM doctor, may actually be a result of weakness in the Kidneys! (Water is not able to control the fire.) Health requires the 5 elements to be balanced. By balancing the energies of each Organ, wholeness can be restored.

Element	Season	Organs
Metal	Autumn	Lungs/Large Intestines
Water	Winter	Kidneys/Urinary Bladder
Wood	Spring	Liver/Gall Bladder
Fire	Summer	Heart/Small Intestines
Earth	Later summer	Spleen/Stomach

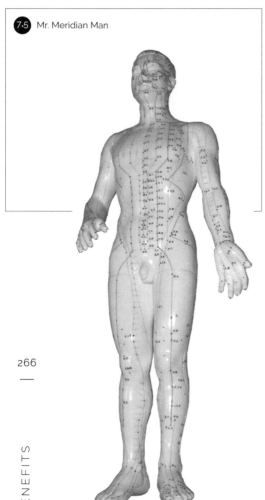

THE MERIDIANS

Meridian is the English translation of the Chinese word for the channels that conduct energy throughout the body. These conduits form a network. If the network is disrupted, if blockages occur, the body will not function properly; if chi, jing and shen do not flow as required, the Organs will not perform their functions, and imbalance arises. When the meridians are clear and open, energy flows freely and all is well.

As in India, the Chinese psychonauts realized that not all channels are equally important. In China, there was greater concern over physical well-being and longevity, and 71 meridians were named; of these, 14 were most important. Each of the 10 major Organs has its associated meridian, and the meridian may be yin or yang, depending upon the zang or fu nature of the Organ. The pericardium and San Jiao also have their associated meridians, which, along with the others, make up 12 major meridians known as *Jing Mai*.

It is worth noting that there is another way to look at these 12 lines: they are actually just one large loop! When the loop is descending in one area, it is given a specific name, and when it turns and ascends, it has another name; turning again and going out, a new name; coming back, another name. In this way, while we have 12 named segments, it is all one very long, looping meridian. In addition to these 12 segments, we will later examine 2 additional significant channels that bring the total number of major meridians to 14.

We will limit our investigation to these major meridians. There are 6 that begin or end in the feet. Relative to their position in the body, these can be considered yin meridians, compared to another 6 that begin or end in the hands, which can be considered yang meridians. As yin meridians, these lower ones are more strongly affected during a Yin Yoga practice than the higher yang meridians. Our investigation begins with these 6 lower lines.[34] We will describe each meridian as a single line, but they are bilaterally symmetric: there are 2 meridians, one for each side of the body.

THE ENERGETIC BENEFITS

The Lower Body Meridians

These 6 meridians are the lines affected most by the yin asanas. This certainly does not mean we cannot stress the other meridian lines during our Yin Yoga work; we can and do, but since Yin Yoga primarily affects the region from the navel to the knees, these lower 6 are affected more frequently.

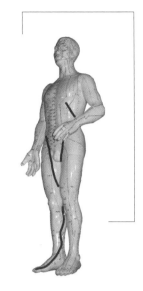

The Liver Meridian

The Liver meridian begins at the inside of the nail of the big toe and runs along the top of the foot. It climbs the front of the ankle and then runs up the inside of the leg until it reaches the pubic area. From here it curves around the external genitalia and goes into the lower abdomen, where it enters the liver and gall bladder.[35] Rising higher, it branches in several directions, with one branch connecting to the Lung meridian. Rising still higher, it follows the throat and connects with the eyes before branching again. One branch reaches down across the cheeks and circles the lips, while a higher one crosses the forehead to the crown, where it links with the Governor Vessel meridian.

Low back pain, abdominal pain or mental disturbances may be a sign of disharmony of the Liver. Frequent or unreasonable anger or irritation may also be a sign of dysfunction here.

The Gall Bladder Meridian

The Gall Bladder meridian begins at the outer corner of the eye and immediately branches into two lines. A main branch remains on the surface and winds back and forth across the side of the head and above the ear before turning downward along the side of the neck. After following the top of the shoulder, it passes under the arm and zigzags along the side of the ribs to the hips. The other branch goes inside the cheek and descends to the liver and gall bladder. From there it descends farther and rejoins the first branch at the front of the hip. The single line then descends, running along the outside thigh and knee until it reaches the ankle. It runs across the top of the foot until it reaches the fourth toe; another branch leaves at the ankle to run across the top of the foot and join the Liver meridian at the big toe.

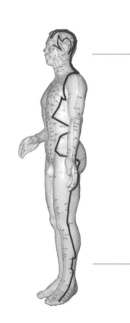

Headache, blurred vision and pains along the side of the body, including the eyes, ears and throat, may be an indication of problems with the Gall Bladder meridian.

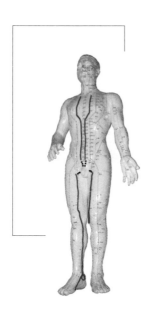

The Kidney Meridian

The Kidney meridian begins at the outside of the little toe, but it stays inside the foot until it surfaces in the sole of the foot, just below the third toe, behind the ball of the foot. From there it follows the sole, makes a circle around the inner ankle, runs through the heel, and comes up the inmost side of the leg and into the tailbone. It follows the spine to the kidney and then branches. One branch heads to the urinary bladder, where it comes back to the surface of the abdomen and up the chest, ending at the clavicle. The other branch touches the liver and diaphragm and moves up through the lungs and throat until it ends beside the root of the tongue.

Disharmony here is suggested by gynecological problems, genital disorders, and problems in the kidneys, lungs and throat. Examples may include impotence, frequent urination and weakness in the lower limbs. Anxiety and fear may also occur.

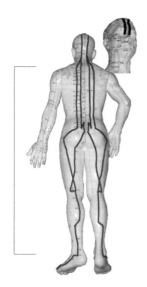

The Urinary Bladder Meridian

The Urinary Bladder meridian starts at the inner eye and then goes up, across the forehead, and to the crown. One branch splits here, enters the brain, and then reemerges at the scapula and runs just inside the line of the scapula, down the spine to the buttocks, where it reenters the body and runs to the urinary bladder and the kidney. The second branch from the crown flows down the back of the neck and shoulder and runs just outside and parallel to the first branch. This branch continues down the back of the buttocks and legs, circles the outer ankle, runs along the outer edge of the foot and ends in the small toe.

Signs of disharmony in the Urinary Bladder may include backaches, headaches, an inability to urinate, mental problems and disease of the lower limbs.

The Spleen Meridian

Starting at the medial side of the big toe, the Spleen meridian runs along the inside of the foot, then turns and runs up the inside of the ankle and the shin. Up to the knee, it runs just above the Liver meridian, then it runs along the top of the thigh and enters the abdominal cavity, just above the pubic bone. It connects to the spleen and then the stomach, where it branches. The main branch comes to the surface and runs up the chest to the throat, where it again enters the body, going to the root of the tongue, where it spreads out. The second branch remains internal and reaches the heart, connecting to the Heart meridian.

Indications of Spleen disharmony include stomach problems, flatulence, vomiting and bloating. Unreasonable worry may also arise.

The Stomach Meridian

Beginning at the side of the nose, the Stomach meridian rises to the corner of the eye before descending along the side of the nose. Entering the upper gum, it follows the outer lips to the lower jaw, toward the joint of the jaw. Here one branch ascends along the front of the ear to the forehead. The other branch descends through the body to the diaphragm and runs to the stomach and spleen. A third branch emerges from the lower jaw and runs across the outside of the body, crossing the chest and belly and terminating in the groin. The line that runs through the stomach reconnects with this third branch and runs downward along the front of the leg, reaching the top of the foot. Here it splits again, with the main branch ending in the outside tip of the second toe. The other branch reaches the inner side of the big toe. Just below the knee, an additional branch splits off and runs to the lateral side of the third toe.

Problems with the Stomach meridian may be indicated by bloating, vomiting, pain in any of the areas the meridian passes through (mouth, nose, teeth, etc.) and mental problems.

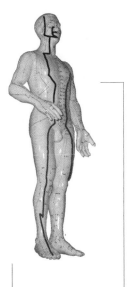

269

The Upper Body Meridians

There are 6 meridians that begin or end in the fingers. They all pass through the shoulder or armpit. While our normal Yin Yoga practice does not target these lines specifically, it is possible to affect all our meridians during a Yin Yoga practice, as described in Chapters 3 and 4.

The Heart Meridian

The 3 branches of the Heart meridian begin in the heart. One branch flows downward through the diaphragm to meet the small intestines. Another rises up alongside

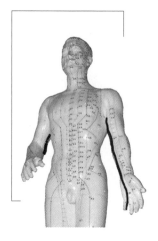

the throat and ends in the eye. The third runs across the chest, through the lungs, and comes out through the armpit. It flows along the midline of the inside upper arm, through the inner elbow, along the midline of the inner lower arm, until it crosses the wrist and palm and ends in the inside tip of the little finger, where it connects to the Small Intestine meridian.

Disorders of the heart and chest such as palpitations, pain, insomnia, night sweats and mental problems may signal problems with this meridian.

The Small Intestine Meridian

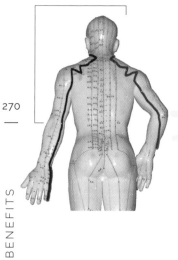

The Small Intestine meridian begins at the outer tip of the little finger. It runs along the back edge of the hand, through the wrist, upward along the outer forearm and upper arm, to the shoulder. After circling the back of the shoulder, it meets the Governor Vessel meridian. Here it branches, with one branch going inside the body and descending through the heart, diaphragm and stomach before ending in the small intestine. Another branch ascends along the side of the neck to the cheek and outer corner of the eye and then goes to the ear. Another small branch leaves the cheek to run to the inner eye, where it meets the Urinary Bladder meridian.

Disharmony may be indicated by ear, eye or stomach problems, such as deafness, pain in the lower abdomen or pain in the shoulders or neck.

The Lung Meridian

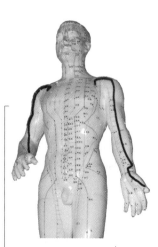

The Lung meridian begins inside the belly just above the navel and drops down to the large intestines. From here it comes back up through the diaphragm and connects to the stomach. It ascends through the lungs and follows the throat before coming to the front of the shoulder from under the clavicle. From here it runs along the outer, thumb side of the upper arm and the front of the lower arm. It crosses the wrist and ends at the outer tip of the thumb. A small branch goes from the wrist to the tip of the index finger, where it connects to the Large Intestine meridian.

Respiratory problems such as coughs, asthma and chest pains may signify dysfunction. Extreme and persistent sadness and grief may also indicate problems here.

THE ENERGETIC BENEFITS

The Large Intestine Meridian

Beginning at the tip of the index finger, the Large Intestine meridian runs between the thumb and forefinger and along the outside of the arm. It comes over the outside top of the shoulder and along the back of the shoulder blades to the spine. Here, one branch descends through the lungs, diaphragm and large intestines. The second branch ascends along the neck and lower cheek and enters the lower gum, circling the lower teeth. On the outside, this line also circles the upper lips, crosses under the nose and rises up to join the Stomach meridian.

Problems in the mouth, teeth, nose and throat, such as toothaches and sore throats, as well as problems with the neck and shoulders, may indicate disharmony.

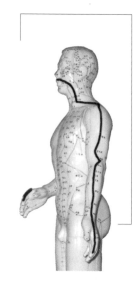

The Pericardium Meridian

The pericardium is a bag of fascia that envelops the heart. Chinese medicine considers it an Organ of its own. The Pericardium meridian begins in the chest and connects to the pericardium. From here it moves down the chest, connecting the 3 sections of the San Jiao meridian. Another branch moves horizontally across the chest, coming to the surface of the ribs, up and around the armpit, and down the front of the bicep and forearm to the palm, ending at the tip of the middle finger. A small branch leads from the palm to the tip of the ring finger, where it connects to the San Jiao meridian.

Pain in the heart area, poor circulation, stomach problems and mental problems may indicate disharmony of the Pericardium meridian.

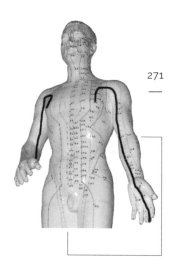

271
—

The San Jiao Meridian

The San Jiao meridian is often called the Triple Burner or Triple Energizer. It begins in the ring finger, where the Pericardium meridian ends. It runs over the back of the hand, wrist and lower arm. It passes the outer point of the elbow and the back of the upper arm to the posterior shoulder. From here it comes over the shoulder to the front of the body and enters the chest beneath the sternum. It branches, with the main branch running to the pericardium and continuing down through the diaphragm to the 3 burners: upper, middle and lower. The second branch ascends along the side of the neck, circles the back of the ear, and then circles the side of the face. Another small

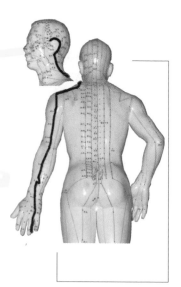

branch emerges from the back of the ear and connects to the Gall Bladder meridian at the outer corner of the eye.

Problems associated with this meridian may occur in the side of the face, neck or throat, or in the abdomen. Examples include deafness, ringing in the ears, bloating and urinary difficulties.

The Extra Meridians

The meridian system is made up of the lines connecting the 5 yin and 6 yang organs, plus the pericardium line. Beyond these 12 are 8 additional meridians that a Chinese doctor must know. We will visit the two most important: the Governor Vessel and the Conception Vessel meridians. These are important because they have acupuncture points separate from those on any of the other 12 main meridians. All the other extra meridians share points with the meridians already mapped out.

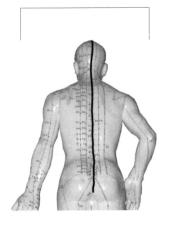

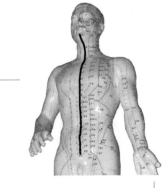

The Governor Vessel

The Governor Vessel begins within the lower belly and splits in 3. Two smaller branches ascend to connect to each kidney. The third and main branch descends to the perineum,[36] where it enters the tip of the spinal cord and rises up to the brain. This branch comes over the top of the skull, down the middle of the forehead and nose, and terminates in the upper gum. Dr. Motoyama recommends the practice of nadi shodhana to purify this meridian.

The Conception Vessel

This meridian also begins in the lower abdomen next to the Governor Vessel. It has only one branch, and it too descends to the perineum. Emerging from the muladhara, it ascends along the front midline of the body through the neck and chin to the mouth. At the mouth, it splits and goes around the lips before sending branches to the lower eyes.

The Governor Vessel and Conception Vessel run along the front and back of the torso. These lines also contain the front and back of each chakra. When we breathe and draw energy up the Governor Vessel and down the Conception Vessel, we are completing the microcosmic orbit.

The Microcosmic Orbit

Pranayama is an Indian yogic way to stimulate and move energy through the nadis. The Daoists have their own ways to move chi, including ch'i-kung and t'ai chi ch'uan. They also use a meditation called the microcosmic orbit, which is a translation of the Daoist term for a full orbiting of energy through the front and back body. In Japanese, it is called "*shoshuten,*" which means a "circling of light."[37] The microcosmic orbit is a way to gather and channel all the stray energies in the body and raise them up from the muladhara to the ajna. This activation of energy is a key preparation for many advanced Daoist practices. Through activating the microcosmic orbit, the reservoirs of the Governor Vessel and Conception meridians are refilled, which means this energy is available to all other meridians and Organs. This is perhaps the best way to cultivate health and long life while at the same time preparing the way to a deep spiritual understanding.

Circulating energy through the microcosmic orbit can be done even during a yoga practice: perhaps prior to asana practice, just before meditation, during the long holds in the yin poses, or even at the beginning of Shavasana as we lie on our backs. The following instructions are fusions of both Daoist principles and yoga philosophy, but the results may prove beneficial to you.

To employ the microcosmic orbit while in Shavasana or in a seated meditation, bring your awareness to the second chakra on the front of the body. This is the *svadhisthana,* which is about halfway between your navel and pubic bone. Feel, or imagine you feel, energy there. Exhale completely. As you inhale, follow a flow of energy down the midline of your body, under the pubic bone to the tailbone, and then upward, along the spine, the back of the neck, over the top of your head, and right to the ajna point between the eyebrows. Pause here at the top of the inhalation for 2 or 3 seconds. As you exhale, slowly feel the energy descend inside the face and throat. Continue to follow the midline of the body down to the sternum, to the navel, and right back to the svadhisthana. Pause here for 2 or 3 seconds before beginning a new orbit. (See figure 7.22.)

As you orbit the body, mentally touch each chakra on both the yin and yang sides (front and back) of the body; feel the energy at those points. Two or 3 minutes of orbiting the energy should be sufficient. When you have finished, release the effort and let the breath be whatever it wants to be. Watch closely how you feel, without reacting to anything.

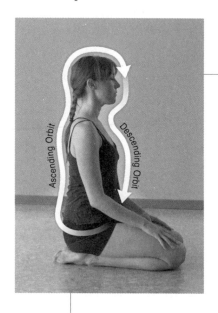

7.22

A Simpler Orbit

Ultimately, we would like the energy in our central channel (the *sushumna* nadi or Governor Vessel) to flow freely, unobstructed. Before this happens, we need the meridians flowing beside the central nadi to be open—the ida and pingala nadis. Indian yogis might use nadi shodhana to open up both channels. We can achieve the same effect by mentally circulating energy through these 3 channels as we breathe and hold our postures.

Begin by feeling the heart center. Sit comfortably and close your eyes. Exhale. Start when the lungs are empty. As you inhale, feel or imagine energy flowing down your spine to the tip of the sacrum. As you exhale, reverse this, and follow the energy as it flows back up to the heart space. Repeat this a few times. Slow the breath down to at least 4 counts for each inhale and exhale. (See figure 7.23.)

At first, there will be no sensation of anything flowing anywhere. Don't be discouraged; this type of sensing takes practice. For now, just pretend you can feel it. It may be helpful to imagine someone running a finger along your spine, down from the heart on inhalations and back up to the heart on exhalations.

Once you can follow this flow, even if only in your imagination, add a short pause at the end of the inhalation. The energy now is in the *muladhara* chakra, at the base of the spine. Leave it there for a moment, but bring your awareness to the *ajna* chakra, between the eyebrows. Just feel, or pretend to feel, energy there. After a second or so, exhale, following the energy back up to the heart.

Try this for a few cycles. If you can follow the energy without distraction for a few cycles, add this final variation: continue to pause at the end of the inhalation but add a short pause at the end of the exhalation as well. By the end of the exhalation, the energy will have returned to the heart space. Leave it there, but bring your awareness back to the muladhara chakra. Feel the perineum and notice the energetic lift there. Hold for just a moment, and begin the next inhalation by returning your awareness back to the heart. All of this can be done with the ocean breath. Remember: a 4-count inhale, 1-count pause, 4-count exhale and a 1-count pause.

When we allow energy to descend on the inhalation, we are joining the prana from the in-breath to the apana in the lower belly. When we reverse this, we are joining the apana from the out-breath to the prana in the upper body. This simple work with the breath moves us toward this ultimate goal.[38] We can do this while we hold a pose. All it takes is intention and attention.

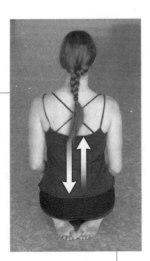

7.23

Orbiting Energy While in a Pose

Backbends are naturally more energetic than forward bends; forward bends are naturally more calming than backbends. We can practice the simple orbiting of energy in any asana, but when we are in backbends, it feels more natural to pause only at the top of the inhalation and bring awareness to the ajna chakra. When we are in forward bends, it feels more natural to hold the breath only at the end of the exhalation and bring our awareness to the muladhara chakra.

When you come into backbends like the Seal, Sphinx or Saddle poses, orbit the energy as discussed above, but only hold the breath at the end of the inhalation. Bring awareness up to the ajna. Pause for a few seconds, then complete the orbit. Do this for approximately half of the time you are holding the pose. For the second half, simply release and follow the breath's natural rhythm, or come to an awareness of the predominant sensation in your body.

When you come into forward bends like the Butterfly, Dragonfly or Snail poses, again orbit the energy, but this time, hold the breath only at the end of the exhalation. Bring awareness down to the muladhara. Engage your chi bridge there.[39] Pause for a few seconds, and then complete the orbit. In any other posture where you are in neither a forward bend nor a backbend, you can continue with holding the breath at the end of both inhalation and exhalation.

A Simple Variation

Now that you have mastered a basic orbit, you may choose to add the side channels. Here we draw the energy down, as before, on the inhalation, but as we hold the breath for a couple of seconds, we send the energy up the left side of the torso, through the heart space, and down the right side, back to the base of the spine. We just hold at the end of the inhalation; there is no retention at the end of the exhalation. On the next cycle, circle the energy up the right side and down the left side while you retain the breath. (See figures 7.24 and 7.25.) Cycling the energy through the left and right sides of the body stimulates and balances the flow of energy through the ida and pingala nadis. In all these variations, you may wish to add the hamsa, so'ham or ocean breaths.

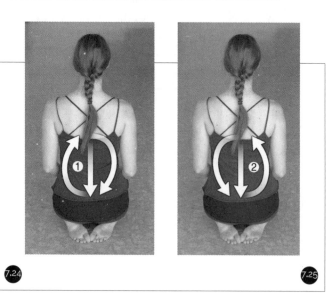

7.24 7.25

There is a yang variation to the orbiting breath: breathe very *deeply*, and hold for a long time with full lungs. This is energizing. In the yin variation, breathe much more quietly and shallowly, and hold with empty lungs for only a few seconds. This is calming.

Acupuncture and Acupressure

The meridian lines flow along the surface of the body and deep inside as well. The interior lines are more important than those on the outside, but along the exterior paths there are special locations, known as acupuncture points, where stimulation is believed to increase or enhance the flow of the various textures through the meridians. There are two ways we can stimulate these points: acupuncture and acupressure.

The practice of acupuncture goes back over 2,000 years. While many high cultures utilized massage, breath work, exercises, special herbs and other dietary prescriptions to enhance health and longevity, the Daoists are unique in their use of needles. The earliest needles were probably bone or bamboo, but it didn't take long for metal needles to come into vogue, with silver and gold being the favorites. In modern times, disposable stainless steel needles are used.

How deeply the needles are inserted depends upon where they are being used: a few millimeters may be enough in the hands, but 2 or 3 inches may be required in the buttocks. Often a dozen or more will be required in any one session. Sometimes the needles are just left in, quietly, and other times they are jiggled, twisted, electrified or heated. They can be left in for just a few seconds or for a few days! But usually they are left in from 20 to 40 minutes. Generally, a dull, achy sensation is felt: this shows that the needles are in fact doing something. What they are doing is rebalancing the energies: what is stagnant will circulate, what is deficient will increase, what is cold will be warmed. Chi and Blood will be affected, and thus all the textures of the body will be affected. Each meridian line upon which the acupuncture points lie pertains to a specific Organ pair, so these Organs also benefit from the procedure.

There are 3 other ways to stimulate the flows of energy beyond acupuncture. In our Yin Yoga practice, we stimulate the flow of chi through acupressure, awareness of sensations and directing the breath. Acupressure, while not as precise as acupuncture, is a simple massaging (compressing or stretching) of the tissues that lie along the meridian lines. Like acupuncture, this can also stimulate energy flow and rebalance our systems. For example, if we feel a strong tugging along the inner groin while in Straddle Pose, we may be stimulating the Liver and Kidney meridians. If we feel a tugging along the outside of the hips in full Swan and compression along the lower back due to the backbend, we may be stimulating the Gall Bladder and Urinary Bladder meridians.

In general, every time we come into a Yin Yoga pose, we should pay attention to where we are feeling the stress. Check the pictures shown earlier to see which meridian lines run along the areas where the stress is significant, and you will discover which meridian lines you are affecting. You will find that we often are stimulating several lines at once. Remember too that the meridian lines will feed more than one Organ. We stimulate yin/yang Organ pairs—for example, stimulating the Gall Bladder in Swan also benefits the Liver. And any time we stimulate the Kidneys, because they are the home of jing, we benefit all other Organs.

Pay attention to the sensations. If you are feeling it, you are doing it! Notice where you are feeling it. Bringing awareness to an area can stimulate energy to flow there. You can test this out for yourself: concentrate on the tip of your thumb for 1 minute. Feel it. You will notice it growing measurably warmer. Where our attention goes, energy flows! Blood vessels dilate, allowing nutrients and healing to increase.

The final way to stimulate energy flow is through directed breathing. Not only does our breath bring oxygen into our system (which our cells use to burn their fuels and release energy), but the very act of breathing can also be stimulating. If we combine a slow, steady breath with an awareness of what that breath feels like in a targeted area (or along a meridian line), we can also enhance the flow of energy to that region. Of course, we don't have lungs all over our body, but we do possess a body-wide fascial network. Each breath stresses that network, and if we are very attentive, we can feel this stress in the targeted area of each posture.

To summarize: there are 4 ways to turn on the tap (to stimulate energy flow in the body):

1. Acupuncture
2. Acupressure
3. Awareness
4. Directed breath

Acupuncture is the only procedure we do not use in a Yin Yoga practice. The other 3 can be consciously adopted to enhance your energy flow.

Emotions

Sometimes what we are feeling is not just physical sensations in the body, but strong emotions. The Daoist yogis noticed that our emotions are embodied. Modern yogis have noticed the same thing and coined the phrase "issues in our tissues." Our Organs are the home of emotions: the Heart contains both love and exuberance. Our Liver contains kindness and anger. Our Kidneys can be the source of fear or the source of deep-seated wisdom. The effect is circular: each Organ not only houses certain emotions, but our emotions can affect the pertaining Organs. Too much fear can deplete Kidney energy (jing). Conversely, if we have too little jing, we may become fearful. The following table shows the positive and negative emotions associated with specific organs, along with their base element.

Organ Pair (Yin/Yang)	Negative/Positive Emotion	Element
Spleen/Stomach	Worry/Creativity	Earth
Liver/Gall Bladder	Anger/Kindness	Wood
Kidneys/Urinary Bladder	Fear/Wisdom	Water
Heart/Small Intestines	Elation or Inappropriate Joy/Love	Fire
Lungs/Large Intestines	Sadness or Grief/Beauty	Metal

Due the circular effect of Organ health and emotions, you can decide to create a Yin Yoga practice to specifically address an emotional issue by targeting the appropriate Organ pair. If you are sad, work the Lung meridians or seek out beauty in the world. If you are fearful, target the Kidneys and Urinary Bladder or cultivate wisdom. Angry a lot? Target the Liver and Gall Bladder, or perform random acts of kindness. Stomach issues? Be creative: write a poem, paint a picture, create a song.

The Indian yogis also noticed a correlation between our bodies and our heart/emotions; so don't be surprised if, during a deep Yin Yoga practice, emotions start to surface. This is part of the practice. Just as we can have physical scar tissues that need to be broken through, we may also have emotional scar tissue to work through. Hip openers will often elicit feelings of frustration, annoyance and anger. Hip openers tend to stress the Gall Bladder meridian and its partner, the Liver, which is the home of anger and frustration. Deep backbends may create feelings of fear or anxiety: here we are working deeply into the Kidneys, which are the home of fear and wisdom. If you can acknowledge your fear, wisdom will grow. If you can be with your anger, kindness may blossom.

Remember to play your edges: don't push too far, too fast. If you are not ready for an emotional release, don't force it. Wait for the heart to open over time. If the emotional sensations are manageable, then let them marinate. We don't have to react to the emotions that arise during our practice; we just need to notice them. Acknowledge what you are feeling and be curious. Yin is allowing: allow what is surfacing to be there, without running away from it or trying to change it—if that is the appropriate response.

If we heal the body, we also heal the heart. Emotional imbalances can be addressed through our practice, which in turn may cure some physiological imbalances. The Daoist maps explain how this happens: our emotions are rooted in the organs, and our organs affect our emotions. What we do to one, we do to the other. Yin Yoga works the total person: our body, heart, mind and soul.

A WESTERN VIEW

To a Western scientist, the purpose of energy is to do work.[40] In the East, energy is much more than this—energy is life! Prana or chi is needed for life's activities. Without prana, there is no life.

In India, the yogic sages observed 10 forms of prana through subjective experience. In China, the Daoists mapped 32 forms of chi. Some seers have intuited even more than this number. To our Western ways of thinking, these subjective claims seem fanciful and unsubstantiated. In the West, we can surmise that the body uses 3 kinds of energy:

1. Transportation energy
2. Transformation energy
3. Communication energy

We use energy to move things around in the body, via the blood system, the digestive system and the lymph system. This is the energy of transportation. We use energy to change materials from one form to another: refining raw food into nutrients and then into cells and tissues. This is the energy of transformation. These 2 forms of energy are gross (meaning not subtle), obvious and easy to measure. The third kind of energy is the energy of communication, of sending information throughout the matrix of the body. Because communication energy is subtle, it is much harder to detect.

Communication occurs chemically via the blood system and electrically along nerves, but there is much more going on than just this. Consider a primitive amoeba: it has no internal vascular system, but if it is injured, it will repair itself. A primitive animal, such as a sponge, will heal even though it has no central nervous system. Obviously, long before there were blood systems and nervous systems, communication and healing were possible within an organism. There is more going on within our bodies than is yet mapped in our Western models. Fortunately, many researchers are hard at work extending our maps to include energy features that the yogis in the East may have been describing.

In this section, we will review just some of the findings in a field called energy medicine. We will begin with a brief primer on electricity and magnetism.

New Paradigms

Wholeness—health—requires communication internally, the ability to move substances and the ability to transform substances. The cells of the body need to communicate with each other. When this communication breaks down, we cannot remain whole. The same point applies to transporting and refining materials within the body. Consider the example of a city during a blackout. When the power is down, transportation is shut down, manufacturing shuts down and communication ceases: the city stops functioning. The body is similar; if we can't communicate information properly, if materials don't flow, if the factories creating tissues are off-line, we are not healthy. In this model, ill health can be considered a failure in communication, transformation and transportation.

For more than five hundred million years, complex life has been evolving and finding ways to improve the ability to communicate, transform and transport. Through trial and error, life has found ways to do this better and better—which means faster, more accurately and with backup systems in case of problems. Nature and her laws of physics provide many possible methods to choose from. The most successful forms of life would naturally adopt as many of these as possible. For our purposes, we will look at the most subtle of these 3 broad forms of energy: the energy of communication.

The earliest multicellular life forms used chemical means to communicate. Materials were physically passed from one cell to the next. Then conduits were created within which these substances could travel farther, faster and more surely. These conduits evolved into our blood vessels. The nervous system evolved in a similar manner.

A new paradigm is evolving in the West, one that broadens the scope of communication far beyond simple chemical and electrical models. This new paradigm includes many other forms of communication that were hinted at by doctors in centuries past.[41] With our modern, sensitive instruments, capable of detecting minute levels of energy, we are able to test these new models. We are going to explore just a couple of these new models, starting with bioelectricity—electricity created by the body.

Bioelectricity

Have you noticed the shoes worn by children that light up as they run? Kids love the flashing light show put on by their shoes, and parents love the fact that no batteries are needed. Where does the electricity come from to spark the lights? The answer is piezoelectricity—electricity created by pressure. The word comes from the Greek *piezein,* which means to squeeze or compress. No batteries required.[42]

Certain kinds of crystals, when subjected to deforming stress, create electrical fields or cause electricity to flow, as shown in figure 7.26. The reverse can also happen:

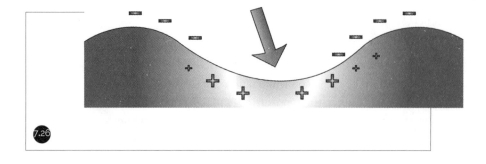

7.26

when an electric field is applied to these crystals, they will bend in response—the stronger the field, the greater the deformation; the greater the stress, the stronger the field.

Piezoelectric crystals do not need to be recharged. When they resume their original shape, the energy potential ends, and when they are deformed again, the field is regenerated. This wonderful ability of some crystals has been exploited in many technologies. From the light show in shoes to barbecues' ignition, microphones and sophisticated sonar systems, piezoelectricity has become commonplace.

A crystal is a structured array of molecules repeated throughout a material. Often overlooked is that tissues in our body are also aligned in structured, repeating patterns. The molecules of our muscles, bones, eyes, cell membranes, collagen, elastin, even our DNA—all have crystal-like structure.

James Oschman in his books summarizing scientific research and energy medicine states that the living tissues of our bodies are best described as liquid crystals. These are materials that are intermediate between solids and liquids and display properties of both.[43] He explains that virtually the whole body is composed of materials arranged in a liquid crystal form and cites several studies confirming this model.

When our liquid crystalline tissues are subjected to deforming stress, they generate piezoelectric potential energy and tiny electric currents. Just like in the children's shoes, every move we make, every breath we take (to paraphrase Sting) creates tiny currents of energy. Let me emphasize—these currents are tiny! No wonder scientists missed their existence and, once they finally were discovered, dismissed their importance.

If these piezoelectric energies we are discussing were expected to transport or transform materials in our body, we would be right to think they have no chance of affecting us. They are too tiny. But consider this metaphor. Suppose that you are cooking a big Thanksgiving turkey (or, for vegetarian yogis, a Tofurky™). You need to preheat the oven, but you don't know how high to set it. You call your mother on your cell phone, and she tells you to try 400 degrees Fahrenheit. The cell phone consumes a very small amount of electricity, say 50 milliwatts. The oven produces a great deal of heat and requires 1,000 watts to run properly.[44] And yet, until the small current in the cell phone gives you the information you need, all that power in the oven is dormant. Certainly the cell phone could not hope to power the oven. But without the information transmitted via the cell phone, the power in the oven would never be activated. A small amount of information can create big changes, and this small amount of information requires very little power compared to the large effect it stimulates. The tiny currents of piezoelectricity are not too small to have effects; they are just what we need to turn things on or off.

If our bodies can be considered like liquid crystals, and if even small movements create electric fields and currents, this could provide a basis for scientific models of information and energy transfers beyond purely chemical or electrical mechanisms, which solely rely on our nervous system or blood system. With such models we can begin to see how modalities that manipulate the body physically, such as yoga and massage, might have an effect on the functioning of our bodies and our health.

Bioelectricity and Our Bones

We have already seen that Yin Yoga can fight degeneration of our bones. One of the many tissues structured in a crystalline array is our bone tissue. When we stress our bones, we create little piezoelectric currents within the bone itself.[45] This current signals the cells within the bones and affects their behaviors. There are cells in our bones whose job it is to create new bone, called osteoblasts, and there are cells whose job it is to clean up old, worn-out bones, called osteoclasts. If we actively stress our bones, through yoga, walking or other weightbearing exercises, we may be telling our osteoclasts to slow down their destruction of older bone, while allowing the osteo-blasts to continue to build new bone, thus making our bones thicker and stronger. Without stress on the bones, they become hollowed out by the continuous action of the osteoclasts. We need to stress the bones so that we create electrical currents that slow down degeneration.

This is not just happening within our bones: these piezoelectric currents are occurring all over our body, guiding our cells to either get busy or slow down. Another form of electrical signaling, again occurring outside our central nervous system, is the injury-repair current. This is a small current created in our tissues when they are damaged, and it is used to signal to various cells that help is needed. This current does not flow through our nerves but through the water-filled spaces within our tissues. The signals are able to attract immune cells, fibroblasts, stem cells and other cells needed to repair the damage. When the repairs are completed, the current ceases.

Electromagnetism

There are two basic kinds of magnets: permanent magnets and electromagnets. The permanent magnets are familiar to everyone; they're what attach notes to the door of your fridge. Electromagnets have a magnetic field only when an electric current is present. When we pass a current through a wire, a magnetic field is created all around the wire. If we reverse the direction of the current, the orientation of the magnetic field also reverses.

A moving electron creates both electric and magnetic fields. It is therefore better to consider electric and magnetic fields as aspects of a more general type of field, known as the electromagnetic field. When we use this term, we are referring to the electrical field, the magnetic field or both.

There are naturally occurring electromagnetic fields and artificially created ones. The earth has a very large magnetic field compared to the fields inside our bodies. The electrical wires outside and inside your home also have electromagnetic fields. These fields also arise from your fridge magnets, stereo speakers and computer power supplies. Some household fields can be far stronger than the earth's magnetic field but are not as pervasive.

Our heart has electric currents regulating it, and as a result it has an electromagnetic field. The size of our heart's magnetic field is one million times smaller than the earth's magnetic field, and it too can vary from person to person and from time to time within the same person. Despite its weakness, the electromagnetic field of the heart is measurable. Electrocardiograms (ECGs) are used to measure the electrical force at various locations throughout the body.[46] Our brains are also a source of electrical activity and have a measurable field. The brain's magnetic field is around a thousand times weaker than the heart's and naturally was not detected until long after the heart's field was discovered.

Any electrons in motion will give rise to an electromagnetic field. What about those tiny piezoelectric fields discussed in the previous section? Do they create electromagnetic fields and, if so, can they be measured? These tiny fields, while too small to have been detected until recently, do exist, and their associated electromagnetic fields have been measured thanks to the invention of a cool-sounding device known as a SQUID.[47] Invented by John Zimmerman in the early 1970s, a SQUID allows magnetometers to detect very small electromagnetic fields. Using this device, Zimmerman and others after him were able to detect an increase in the electromagnetic field of a therapeutic touch from a practitioner's hands.[48] The study of these generated electromagnetic fields is called bioelectromagnetism.

Bioelectromagnetism

Our blood is mostly water with a lot of salts and minerals dissolved in it. Water saturated like this turns out to be an excellent conductor for electricity. It is not surprising that an ECG will pick up signals from the heart throughout the body: the field is propagated via the blood system and the water in our fascia. The heart's electrical field touches every part of us, and its magnetic field is also pervasive. The signals from the heart have been speculated to send information throughout our matrix. The heart is not just a pump: it is the center of a communication system that can let the whole body know what is happening. Unfortunately, in earlier standard medical paradigms, the presence of the body's electric fields was used only as a diagnostic tool; these models could not predict any therapeutic procedures that could utilize the electric or magnetic fields of the body. As we will see, alternative medicine practitioners have used this knowledge in a therapeutic way.

So far we have discussed only how an electron in motion gives rise to a magnetic field. The reverse is also true. A moving magnetic field can create an electrical current. This is how an electric generator works. A magnet is placed within a coil of wires. When the magnet is rotated, electricity is created. Conversely, if electricity is run through the coil, the magnet rotates. That is the basis for an electric motor.

Not only do our bodies create magnetic fields, they can also be affected by them. After inventing the SQUID, John Zimmerman began some interesting research on the magnetic fields of touch therapists. A similar but more detailed study was done later in Japan.[49] The Japanese study included not just therapists but also ch'i-kung masters, Zen masters, yogis and meditators. The results of these studies showed that a therapeutic touch specialist emitted from her hands magnetic fields that were 100 to 1,000 times stronger than our heart's field. The studies also revealed that the magnetic fields were pulsating at low frequencies, ranging from 0.3–30 Hz.[50] Most of the magnetic field frequencies centered around 7–8 Hz, but the fields continuously spanned the range of frequencies. Of course, the therapists had no idea of this; they were just doing their thing.[51]

Bioelectromagnetic Healing

All of this is fascinating, but why is it important? Since the early 1800s, scientists and doctors have experimented with magnets for their possible therapeutic benefits. In the late 1800s, when medicine became standardized, this research was abandoned. Recently, however, it has begun again. The findings of modern researchers have vindicated the earlier beliefs that magnetism can help people heal in certain situations. One therapy is called pulsed electromagnetic field (PEMF) therapy.

Here's how it works. Occasionally, when someone suffers a broken bone, the bone doesn't heal. The doctor sets the bone, perhaps applies a cast, but after several months, the bone is still fractured. After several years, it is still broken! This is known as a "non-union fracture." Somehow, something has gone wrong with the repair mechanism in the body. The information needed to heal the fracture is not getting to the tissues responsible for fixing the break. Today, many doctors know that PEMF will help. A magnetic field generator is placed around the broken bone, and a pulsating magnetic field is applied for 8 to 10 hours every day. Clinical tests have shown that even broken bones that have remained unhealed for 40 years can be repaired with this technique.[52]

The frequency of the magnetic field applied to a broken bone is 7 Hz. This healing frequency is called the "frequency window of specificity" (FWS). Different frequencies can affect different tissues, as shown in the following table.

Frequency	Effects
2 Hz	Nerve regeneration
7 Hz	Bone growth
10 Hz	Ligament repair
15–20 Hz	Skin repair
25 and 50 Hz	Assistance with nerve growth

While Zimmerman's investigations of the magnetic fields emitted by touch thera-pists did not prove that healing was occurring, he did discover that the therapists were emitting fluctuating magnetic fields that spanned the same frequencies that other scientists had discovered stimulated healing. Future studies are required to prove that healing touch can actually heal, but these results have pointed to a prom-ising area of investigation.

Let's reflect for a moment on what this means to us as we do our yoga practice. All yoga practices stress our tissues, and this pressure creates piezoelectric currents. These currents send information through our tissues and communicate what is happen-ing so that proper cellular responses can occur. These currents also create magnetic fields, which can also trigger healing responses. As we stretch, twist and compress our muscles and connective tissues we are energetically turning ourselves on, literally.

Energy Pathways

When the required information is not provided to an injured or sick area of the body, the body's own resources are not mobilized to respond, or the body responds inef-fectually or even inappropriately. Alternative healing modalities such as yoga, t'ai chi ch'uan, massage, energy manipulation therapies and many others could be ways of injecting the missing information through very weak, low-frequency electromagnetic field generation. Let's complete the construction of a possible model by looking more closely, at the cellular level, at how this information may be transmitted.

Electrical fields follow the flow of electricity. As we have seen, the nerves are not the only conductors of electricity in the body. An ECG measures the electrical activ-ity of the heart in places far away from our chest. These signals are possible because the blood system itself conducts electromagnetic information. So the circulatory sys-tem is one possible channel for electromagnetic energy, not just chemical energy. Interestingly, the Daoists long ago identified the Blood system as a conduit of chi. If chi is not simply chemical energy, perhaps they were sensing this conductance of electromagnetic energy through our blood vessels. Or perhaps the definition of chi needs to be broadened to include all these forms of energy: chemical, electrical and electromagnetic.

Does it stop there? Does our circulatory system feed every part of the body? What about inside the cells? How can information be transmitted to the insides of the cells themselves? To answer this question, we need to look at the current and evolving models of the cell.

The Bag of Soup Model

In most books that describe the anatomy of a cell, you will find lovely diagrams showing all the organelles, the major components of a cell, floating in a pool of liquid. These models are very elegant and detailed, but what is that water-like substance inside the cell? Soup! In an early, popular model of the cell, all the internal apparatus float in this soup. Materials from outside the cell ease their way past the permeable cell membrane and then drift around in the soup until they happen to bump into something important. The chemical energy model of communication requires a random movement of these substances until they find and latch onto their destination.

This is not a very satisfying model, relying as it does on random timing for information transfers to occur. James Oschman notes that many cellular activities happen much faster than a random walkabout would allow. Something is missing in this model.[53]

When we look in most anatomy books and see the way the body is depicted, we find a similar "something missing." The pictures will show in wonderful detail the circulatory system, or they may trace the skeletal system or the muscular or nervous systems. But all these models omit the material that these systems are embedded within. What is missing is the fascia! Fascia joins the circulatory system to the nervous system to the muscular system and so on. Our fascia is ubiquitous and, as we have seen, is formed of collagen fibers, elastin fibers and many other components arrayed in crystalline matrices. These matrices form the piezoelectric crystals that create and conduct the electrical energies we were discussing in the previous section. These matrices are exactly what are missing in the bag of soup cellular models. We need a new model that fills in the gaps and explains the cellular processes more completely.

The Cytoskeleton

Newer models of the cell's anatomy recognize that the cell is not just a bag of goo. There is a structure inside it. As shown in figure 7.27, the cell is filled with fibers, filaments and tubes. Collectively this structure is called the cytoskeleton or the cytoplasmic matrix and, just like our body's bony skeleton, it provides rigidity and support to the whole cell. More than that, the cytoskeleton provides pathways for information to flow along. No longer do we have to imagine chemical information just floating around in the sea of soup, waiting for a chance encounter. Now we find that chemical information can be guided to its destination by enzymes and proteins that lie along the cytoskeleton.

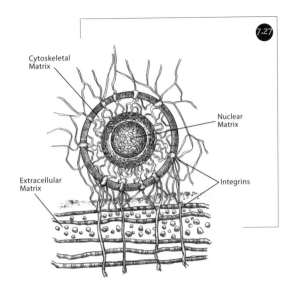

Notice that the lines forming the cytoskeleton extend out beyond the cell walls. These linking elements are called integrins, and they connect the inner and outer worlds of our cells. We have already seen that the extra-cellular matrix (ECM) is networked via our fascia throughout our whole body. With each cell connected inside and outside and to the 3-D fascial stocking we all wear within, we find that every cell has a connection to every other cell in our body. There is no place that is not connected to every other place within us. Looking even more closely, we see that these mechanical connections extend right down into the DNA of our cells.

I have postulated that illness is a blocking of information, an inability of the body to transmit healing signals to the affected area. If a problem isolates one region of the body from the others, information may not get through. Like a city suffering a power outage, communication lines may be out of service, transportation systems may fail. The city may survive for a short time, but unless outside help arrives, the city is doomed. Our body is not very different. Health means wholeness. If one part of the body is cut off from the information flow throughout the body, illness arises.

Mechanotransduction

So far, we have been looking at bioelectromagnetic communication flowing through the body, but there are many other pathways that information can flow through. The relatively new science of cellular signaling has uncovered dozens of different ways that cells talk to each other. These pathways can be biochemical, viral, electromagnetic or even mechanical. Mechanical stresses, when of sufficient strength and frequency, are another form of communication. This has been known for over 150 years. In the mid-1800s it was given the name *mechanotransduction*. This occurs when cells convert mechanical stress into biochemical and electrical signals. When the cells' membranes sense physical pressure, a cascade of events occurs within the cell.

Look again at the above picture of the cell and notice that there is a physical continuity from the fascia above, through the cell membrane and into the nucleus. Stress on the fascia creates a tugging on the cell membrane, which acts like the brain of the cell. It is the membrane that evaluates what is happening in the outside world and then decides what signals to allow to go to the nucleus.[54] If we want to regrow tissues—say, cartilage to replace a torn meniscus—an artificial scaffold is necessary. This scaffold guides stem cells to reproduce new cartilage in the right location.

There was a mystery in medical science: Why do some injuries heal but not fully? Why do injuries get better for a while, but the job remains unfinished, and some weakness or infirmity lingers? The answer to this mystery is starting to be discovered: stress! The body needs stress in order for our cells to receive communication.

Our extracellular matrix is under constant tension. When researchers apply stress to the ECM, stem cells begin behaving in the most remarkable ways. They multiply and migrate to the right places on the scaffold where they can be most effective. But there is another surprise: different levels of stress on the matrix cause the stem cells to differentiate into different tissues! A single scaffold can initiate stem-cell differentiation into a wide variety of different tissue types, because at different locations within the scaffold's matrix, there are different levels of stress.[55]

Stress is needed to stimulate our stem cells to be active, and depending upon the degree of stress, the cells can become the kind of tissue needed for the occasion. When a stem cell senses flowing movement, it will become a blood vessel. If the amount of stress is very slight, it becomes a nerve cell. If the stress is a bit stronger, it becomes a fat cell. Stronger still and the stem cell will become a muscle cell. With even more stress, it becomes bone. Too much, too little or no stress and the stem cell doesn't respond at all.

To quote science writer Bob Holmes, "This may explain why exercise and physical therapy are so important to health and healing—if cells don't get the right physical cues when you are recovering from an injury, for instance, they won't know what to do."[56] And this brings us back to yoga's magic ingredient: stress. All tissues need stress to remain healthy; remember our fragility curves. Sometimes the stress is blocked from reaching the cells: this can be the case when scar tissue has replaced the normal ECM structure. The tissues are too stiff. Cells may also not get the message when the stresses are too slight; instead of muscles, bones or fascia being regenerated, only fat is created, which does not help restore strength or range of motion to the injured area. We need to stress our tissues, but we need to do it in the right way and to the right degree.

MERIDIANS REVISITED

Western scientists who originally investigated the Eastern claims of meridians and nadis went back to their dissection tables, looking for physical manifestations of these channels. Their dissections discarded the supposedly inert fascia. They looked past these tissues, searching for something that just wasn't there. They looked for channels and conducting tubes similar to nerves and blood vessels but could not find them. Their conclusion: no channels, no meridians. Ironically, they discarded the very tissues that may form the channels they were seeking. Energies flow through our fascia!

The ancient sages told us there are 72,000 nadis. Some said 300,000, others 350,000. How many connecting pathways are actually in the body? Beyond counting![57] Perhaps these connecting fibers of the fascia are, in part, the nadis and the meridians that the sages experienced. It is interesting to speculate that they are the conduits of the energies of prana and chi. Perhaps these are the energies and channels that the early psychonauts were trying to map with the cultural concepts they had at their disposal.

What about the 32 different forms of chi that the Daoists detected? We have just seen that in the realm of cellular signaling, there are many dozens of forms of communication at our cells' disposal. In his studies, Dr. Oschman also investigated gravitational information as well as infrared, photonic, microwave and many other forms of energy that the body seems to employ to send and receive information. It does indeed seem likely that, over hundreds of millions of years of evolution, life on earth has adapted to, and adopted, everything Mother Nature has made available to us. Rather than assuming that the Indian and Daoist yogis were exaggerating, we can speculate that they were trying to explain their experiences in the only language they had available. Thus, they used analogies to our breath, where today scientists use analogies to physics and chemistry.

Fascia and the Meridians

Our fascia surrounds and invests all of our tissues, including the muscles and organs. Water lubricates the surfaces of the fascia, allowing for easy gliding of one layer over another. But water is also a great conductor of electrical and magnetic fields and currents. And fascia is piezoelectric. The bags and tubes of fascia form while we are embryos, folding in on themselves and enveloping the tissues and organs. The interfaces between these bags turn out to map very closely to the standard map of meridians the Daoists intuited. If you go back and look at the exterior meridians in the legs, you will see that they correspond very closely to the fascial boundaries of the major muscle groups.

Examples can help to explain this. The Kidney meridian follows the bags surrounding the muscles in the legs (the deep fascia and epimysium). Specifically, it follows the adductors to the lower hamstrings (semimembranosus), down to the calf (between the gastrocnemius and tibialis posterior), along the Achilles tendon to the deep muscles of the foot.[58] The Spleen follows the medial line of the rectus femoris at the top of the thigh, while the Stomach meridian follows the lateral edge. The Liver lies between the middle adductors. The Urinary Bladder follows the hamstrings. The Gall Bladder meridian lies between the medial hamstrings and the back of the medial quadriceps. The same relationship can be seen in the rest of the body as well. For example, the Stomach meridian runs alongside the fascial lining of the rectus abdominis in the front torso. The Urinary Bladder follows the erectors spinae in the back. These are merely the external lines; there is also a continuity of these fascial planes deep into the body, right to the bags that envelope the organs.

Fascia can not only create electrical currents, it can conduct them throughout the body. Fascia is the tissue that joins Eastern and Western views of energy and anatomy for it is through the fascial boundaries that continuity is found and communication flows.

Acupuncture Revisited

In 1997, the National Institutes of Health (NIH) removed the "experimental" label from the use of acupuncture and noted that acupuncture can be effective at reducing nausea that occurs after chemotherapy and during pregnancy. Acupuncture also yields some pain relief for certain conditions. The NIH conducted a multi-year study into the many claims of acupuncture benefits and found that while there were some scientific studies done with proper controls, most studies lacked controls and were inadequate. While acupuncture was found to be efficacious for pain and nausea, conventional Western medical treatments such as analgesics also dealt with these conditions without having to subject patients to the pain and trouble of being "needled."[59]

By 2009, several rigorous studies had been conducted that showed acupuncture can indeed change the brain's perception of pain, and there are some indications that acupuncture can help with other conditions, such as irritable bowel syndrome and depression.[60] Another study showed that acupuncture can be effective even without the needles![61] All we need to do is stress the acupuncture point, which of course is acupressure. In some cases, it was found that just a simple pinch was needed to stimulate endorphin releases in the brain.[62]

Clearly the Western point of view about acupuncture is still evolving. It is doubtful that all the extravagant Eastern claims of the vast array of benefits from acupuncture will remain when more research is done, but it is also quite clear that something is happening when we stimulate these acupuncture points and meridians, whether with or without needles. What could this "something" be?

There is, again, no consensus on how acupuncture works, and there may indeed be several mechanisms involved. One speculation is that acupuncture needling simulates an injury, which causes an injury-repair current to be generated. If this current is generated in a place where there is a communication channel, perhaps some low-resistance pathway through the water-filled extracellular matrix, then this current can travel through the body to some other place where it can stimulate a healing response.[63] Another speculation is that when we compress a point (acupressure), or when the acupuncture needle is jiggled or twisted, it mechanically tugs on the collagen and elastin fibers in the connective tissue. The mechanical tugging affects the nearby cells and their integrins, so in effect, the stress goes right inside the cells—this is what we called mechanotransduction earlier. Reorganization of the cytoskeleton can cause cell migration, contraction and secretion of various proteins. All of these changes can create a cascade of effects within the extracellular matrix.[64]

Do you recall the researcher mentioned in Chapter 6 who was looking into the effects of very long stresses on fascia (similar to Yin Yoga stresses) and discovered that a whole-body stretch held for 10 minutes twice a day reduces acute inflammation? Her name is Helene Langevin, and she is a world-renowned fascia researcher who is also fascinated by acupuncture. Her studies have shown that through mechanotransduction, cells are activated by the long-held stresses placed upon them. It her speculation that yoga has a similar effect.[65] However, yoga postures are not held nearly as long as needles are normally left in an acupuncture patient (in her experiments, she left needles in for 20 minutes). But a Yin Yoga student may apply an equally long mechanical stress to her cells through repetition. For example, spinal flexion for 20 minutes may occur if a student does Butterfly for 5 minutes, Half Butterfly over each leg for 5 minutes and then Straddle for 5 minutes. It is not a leap of logic to see why yoga, through long periods of acupressure, can have similar effects as acupuncture.

Whether we understand the mechanism or not, our own experience is what is most important. Sometimes there is no map for where we are going, and we will just have to create our own. Don't ignore your experience just because there is no current scientific map explaining it. There is evidence of some benefits from acupuncture and acupressure acknowledged in the West. There are many more anecdotal reports of benefits from the East. When we practice Yin Yoga, we should be open to and aware of the changes we are experiencing, both during the practice and in the days that follow. Be open to the reality of your own experience.

Here is some great news: you do not need to memorize the exact location of the acupuncture points to benefit from the practice! You do not even need to know the exact routing of each meridian (and since everybody is different, these lines will not be in exactly the same place on everybody anyway). We don't use acupuncture in our yoga practice, but we do use acupressure. As long as the stresses are applied to the tissues (tension or compression—it doesn't matter), then the mechanical stress and piezoelectric effects will occur. This means that if you sense a stress anywhere in a broad range within which the meridian line lies, then you will get the acupressure response. For example, if you feel a stress on the top of the thighs, you will probably be stimulating the Spleen and Stomach meridians. If you feel a stress along the spine or the back of the legs, you will probably be stimulating the Urinary Bladder meridians. Inner legs? Kidney and Liver. Outer hips? Gall Bladder. If you are feeling it, you are doing it!

Pranayama Revisited

The Indian yogis were quite clear that the nadis they were mapping for us were part of the subtle body, not easily detected and obviously not our nerves. The Daoists were equally certain that the meridians they were stimulating through acupuncture were also not nerves. But what about our nerves? If yoga is good for all our tissues, how does our nervous system benefit from the practice? It turns out that some of the pranayama practices already discussed, like the ocean breath and nadi shodhana, affect us in ways well known and understood by Western science—by influencing our nervous system.

Scientists love to break things down into components. It is easier to study subsystems and from there try to work out what the whole system does. Our nervous system consists of 2 main subsystems: the central nervous system (CNS), which includes the brain and the spinal cord, and the peripheral nervous system, which includes the nerves that innervate our body and which connects to the CNS. The peripheral nervous system in turn divides into the somatic nervous system, which allows conscious control over our muscles, and the autonomic nervous system (ANS), which provides involuntary control over our viscera: our organs, glands and smooth muscles. A map of the ANS shows it consisting of 3 more subsystems: the enteric nervous system, which controls our digestive tract; the sympathetic nervous system (SNS), which is responsible for our fight-or-flight response; and the parasympathetic nervous system (PNS), sometimes called our rest-and-digest response. That's a lot of capital letters, but we only need to understand the last 2 in detail.

The Sympathetic Nervous System

"It can be argued that stress is the number one killer in the Western world today." This quote is from Dr. Timothy McCall. In his book *Yoga as Medicine*, McCall relates that stress fuels some of the biggest health problems of our day, including diabetes, depression, osteoporosis, heart attacks, strokes and autoimmune diseases such as multiple sclerosis and rheumatoid arthritis.[66] He also says that while there isn't a lot of evidence that stress causes cancer, it appears to increase the odds of dying from it.[67]

Stress is unavoidable in our culture, and some amount of stress is actually needed for our bodies to be strong and healthy. All exercise needs to include the dual components of stress and rest. However, when we experience too much stress and not enough rest, problems arise. In physiological terms, we are hyperactive in our SNS and hypoactive in our PNS.

The SNS is our basic fight-or-flight system: it is yang-like. When our ancestors were being chased by a saber-toothed tiger or attacked by the tribe in the next valley, their SNS would strongly activate and give them the energy and focus needed to flee or fight. The brain's amygdala recognizes the threat and stimulates the hypothalamus, which in turn releases hormones that activate the pituitary gland. The pituitary then releases hormones that cause our adrenal glands to release several other hormones, including adrenaline, which speeds up our heart and respiration rates, and cortisol, which activates many systems, such as our frontline immune system and the liver's production of glucose. Stimulating the SNS also diverts blood from the digestive organs and the reasoning centers of our brain to our muscles; who needs to digest or remember the 12-times table when the most important thing is to run for our lives?

Today, our bodies react in the same way to threatening signals from our environment, but the saber-toothed tigers are gone. Our stresses are mostly caused by our way of viewing our life, not by actual external threats. The neighboring tribe may be your ex-mother-in-law, your boss or an angry customer. Where our ancestors might have encountered a stressful situation once or twice a week, we are faced with stressful situations constantly. Simply listening to loud music, watching the news, listening to a friend complain about her life, viewing commercials, arguing with a family member, commuting to work, eating hot or spicy foods or watching action movies can all trigger our SNS. We are in a constant state of SNS activation—we are overstressed.

The result of chronic stress is chronically high levels of cortisol. High cortisol levels are linked to elevated fasting-blood-sugar levels, higher blood pressure, insulin resistance and a reduction in our backline immune system.[68] We may begin "food-seeking behavior" due to our stress: Dr. McCall noted a study that found stressed-out children will consume more than twice as much food as their calmer fellow students.[69] While a temporary spike in cortisol can sharpen our mental focus, a continually elevated cortisol condition will lead to poor mental abilities, decreased memory and a depressed immune system. Our blood viscosity remains too high, causing many heart problems. Bone loss, insomnia, poor wound healing, weight gain, depression and fatigue are all consequences.

The Sympathetic Nervous System	The Parasympathetic Nervous System
Dilates pupils	Constricts pupils
	Stimulates tear glands
Reduces salivary flow	Stimulates salivary glands
Accelerates heart rate	Reduces heart rate
Constricts arterioles	
Dilates bronchi	Constricts bronchi
Inhibits stomach secretions	Stimulates stomach secretions
Relaxes urinary bladder	Contracts urinary bladder
	Stimulates sexual arousal

The Parasympathetic Nervous System

The PNS is more yin-like and works as a complement to the SNS: it is our rest-and-digest response. Through stimulation via the nerves running to our internal organs (primarily the vagus nerve), and through the release of acetylcholine, our heart rate slows and blood pressure drops. Blood flow that was diverted away from the intestines, brain and reproductive organs, whose function isn't essential in an emergency, returns. When we relax, our tears can flow. Our short-term memory returns, and we can think clearly. In sum, once our SNS is turned off and our PNS turned on, we rebuild and recover our health.

The key activities that turn off the fight-or-flight system and activate the rest-and-digest system are breathing and thinking. Not just any old breath, but a proper yogic breath. A slow, deep, even breath, the ocean breath, will create a relaxed nervous system, yielding a calm mind, which in turn will help the breath become slower and more even. Not just any old thinking either: our thoughts need to be calm. A positive feedback loop between the breath and our thoughts can be established that increases the effectiveness of the PNS and boosts the production of a neurotransmitter known as GABA.

The Brain on Yoga

The second most common neurotransmitter in our central nervous system is called GABA.[70] GABA decreases brain activity: it helps to turn off the lights when we are no longer home. If we are stressed, all the lights are on, even if we are not home. Similar to the PNS, GABA helps to reduce our stress response. People with low levels of GABA can suffer from depression and mood and anxiety disorders; drugs are often prescribed that increase GABA. Our yoga practice, when done properly, can increase our GABA levels and turn on the PNS.

Boston University Medical Center reported in August 2010 that GABA levels and mood are positively affected by yoga practice.[71] The researchers' study showed that yoga increases GABA levels in the brain and improves our mood. But we don't need a study (and there have been several[72]) to tell us that we feel better when we do yoga. We just need to know how to tap into the practice more deeply. What is it about yoga that makes us feel so good? One factor that has been proven to make us feel good is the already mentioned ocean breath.

Professor Luciano Bernardi, at the Italian University of Pavia, reported in a 2001 study that slowing our breath rate down positively affects our heart rate variability[73] and increases baroreflex[74] sensitivity. He studied the effects of chanting the Tibetan mantra "Om Mani Padme Hum," and he discovered the benefits were identical for people who chanted "Ave Maria." In both cases, the chanting slowed the breath down to only 6 breaths per minute. Bernardi's conclusion was, "Rhythm formulas that involve breathing at 6 breaths per minute induce favorable psychological and possibly physiological effects."[75]

If we can allow our breaths to be 10 seconds long (6 per minute), we will get the same benefits described in Bernardi's study. We can turn off the SNS and activate the PNS very quickly and simply. When you settle into your Yin Yoga pose, begin the ocean breath: count to 4 as you inhale, pause for 1 count, count to 4 as you exhale, and again pause for 1 count. This is a 10-second breath—proven by Bernardi's study to be great for our heart, lungs and minds. You don't have to keep doing it either. Like a light switch, once it is turned off, you don't have to keep tugging on the switch. It is off. Once you have turned off your SNS, it is off. Unless you turn it on again with unhelpful thoughts, you can stop your ocean breath after a few minutes.

No matter whether the Indian, Daoist or Western view resonates most for you, slow ocean breaths while you are holding your Yin Yoga poses will reduce stress, activate your rest-and-digest system, improve your heart and lung function, and improve your blood pressure.

SUMMARY OF ENERGETIC BENEFITS

There are 2 ways yoga affects energy (we turn on the tap and remove blockages); there are 3 forms of energy we use in our body (the energies of transportation, transformation and communication); and there are 4 ways we can turn on the tap and stimulate energy to flow (acupuncture, acupressure, directed awareness and the breath). An easy way to remember this? Just think: *Energy 2-3-4.* Once we do these things, we obtain many benefits, regardless of which map you choose to explain the results.

From an Eastern perspective:

- Awaken, enhance and balance prana.
- Slow the whirling thoughts of the mind.
- Stimulate and awaken the kundalini serpent, leading toward eventual liberation and enlightenment.
- Stimulate the production and flow of chi and jing energies.
- Nourish the Organs through acupressure via stimulation of the meridian lines.
- Replenish the store of jing in our Kidneys, which in turn helps all our Organs function properly.

From a Western perspective:

- Through acupressure stress, we create tiny piezoelectric currents that stimulate optimal cellular responses.

- We create internal pulsed magnetic fields that can restore cellular health.

- These communications can flow through the fascia to the organs, perhaps stimulating optimal performance and health.

- We create mechanotransduction stresses, which physically stimulate cells.

- We reduce acute inflammation and balance immune system responses.

- Through mindful, slow breathing, we improve heart rate variability and baroreflex.

- We can turn off the sympathetic nervous system (fight-or-flight) and turn on the parasympathetic nervous system (rest-and-digest).

- We may increase levels of the neurotransmitter GABA.

Endnotes

1   See Davie Gordon White, *Sinister Yogis* (Chicago: University of Chicago Press, 2010) for more detail on the breadth of yoga that has existed.

2   The roots of classical yoga go deeply into the forest, and many of the practices described in the Yoga Sutra existed for centuries before the text was compiled. For more on the history of the Yoga Sutra, see David Gordon White's *The Yoga Sutra of Patanjali: A Biography* (Princeton, NJ: Princeton University Press, 2014).

3   This form of disembodied liberation is known as videha-mukti.

4   Prakriti is everything outside of pure consciousness: everything we see, touch, feel, think, remember or sense in any way is prakriti. From the most obvious element, earth, to the most subtle thought, emotion, sense of self (ego) or intelligence, all we can discern is prakriti.

5   Yogis call this a science because it meets the requirements of a scientific investigation: a model is posited that predicts certain testable behaviors, which can be verified by anyone who duplicates the conditions of the inquiry. The challenge is that very few people are equipped with, or can develop, the abilities to meet these conditions of inquiry.

6   Purusha here refers to the cosmic man or the original Self from which all comes. During the classical yoga era, and especially in the Samkhya philosophy of that time, it came to signify our own individual consciousness, separate from all other purushas. Great debates raged over whether there were many purushas or only one great purusha, known later by various names such as brahman, Ishvara, paramatman or one of the great gods, Vishnu or Shiva.

7   As in English, putting the letter "a" in front of a Sanskrit word negates it, so ayama means "not yama" or "not controlled."

8   The 5 minor pranas are not important unless the student is going into advanced practices. This is fortunate as different sages describe different and conflicting effects of these minor energies. The 5 minor pranas and their effects are: naga, causing salivation and hiccups; kurma, causing opening of

the eyes and blinking; krikara, causing sneezing and sensation of hunger; devadatta, causing yawning and sleep; and dhanamjaya, causing hair growth and lingering even after death.

9 Vayu means "wind" or "air."

10 See Dr. Hiroshi Motoyama's *Theories of the Chakras: Bridge to Higher Consciousness* (Wheaton, IL: Quest Books, 1988).

11 We will learn more about the Governor Vessel later in this chapter.

12 Georg Feuerstein, *Shambhala Encyclopedia of Yoga*, 162.

13 Vibhutis are special powers obtained via yoga that give the yogi magic abilities. They are also called siddhis.

14 The two words that make up the word "hatha" are ha and tha. Most teachers interpret ha to mean the sun and tha to mean the moon. However, as usual in the world of yoga, there is no unanimity. T.K.V. Desikachar in his book *The Heart of Yoga* defines ha to be the moon and tha to be the sun. But even he admits the left nostril is the lunar channel.

15 There are ways to change the flow of the breath so you won't have to tell your anxious lover to wait for a couple of hours. A sinus reflex can be stimulated, allowing the breath to switch sides within a few minutes. There are a couple of ways to tap into this reflex. One is to lie on your side that is already open, with that arm extended under your head and used as a pillow. Another is to sit and shift your weight to the buttock of the open nostril. If neither intervention works, please do not blame yoga for your lover's frustration.

16 In Sanskrit, these blockages are known as granthis (pronounced "grunties"). You can tell from the sound of this word that you don't want grunties in your body! Granthis bad!

17 The *Hatha Yoga Pradipika* (2.15) warns, "Just as lions, elephants or tigers are tamed gradually, so the life force is controlled gradually or else it will kill the practitioner himself."

18 This means "against the grain."

19 Ajapa means "unpronounced," so this is a silent mantra. Another translation is "muttering." See Feuerstein, *Shambhala Encyclopedia of Yoga*, 14.

20 It is from this hierarchy that we derive the phrase "in seventh heaven" to signify experiencing the greatest joy.

21 Georg Feuerstein, *Tantra: The Path of Ecstasy* (Boston: Shambhala, 1998) has a good introduction to this topic. Another source that can be investigated is Joseph Campbell's *Transformation of Myth through Time* (New York: Harper Perennial, 1999).

22 See Hiroshi Motoyama, *Awakening of the Chakras and Emancipation* (Tokyo: Human Science Press, 2003). Also of interest is his book *Theories of the Chakras*. Another good introduction to this view of energy and chakras is Paul Grilley's DVD *Chakra Theory and Meditation*.

23 When immortality in this present body became rather elusive, the practitioner's intention evolved into seeking spiritual immortality.

24 It should be noted that what today we call Traditional Chinese Medicine is not actually the original Chinese medicine! For more information on this, read Mark Seem's book *Acupuncture Imaging: Perceiving the Energy Pathways of the Body* (Rochester, VT: Healing Arts Press, 2004).

25 Our use of the term meridian is not a great choice. The Chinese word is jing-luo, which may better be translated as a channel. Jing here means "to go through," and luo means "like a net," so jing-luo is more like a network that allows chi to flow through our body. The word "meridian" invokes a sense that the lines are imaginary, like the meridians found on our maps of the world, without conveying the channeling of energy.

26 A more complete introduction to chi can be found in Ted Kaptchuk's book *The Web That Has No Weaver: Understanding Chinese Medicine* (New York: McGraw-Hill, 2000) as well as Daniel Keown's *The Spark in the Machine: How the Science of Acupuncture Explains the Mysteries of Western Medicine* (London, UK: Singing Dragon, 2014).

27 See Keown, *The Spark in the Machine.*

28 Good foods are "chi-full" foods as opposed to so much of the "chi-free" foods we consume in our typical Western diet. Fast food is chi-free. Similarly, we all know people who are chi-full and others who drain us, who are chi-free. There are chi-full and chi-free jobs, books, movies, locations, etc.

29 For completeness, we would need to investigate the 5 subcategories of shen: yi, which means consciousness of potential; hun, our non-corporeal souls; zhi, our will; shen again, but this time as our spirit; and po, which is our animal soul, which dies when the body dies. Unfortunately, this level of investigation is beyond our scope. See Kaptchuk's *The Web That Has No Weaver* to learn more.

30 There used to be a belief in the West that constant worry would lead to ulcers in the stomach. Then scientists discovered that the source of ulcers was a bacterium called helicobacter pylori (H. pylori), not worry per se. However, in Japan, after a severe earthquake in Kobe in 1995, the incidence of ulcers skyrocketed; there was not a big increase in H. pylori in the people's stomachs, but the stress of worrying about their homes, jobs and families made the conditions in the stomach hospitable to the bacteria, which then multiplied and caused an increase in ulcers. See the study by Nobuo Aoyama et al., "Peptic Ulcers After the Hanshin-Awaji Earthquake: Increased Incidence of Bleeding Gastric Ulcers," *American Journal of Gastroenterology* 93.3 (1998): 311–16.

31 The Chinese never developed the concept of glands, but what they ascribe to weakness in the Kidneys doctors in the West would ascribe to adrenal exhaustion.

32 Consider, as one example, alcoholics who eventually destroy their liver: many suffer from anger management problems.

33 Another name for these locations is the tan-t'iens, which we discussed in Chapter 1.

34 Within these 6 lower body meridians we will discover that 3 are more yin-like (those that run along the inner legs), and 3 are more yang-like; again, we see that there is yang within yin and vice versa.

35 Unfortunately, in these pictures we can't see the inside lines on Mr. Meridian Man, so it is not possible to visually follow these interior routes for the meridians.

36 The perineum is the spot at the base of the torso halfway between the anus and the genitals.

37 This circling of light is an alchemical or transforming process. When the light circles long enough, it crystallizes and the body is transformed. We attain the natural spirit-body, and this body is formed "beyond all heavens." The sages claim in *Secret of the Golden Flower* that the only tool we need to master is this concentration of thought on the circling light.

38 We are moving a bit beyond the practice of Hatha Yoga now, into the practice of Tantra Yoga, in which the ultimate goal is to awaken shakti (also known as the kundalini energy) and send it up along the completely opened sushumna nadi so she can join with Shiva, who is awaiting her at the seventh chakra, just above the crown of the head.

39 Tighten your perineum.

40 In physics, this is defined by a formula of force times distance (W = FxD).

41 James Oschman's book *Energy Medicine in Therapeutics and Human Performance* (Waltham, MA: Butterworth-Heinemann, 2003) has a brief but interesting review of the history of Western medicine and of the use of magnets and electricity by doctors in the 19th century.

42 The piezoelectric phenomenon has been known for over a hundred years and was given its name in 1824 by David Brewster.

43 Oschman, *Energy Medicine*, 87.

44 This is 20,000 times stronger than the cell phone.

45 The mineral component of bone, hydroxyapatite, also creates piezoelectricity under stress and may play a facilitating role in the creation of piezoelectricity in the collagen fibers within bone. For a more complete discussion of electrical signals generated in and flowing through bones, see Andrew C. Ahn et al., "Relevance of Collagen Piezoelectricity to 'Wolff's Law': A Critical Review," *Medical Engineering and Physics* 31.7 (2009): 733–41.

46 If you have ever had an electrocardiogram, you may have noticed that the electrodes were placed over the heart and in more distant locations, sometimes on the ankles or wrists. These electrodes pick up the electromagnetic field of the heart as it moves over the whole body.

47 SQUID stands for Superconducting Quantum Interference Device. Through its invention, magnetic resonance imaging (MRI) machines became possible.

48 Such as Kusaka Seto of Japan.

49 See Oschman, *Energy Medicine*, 78.

50 A hertz (or Hz) refers to the number of times each second that the magnetic field pulsates. Thirty Hz means the field pulses 30 times each second. A 0.3 Hz measurement means the field pulses every 3 seconds.

51 One speculation as to how these therapists could generate such large magnetic fields suggests that they were somehow tapping into the earth's own magnetic field. Interestingly, at times, the therapists would lose their abilities. One possible cause for this is the ever-changing frequency of the earth's magnetic field due to solar flares and lightning strikes on earth. Normally the earth's field pulsates at something known as the Schumann frequency, which is in the range of 7–10 Hz. However, at certain times the fluctuations cease, and this may cause therapists and other chi masters to have lesser abilities at those times.

52 See P.R.J.V.C. Boopalan et al., "Pulsed Electromagnetic Field (PEMF) Treatment for Fracture Healing," *Current Orthopaedic Practice* 20.4 (2009): 423–8.

53 See Oschman's *Energy Medicine*, chapter 14, for more details on this topic.

54 The nucleus in this analogy is more the reproductive organs of the cell, not the brain.

55 It is now possible to regenerate a complete organ, with all its complexities of structure, blood vessels and nerve cells, through seeding a scaffold with only a few types of stem cells. Researchers have recently grown a complete kidney, which is a very complicated organ, and successfully implanted it into an animal.

56 See Bob Holmes, "Healing Touch: The Key to Regenerating Bodies," *New Scientist*, February 16, 2010.

57 According to an article in *Science* (February 11, 2011), there are 80 billion neurons in the human brain, communicating with each other through 150 trillion synapses, which are the points of communication between cells. That's just within the brain!

58 See Daniel Keown, *Spark in the Machine*, 164.

59 See C. Holden, "Thumbs Up for Acupuncture," *Science* 278.5341 (Nov. 1997): 1231, and A. Taub, "Thumbs Down on Acupuncture," *Science* 279.5348 (Jan. 1998): 155.

60 See "Study Maps Effects of Acupuncture on the Brain," *Science Daily*, February 5, 2010.

61 See "Acupuncture Just as Effective Without Needle Puncture," *Science Daily*, December 1, 2008.

62 For a more skeptical investigation into the claims of acupuncture, read The Committee for Skeptical Inquiry's report on their visit to China to investigate TCM and acupuncture, entitled Traditional

Medicine and Pseudoscience in China, published in 1996 and available at https://www.csicop.org/si/show/china_conference_1.

63 See Oschman, *Energy Medicine*, 77.

64 H.M. Langevin, D.L. Churchill, and M.J. Cipolla, "Mechanical Signaling Through Connective Tissue: A Mechanism for the Therapeutic Effect of Acupuncture," *FASEB Journal* 15.12 (2001): 2275–82.

65 See Langevin's "The Science of Stretch" at https://www.the-scientist.com/features/the-science-of-stretch-39407.

66 Timothy McCall, *Yoga as Medicine: The Yogic Prescription for Health and Healing* (New York: Bantam Books, 2007), 49.

67 I am aware, however, that many physicians do believe that stress can and does cause cancer. See Gabor Maté's book *When the Body Say No: The Cost of Hidden Stress* (Hoboken, NJ: John Wiley, 2011) as one example.

68 Our immune system has 2 key components: the innate system, which responds quickly to problems, and the adaptive system, which takes time to kick in but is more targeted in response to particular problems. The innate system is our frontline immune response; during times of stress, when the SNS is activated, the frontline immune system increases clotting factors in our blood (in case we get cut), increases cortisol levels (to boost glucose flow into the blood stream and decrease inflammation, which helps to improve blood flow), and releases cytokines, which attract specialized blood cells (such as macrophages and phagocytes) that target anything that is not "you," to combat infections. To assist with the initial response during acute stress, our heart rate, blood pressure and blood volume increase, helping to get the immune system's fighters to the front line. The frontline immune response is very fast but also very generic and often misses things. What gets missed is dealt with by the backline system, the adaptive immune system. The backline immune system adapts to any infections that evaded the frontline system. Specialized white blood cells—called killer T cells and beta cells—are created to hunt for these specific invaders; viruses and bacteria are rooted out from their hiding places. If we've suffered an injury, the damaged area is cordoned off through inflammation, triggered by cytokines, which are small protein messenger molecules that function like hormones but are much smaller and more numerous. Inflammation restricts the infection to one small region and allows the adaptive system to be more efficient in resolving the problem. Inflammation is part of the backline immune system and is turned off by the frontline system.

69 McCall, *Yoga as Medicine*, 49.

70 GABA stands for gamma aminobutyric acid.

71 C.C. Streeter et al., "Effects of Yoga Versus Walking on Mood, Anxiety, and Brain GABA Levels: A Randomized Controlled MRS Study," *Journal of Alternative and Complementary Medicine* 16.11 (2010): 1145–52.

72 Check other issues of the *Journal of Alternative and Complementary Medicine*.

73 Heart rate variability (HRV) refers to the difference in heart rate that occurs as we breathe. You may think that a healthy heart keeps one beat, like a metronome, but a healthy heart speeds up as we inhale, beating faster, and slows down as we exhale. The change in rhythm is the HRV, or the RR interval as it is sometimes referred to. People with heart disease have very low HRV.

74 Our baroreflex helps to maintain our blood pressure. For example, when we suddenly stand up, the baroreflex increases our blood pressure so we don't feel faint.

75 See *British Medical Journal* 323 (2001): 1446–9.

8

THE HEART AND MIND BENEFITS

Remember when we talked about the 3 principles of the Yin Yoga practice in Chapter 2? They were:

1. Come into the pose to an appropriate depth.
2. Resolve to remain still.
3. Hold the pose for time.

Holding the pose for time is the magic ingredient in Yin Yoga that benefits us physiologically; when we hold the stress of a pose for a long time, our tissues deform, reform, and become stronger, thicker and longer. Coming to an appropriate edge is the magic ingredient that benefits us energetically: we stimulate the acupressure points and meridian lines that send energy to our Organs (or maybe we simply create communication signals between our cells via the fascia). Resolving to remain still is the magic ingredient that benefits us mentally and emotionally. This is our final investigation.

Look again at the yin/yang symbol here: notice once more the black yin dot within the white yang swirl. This is the still point. Consider a powerful, destructive hurricane: at the center is the eye—the point of absolute stillness. Think of a top spinning at high speed: at the fastest spin, the apex of the top is completely motionless. Now think of all the drama and activities happening in your life right now. Where is your still point? Where do you go to find the eye of your storm?

We can practice finding the still point at the center of our drama when we hold a Yin Yoga pose long enough that we become challenged. The urge to move is growing

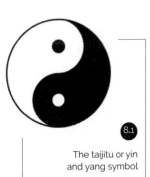

8.1

The taijitu or yin and yang symbol

stronger, and our mind is chattering, but we continue to breathe with awareness until finally, the eye appears. The winds are still flowing furiously all around us, but we have become calm.

When we practice finding calmness in the midst of a fierce storm during our yoga practice, we learn how to find that same centered still point at other times in our lives, when drama threatens to overwhelm us. When we are calm, our vision expands and we can decide more skillfully the course of action we wish to follow. When we are stressed, when the sympathetic nervous system is active, when our mind is frantic with thoughts, when our breath is quick, shallow or uneven, our vision narrows, and we are impelled to take the first and quickest solution in front of us. We have no ability to seek a wiser path; we simply react instead of reflect. When we practice mindfulness, at first within our yoga practice so that we learn how to also practice during the rest of our life, we learn to pause and see what is actually going on, and thus we are open to taking wiser actions.

THE BENEFITS OF MINDFULNESS

There have been many studies over the past few decades showing the physiological effects of mindfulness-based stress reduction (MBSR) practices.[1] Many of these we have already referred to:

- Improved blood pressure and lowered heart rate
- Reduced fight-or-flight stress response
- Activated rest-and-digest response
- Improved digestion
- Lessened inflammation
- Improved immune system

These are some of the physical benefits of mindfulness, and they are great! Who doesn't want a stronger immune system or better cardiovascular health? We have also seen that by paying attention to sensations and our breath, we can enhance the flow of energy through our body, nourishing our organs and improving communication between cells. Mindfulness helps us physically and energetically, but we also gain from this practice emotionally.

Connecting the Dots

The heart, mind and body are not 3 separate things. Scientists like to break a system down into components to understand the whole; however, sometimes this classification technique requires tearing the whole apart in order to create the subsystems. The whole is always greater than the sum of the parts. To investigate the emotional and psychological benefits of Yin Yoga, it is useful to consider a model of the heart, mind and body that is reconnected. Let's consider these to be 3 dots forming a simple triangle.

The first dot is our heart: the seat of emotions. The second is our mind: the seat of thoughts. The third dot is our body: our physical home. These 3 are connected; when we stimulate one of them, the others react. For example, when someone yells at us, we immediately feel an emotion, perhaps of fear or maybe of anger. The emotion arises in the emotional body, which we are loosely calling our heart.[2] The emotional body quickly stimulates our physical body: we begin to secrete hormones from the adrenal glands that get us ready to fight, argue or retreat. Our heart rate rises, we feel flushed, our pupils dilate—we are ready for some sort of action. This physical response generates certain thought patterns within our mind. We start to think about what is happening and how we are right, the other person is wrong, how unfair the situation is, etc.

Emotions stimulate the physical body, the physical body stimulates the mind, and the mind stimulates emotions. This cycle can spiral out of control in a negative feedback loop until a petty annoyance can become a towering rage. It is not possible for most of us to consciously control our adrenal glands or amygdala. It is not possible for most of us to stop strong emotions from arising. It is possible, however, for everyone to change his or her thoughts. We can interrupt this feedback loop by turning off the flow of negative feedback between the mind and the heart, by changing our thoughts. While this is possible, it is not easy.

PAYING ATTENTION

It is possible to change our thoughts, but to do so we first have to pay attention to them. We have to be mindful of what is actually happening right here, right now. In Chapter 2, we looked at how to take an inner inventory of what we are feeling. It begins simply: awareness of present experience with acceptance. With this openness, begin to notice the sensation of breathing; notice what happens as you happen to breathe. Next, become aware of the emotional backdrop that is present in your heart space. You may not notice any emotion, but that is simply a lack of practice and awareness. There is also some emotional backdrop occurring. Finally, become aware of your thoughts. Of course, we always have thoughts coming and going. We are not trying to change what we are experiencing; we are simply open to whatever is arising and passing. This is the beginning of using mindfulness therapeutically, to help us deal with the inevitable dramas that occur in our daily life now and then.

There are 4 reactions we can have to the strong sensations that will arise in a Yin Yoga practice. Two of these are yin-like and 2 are yang-like. Only one is really skillful;

the other 3 occur more out of habit than by choice. The reaction we default to in our practice is most likely the reaction we also default to at other times in our lives when we face a great challenge. The reactions are:

1. Running away from what is happening
2. Trying to change what is happening
3. Giving up and suffering through what is happening
4. Accepting what is happening

During our Yin Yoga practice, when the drama reaches a peak, when we really want to come out of the posture, pay attention to what is happening. Notice your cravings and your aversions. Start to notice how you want something else other than what is happening right now. Are you running away by mentally hiding in some fantasy? Are you moving to a slightly different position? Are you staying still but getting upset and thinking of how this is a stupid pose and a stupid teacher and you don't deserve to be treated like this? Or do you accept that at this moment in your life, this is what you are experiencing?

For some of us, our preferred response is to change the world. This is a highly valued quality in our culture. For others, our preferred response to life's crises is to hide; this is the running away choice. These are both yang strategies that many of us use to deal with challenges. The third choice is a yin strategy: just give up and feel sorry for ourselves as helpless victims.

None of these 3 strategies is skillful, but they are common. The final strategy is also yin-like but very skillful: paying attention and accepting what is happening. This does not mean that we continue to do nothing if doing nothing is inappropriate. We may choose to do something, but it will be a conscious decision based upon our best judgment at that time. In a Yin Yoga pose, after 5 minutes, we may decide, wisely, that it is indeed time to move, but this is a conscious decision and not a default reaction to what is happening. This decision can only happen when we are mindful and paying attention to our breath, our body and our thoughts.

DUKKHA

Dukkha is a Pali word that has been translated in many different ways.[3] It is used frequently in Buddhism, where it is often translated as "suffering."[4] The Buddha noted that all life contains 3 characteristics—*dukkha*, *anicca* and *anatta*: suffering, impermanence and no independent arising or self. Dukkha is part of life; if you are alive, you will experience it.

A better translation of dukkha is *unsatisfactoriness* or *unreliableness*. Life is not always sorrowful or filled with suffering, but there are times when pain will arise, when things will happen that we wish were not happening. That is dukkha. How we react is what creates our suffering and sorrow. Pain is just pain; when we make a drama around it, we turn the pain into suffering.

The difference between pain and suffering is nicely illustrated through a parable that the Buddha once related. One day, the Buddha was sitting in front of a group of monks, and he asked them, "Imagine there was a man, and imagine that this man had just been shot in the thigh with an arrow. How would the man feel?" The monks replied, "Hurt! In pain!" "Right," said the Buddha. "Now, imagine that this man got hit by a second arrow, right in the same spot! Now how would he feel?" "Worse! Agony!" responded the monks. "Exactly," said the Buddha. "And the name of that second arrow is suffering… and it is optional!"

The first of the Buddha's two arrows is dukkha. There will be times in life when pain arises. The second arrow, which he called suffering, is caused by what we do about the first arrow, and that is why it is optional. We can choose to just be with the pain that has arisen in our life, but we don't: we add to it. We love to create drama. A comedian once said that Christmas is a time when dysfunctional families get back together and retraumatize the hell out of each other. This is optional!

The Buddha is famous for being the first, but not the last, to point out that we are what we think. If we allow our thoughts to linger negatively on what is happening—or worse, if we allow our thoughts to remain negatively on what might happen or what has happened—we are striking ourselves with that second arrow. If you want to be unhappy, think about unhappy things. If you want to be content, think of all the things you already have.[5] This may seem, on the surface, to be a variation of the first strategy described earlier, of running away or ignoring what is happening, but it's really the last strategy. We pay attention to what is actually happening, notice what our reaction is, evaluate whether this reaction is a wise one or not, and if not, change it by changing our thoughts.

What does this have to do with our Yin Yoga practice? It is during Yin Yoga that we get to practice this advanced level of paying attention to our life. When we are at our edge and feeling the juiciness of the pose, we are simulating a challenging time. Now we get to notice our habitual pattern of reaction, and if it is not skillful, work to change that reaction, to create a new pattern.

PATHING

Pop quiz: what is the difference between being stuck in a rut and being in the groove? People hate being stuck in a rut, doing the same old same old every day. But being in the groove means you're on a roll. Athletes call it being in the zone; they practice the same movement over and over again until it becomes automatic. Dancers and musicians similarly want to find that place where they can just flow. The only difference between a rut and a groove is our attitude toward what we are doing: if we don't like what we are doing, it's a rut, but if we love what we are doing, we're in the groove.

Our habitual patterns are paths. We can call them grooves or ruts, depending upon whether they serve us well or not. There is an ancient concept called karma that embodies this: our current actions are the results of our past actions. This is exactly how a path is created. To illustrate, think of a beautiful forest. Imagine that you want to get from one side to the other, and you are the first person or animal to have ever traversed these woods. It is not easy to walk through virgin forests; you have to blaze a trail. The first time you walk the trail, it is hard work. You may have to carve out your path, maybe with an axe or a machete. The second time, it is a bit easier. After walking this path 100 times, it is really easy to follow the trail and difficult to leave the path to go in another direction. To go somewhere else requires blazing a new path, with all that effort being redone.

It's no wonder that people stick to their ruts in life—it's hard to create a new path. Athletes and musicians have to work very hard to blaze the new paths in their neural networks so that their performance is easy. But if the path you are following is no longer serving you, get off that path and blaze a new one! Our thoughts create paths in our brains as well. It is not easy to stop thinking in the same old ways we have always thought. If your standard strategy for dealing with challenges in life is number 1, 2 or 3 above, you have created a path that will be difficult to change—but far from impossible!

Yin Yoga is the chance to practice changing our chosen paths. We get to blaze new trails, more skillful grooves to follow. The process is quite simple: notice what is going on, choose not to default to your habitual response, decide what is the most skillful thing to do right now, and then do it.

WATERING FLOWERS

The Zen monk Thich Nhat Hanh has often used watering flowers as a metaphor to illustrate how we default to following a path in our mind that does not serve us well. As we become more practiced at noticing our thoughts and emotional states, we discover that we spend a lot of time watering weeds. Now, if you were a gardener, you'd think this a very silly thing to do. Don't water weeds—water flowers! But the path to your weed patch is well worn from years of walking there. It is easy to get to the weed patch, so we allow our thinking to just go to these weeds.

What are the weeds in your mind's garden? Whenever you allow thoughts of regret, fear, anxiety, anger, frustration, envy, jealousy, sadness or guilt linger inappropriately, you are watering weeds. Whenever you allow your thoughts to remain on things long past that you wished had turned out differently, or fantasize about a future that you know cannot be, you are watering weeds. And of course, the more you water these weeds, the taller and pricklier they become. The more you walk the path to the weed patch, the easier it is to continue to go there. Yin Yoga gives you the chance to stop watering your weeds and start watering your flowers!

Remember: it is not easy to get out of a rut, but it is possible. When you notice that your mind is thinking about weeds, take your watering can and go over to your flower garden. Start watering your flowers. It takes a while to build a new habit and stop an old one. It requires intention and attention. Remember why you are doing this! Use the power of your intention to give you the strength to get out of that old mental rut and blaze a new path to your garden.

When you have left the weed patch, you can direct your mind to linger on thoughts of joy, compassion, kindness, equanimity and love. Everyone has flowers to water. If you have difficulty with this practice, start with the beautiful flower of gratitude. Bring to your mind all the things in your life that you are grateful for. Once you start thinking about gratitude, you will discover so many flowers all around you: think of your parents, your children, your friends, your health.[6] You can meditate on how grateful you are for your job, your home, your city or country, for the hobbies in your life that give you so much pleasure, your books and music, for sports and for the great outdoors, for being able to learn new things—and of course, you can think about how grateful you are for your yoga practice.

If you cannot think of any flower to water right now, a flower that is always with you is your breath: be grateful for this breath that you are breathing right now. Enjoy your breath. Watch your breath. Simply by returning to the flower of this breath, you stop watering weeds. When you stop watering your weeds, they dry up and wither. When you stop visiting the weed patch, the path eventually becomes overgrown and hard to follow, while the path to your flower garden becomes easier and easier to follow. Eventually, you will no longer go to the weed patch, because it is so much easier and more enjoyable to go water your lovely flowers.

MINDFULNESS

Mindfulness simply means to pay attention. This is the practice of presence. During our yoga practice, we build the habit of mindfulness so that we can call upon this skill at any time that we need presence. Thich Nhat Hanh explained it this way:

> Mindfulness is the energy of being aware and awake to the present moment. It is the continuous practice of touching life deeply in every moment. To be mindful is to be truly alive and at one with those around us. Practicing mindfulness does not require that we go anywhere different.
>
> We can practice mindfulness in our room and on our way from one place to another. We can do very much the same things we always do—walking,

sitting, working, eating, talking—except we learn to do them with an awareness of what we are doing.[7]

This is the goal when we hold yin poses in stillness: to awaken to the present moment. We touch what is happening in our body, and in our heart and mind. We don't have to go anywhere; right here, right now—this is life. Remember this little mantra, and use it often in your practice and your life:

Awareness of present experience with acceptance.

ADVERSE REACTIONS TO MINDFULNESS—A WARNING!

Human variation is a reality, even in the fields of psychotherapy and meditation. There is no therapy that will work for everybody. Just as contraindications are offered to yoga students before doing postures, it should be noted that many people have negative reactions to meditation practices and mindfulness. In one study, 63% of meditators in a Vipassana retreat experienced negative effects from the practice, with 7% citing profoundly upsetting experiences. The negative effects ranged from relaxation-induced anxiety to panic, confusion, impaired reality testing, lower motivation, boredom, a spaced-out feeling and depression.[8] There are some indications that too much mindfulness can lead to functional disorders, causing psychosomatic problems from epilepsy to asthma, chest pains and constipation. (Psychosomatic does not mean "made up"; it indicates a disconnect between the mind and the body.)[9] These problems are not due to inexperience. Meditating longer will not make these reactions go away, and there is nothing wrong with people who experience them. It is simply that nothing works for everyone. If you find that meditation or mindfulness does not provide you with the benefits you seek, or indeed makes matters worse, find another approach! Seek out an experienced therapist or teacher who is willing to work with you to find other ways to get where you want to go.

SUMMARY OF HEART AND MIND BENEFITS

The act of practicing presence, of being mindful of what is happening right now, can help us physiologically, energetically and mentally/emotionally. Our stress begins to evaporate as soon as we pay attention to our breath and allow it to slow down. When our stress level declines, we reap many health benefits: our blood pressure drops, heart rate slows, immune system reactivates, digestion improves and inflammation decreases. By paying attention to the sensations within, we can stimulate and enhance energy movement. And by being present, we can choose to change our brain.

We all have habitual reactions to life that we no longer think about. These are unconscious reactions that may have served us well at one time but are no longer the best choices we could make today. Since we are not conscious of these reactions, we don't stop to think about how we could do better: we simply live the way we always have. But if we are finding that life is not as satisfying as it could be or once was, perhaps it is time to take a deeper look at how we are responding to life. Instead of life being something that is just happening, we can discover that we are free to build new, skillful habits that will enhance our enjoyment of life. We do this through mindfulness, which we develop through the stillness of our yoga practice.

In Yin Yoga, we come to an edge in a pose and become still. While we hold the pose, we go within. We start to notice what is going on in life, right here, right now—without adding any drama, without taking anything away from the experience. With clarity, we see what is really needed, beyond the cravings and aversions that normally move us. We are now free to create a new response, and over time build new paths to follow.

The real benefits of yoga are physical, emotional and mental health and well-being. We build habits that last a lifetime. We become present and enjoy this moment, the moment that is happening right now. We become grateful for this wonderful gift— and perhaps we resolve to share what we have discovered with others, so that they too can live well.

Endnotes

1 For a complete investigation into MBSR benefits, check out the work of Jon Kabat-Zinn.

2 In this map, we are not dividing the home of our emotions into all the major organs, as the Daoist maps do. Nor are we looking at the centers in the brain, such as the amygdala, that scientists know start the chain of reactions when we are frightened. We are proposing a much simpler model here, in which we see all emotions arising in the heart.

3 In Sanskrit, it is written duhkha. Since the original Buddhist texts were written in Pali, we are using the Pali spelling.

4 The original use of the word referred to the center of a wheel, such as a potter's wheel or a chariot wheel. If the center was not quite centered, the wheel did not spin well: that was dukkha. If the center was right in the middle of the wheel, the wheel spun nicely: this is called sukha, which is often translated as happiness.

5 Rabbi Schwartz once said, "True happiness is wanting what you already have." That's a quick way to contentment.

6 Even if your health is relatively poor right now, it could still be far worse! Be grateful for what you do have.

7 From Thich Nhat Hanh, *Happiness: Essential Mindfulness Practices* (Berkeley: Parallax Press, 2009).

8 See "Meditation: Concepts, Effects and Uses in Therapy" by Alberto Perez-De-Albeniz and Jeremy Holmes, *International Journal of Psychotherapy*, March 2000, Vol. 5 Issue 1, p. 49.

9 See "The illnesses caused by a disconnect between brain and mind" by Claire Wilson in *New Scientist*, April 3, 2019.

Alter, Michael. *The Science of Flexibility.* Champaign, IL: Human Kinetics, 2004.

Becker, Robert O., and Marino, Andrew A. *Electromagnetism and Life.* Stony Brook, NY: SUNY Press, 1982.

Campbell, Joseph. *Transformation of Myth Through Time.* New York: Harper Perennial, 1999.

Clark, Bernie. *From the Gita to the Grail: Exploring Yoga Stories and Western Myths.* Indianapolis: Blue River Press, 2014.

———. *Your Body, Your Yoga: Learn Alignment Cues That Are Skillful, Safe and Best Suited to You.* Vancouver, BC: Wild Strawberry Productions, 2016.

———. *Your Spine, Your Yoga: Developing Stability and Mobility for Your Spine.* Vancouver, BC: Wild Strawberry Productions, 2018.

Desikachar, T.K.V. *Health, Healing and Beyond.* New York: North Point Press, 1998.

Doniger, Wendy, trans. *Rig Veda.* New York: Penguin, 1981.

Feuerstein, Georg. *Tantra: The Path of Ecstasy.* Boston: Shambhala, 1998.

———. *The Shambhala Encyclopedia of Yoga.* Boston: Shambhala, 2000.

———. *The Yoga Sutra.* Rochester, VT: Inner Traditions, 1989.

———. *The Yoga Tradition: Its History, Literature, Philosophy and Practice.* Prescott, AZ: Hohm Press, 2001.

Freeman, Richard. *The Yoga Matrix Audio CD.* Boulder, CO: Sounds True, 2003.

Grilley, Paul. *Anatomy of Yoga DVD.* San Francisco: Pranamaya, 2008.

———. *Yin Yoga: Outline of a Quiet Practice.* Ashland, OR: White Cloud Press, 2002.

Hedley, Gil. *The Integral Anatomy Series*, vols. 1–4. Beverly Hills, FL: Integral Anatomy Productions, 2005–2009.

Holt, L., Pelham, T., and Holt, J. *Flexibility: A Concise Guide.* New York: Humana Press, 2008.

Iyengar, B.K.S. *Light on Yoga: Yoga Dipika.* New York: Schocken Books, 1979.

Johnson, Robert. *Owning Your Own Shadow: Understanding the Dark Side of the Psyche.* New York: HarperCollins, 1993.

Jois, Sri K. Pattabhi. *Yoga Mala: The Original Teachings of Ashtanga Yoga Master Sri K. Pattabhi Jois.* New York: North Point Press, 2000.

Kaptchuk, Ted. *The Web That Has No Weaver: Understanding Chinese Medicine.* New York: McGraw-Hill, 2000.

Keown, Daniel. *The Spark in the Machine: How the Science of Acupuncture Explains the Mysteries of Western Medicine.* London, UK: Singing Dragon, 2014.

Lindsay, Mark. *Fascia: Clinical Applications for Health and Human Performance.* Clifton Park, NY: Delmar Cengage Learning, 2008.

Mallinson, James. *The Gheranda Samhita.* Woodstock, NY: YogaVidya.com, 2004.

———, trans. *Shiva Samhita.* Woodstock, NY: YogaVidya.com, 2007.

Maté, Gabor. *When the Body Say No: The Cost of Hidden Stress.* Hoboken, NJ: John Wiley, 2011.

McCall, Timothy. *Yoga as Medicine: The Yogic Prescription for Health and Healing.* New York: Bantam Books, 2007.

McGill, Stuart. *Low Back Disorders.* Champaign, IL: Human Kinetics, 2002.

Mohan, A.G. *Krishnamacharya: His Life and Teachings.* Boston: Shambhala, 2010.

Motoyama, Hiroshi. *Awakening of the Chakras and Emancipation.* Tokyo: Human Science Press, 2003.

———. *Measurements of Ki Energy, Diagnosis, and Treatments.* Encinitas, CA: California Institute for Human Science, 1997.

———. *Theory of the Chakras: Bridge to Higher Consciousness.* Wheaton, IL: Quest Books, 1988.

Oschman, James. *Energy Medicine: The Scientific Basis.* Philadelphia: Churchill Livingston, 2000.

———. *Energy Medicine in Therapeutics and Human Performance.* Waltham, MA: Butterworth-Heinemann, 2003.

Powers, Sarah. *Insight Yoga.* Boston: Shambhala, 2008.

———. *Insight Yoga DVD.* San Francisco: Pranamaya, 2005.

Seem, Mark. *Acupuncture Imaging: Perceiving the Energy Pathways of the Body.* Rochester, VT: Healing Arts Press, 2004.

Stecco, Carla. *Functional Atlas of the Human Fascial System.* Philadelphia: Churchill Livingstone, 2015.

Strom, Max. *A Life Worth Breathing: A Yoga Master's Handbook of Strength, Grace, and Healing.* New York: Skyhorse Publishing, 2010.

Swatmarama, Swami. *Hatha Yoga Pradipika.* Seattle, WA: Pacific Publishing Studio, 2011.

Thich Nhat Hanh. *Happiness: Essential Mindfulness Practices.* Berkeley: Parallax Press, 2009.

White, David Gordon. *Sinister Yogis.* Chicago: University of Chicago Press, 2009.

Wilhelm, Richard. *Tao Te Ching.* New York: Prentice Hall, 2002.

————. *The Secret of the Golden Flower.* New York: Harcourt Brace & Co., 1962.

Wong, Eva. *The Shambhala Guide to Taoism Yoga.* Boston: Shambhala, 1996.

————. *Taoism: An Essential Guide.* Boston: Shambhala, 2011.

INDEX

Page numbers followed by "n" indicate notes. Numbers in *italics* indicate photos or illustrations.

Williams, David, 52

Window Pose, 98

Windshield Wipers, 112, *158*, 158–159

Winged Dragon, 41, *90*, 91

Wolff, Julius, 209

Wolff's law, 209

women, 48n11

    pregnant, 203–206

    who have had vaginal birth, 207

Wong, Eva, 17n29

worker's compensation, 49n14

wrists

    flow for the shoulders, arms, and wrists, 172–174

    poses for, *152*, 152–153

Y

yama, 249

yang (surya), 2–5, 252

yang counterposes, 159

yang exercise, 7–8

yang practices, 4

yang tissues, 1, 5–8

Yang Yoga, 234–235

yi, 298n29

yin, 2–5

    chandra, 252

    original, 9–11

yin and yang symbol, *2*, 301, *301*

yin exercise, 7–8

yin tissues, 1, 5–8

Yin Yoga, 1–2, 6

    benefits, x, xii, 21, 22

    cautions, xvi, 2, 19

    energetic benefits of, 247–300

    first principle, 25

    flows, 163–194

    fourth principle, 233

    heart and mind benefits, 301–310

    history of, 9–11

    how to practice, 20–23

    physical benefits of, 209–245

    physiological benefits of, 238–241

    as portable, 33

    poses for upper body, 144–159

    postnatal, 206–207

    practice, 19–49

    precautions, 22–23

    principles of, 301

    reactions to, 303–304

    sensations that can arise during, 42

    tattvas of practice, 25

    wall yin, 185–189

    when to practice, 20–21

    where to practice, 20

    whole body workout, 182–184

    before or after Yang Yoga, 234–235

Yin Yoga (Grilley), 51

ying chi, 259

YIP (Yoga Injury Prevention), 52, 159n2

yoga. *see also specific types*

    definition of, 9, 247, 248

    effects on brain, 294–295

    functional, 23–24, 34

    reasons for doing, 253

Yoga Injury Prevention (YIP), 52, 159n2

Yoga Sutra, 9–10, 17n15, 248, 296n2

yogi, 16n4

yogin, 16n4

yogini, 16n4

yuan chi, 259

Z

zang Organs, 261–263

zheng chi, 259

zhi, 298n29

Zimmerman, John, 283, 284

Zipper, 182

zong chi, 259

zygapophyseal facets, 194n6

OTHER BOOKS
BY BERNIE CLARK

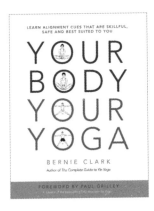

YOUR BODY, YOUR YOGA

Learn Alignment Clues that Are Skillful,
Safe and Best Suited to You (2016)

Your Body, Your Yoga goes beyond any prior yoga anatomy book available. It not only looks at the individual uniqueness of our anatomical structures and what this means for each person's range of motion but also examines the physiological sources of restrictions to movement. Volume 1 proposes a new mantra to be used for every yoga posture: What stops me? The answers presented run through a spectrum, beginning with various types of tensile resistance to three kinds of compressive resistance. The nature of muscles, fascia, tendons, ligaments, joint capsules, bones and our extracellular matrix are examined, along with their contribution to mobility. The shapes of these structures also define our individual, ultimate ranges of movement, which means that not every *body* can do *every yoga posture*. Volume 2 applies these principles to the lower body, examining the hip joint, knee, ankle and foot and presenting how your unique variations in these joints will show up in your yoga practice.

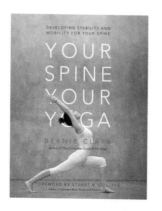

YOUR SPINE, YOUR YOGA

Developing Stability and Mobility for Your Spine (2018)

Your Spine, Your Yoga is the second book in the *Your Body, Your Yoga* series and is arguably the first book that looks at the spine from both the Western anatomical/biomechanical point of view and the modern yoga perspective. It focuses on the axial body—the core, from the sacral complex, which includes the pelvis, sacrum and sacroiliac joint, through the lumbar and thoracic segments of the spine, to the cervical complex, which includes the neck and head. It is filled with detail, discussion, illustrations and practical advice for spines of all types. No two spines are exactly alike, and no two people have the same biology and biography. What your spine is able to do may be vastly different from what other yoga students' or teachers' spines can do.

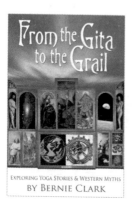

FROM THE GITA TO THE GRAIL

Exploring Yoga Stories & Western Myths (2014)

What is the meaning of Shiva dancing on a dwarf named Avidya? Why does Vishnu sleep upon an endless snake? To what did the Buddha awaken? What do we mean by soul? The practice of yoga has become quite common and popular in the West; however, the stories of yoga are still strange to Western ears. What do these ancient symbols mean, what are they trying to teach us, and how should we incorporate the knowledge skillfully into our Western lifestyle? By looking at the myths of yoga along with the stories that have influenced Western culture, we are presented with opportunities to select the best of both worlds and create new maps to help guide us through the uncertainties of modern living.

"In this insightful book, Bernie reminds us that we have a choice in how we live our lives; we can hold tight to our beliefs, allowing them to dictate our reality, or we can invite every story (or even encounter) to be a gateway into the poetic, multifaceted dimensions of truth, and the fluid nature of reality."
—*Sarah Powers, author of* Insight Yoga *and founder of the Insight Yoga Institute*

YINSIGHTS

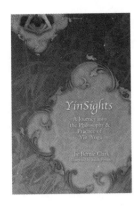

A Journey into the Philosophy & Practice of Yin Yoga (2007)

Why practice yoga, Yin Yoga in particular? *YinSights* has the answers. *YinSights* explores the benefits of yoga as viewed in the Eastern and Western worlds and relates how it affects the body and mind. *YinSights* serves as a practical guide for students interested in understanding Yin Yoga. The first half of the book investigates the benefits of yoga on the physical body, the energetic body and the mind/emotional body. Presented are three points of view: those of the yogis in India, the Daoists in China, and the medical and scientific researchers of the West. The second half is Bernie's earliest exploration of the practice of Yin Yoga and offers several flows, each with different themes. Slower versions of the normally active, or yang, Sun Salutations are provided, as well as even gentler ways to stimulate the flow of prana, chi or energy. While *YinSights* illustrates how to practice Yin Yoga, it is not just for those seeking knowledge about Yin Yoga in particular. The book also discusses the advantages of all styles of yoga and will be of interest to every yoga student.

ABOUT THE AUTHOR

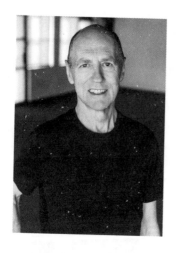

Bernie Clark loves learning about and then sharing the things that fascinate him. As a child, he enjoyed studying the world and how it works, and as a teen, he loved thinking about the mind and the soul. These seemingly contradictory interests in science and spirituality continued to shape his philosophy of life well into his adult years. With one foot in the commercial world of space and computer technologies and another in the realm of meditation and yoga, he sought bridges between Eastern and Western maps of reality. These maps and bridges are described in his teachings and writings with the hope that others who share his fascinations will be able to enjoy what he has learned, without having to go through the labor of detailed research.

Bernie has a degree in science and spent 30 years as a senior executive in the high-tech/space industry. He embarked upon meditation in the 1970s and began teaching yoga in the 1990s. He conducts yoga teacher trainings several times a year in Vancouver, Canada. To stay informed about Bernie's activities, visit his website, www.YinYoga.com, where you can subscribe to his *YinSights* newsletter.